PASSAGE to POWER

ALSO BY LESLIE KENTON

Nonfiction

The Joy of Beauty
Ultrahealth
Raw Energy (with Susannah Kenton)
Raw Energy Recipes (with Susannah Kenton)
Ageless Aging
The Biogenic Diet
10-Day Clean-up Plan
Cellulite Revolution
Endless Energy (with Susannah Kenton)
Nature's Child
Lean Revolution
Ten-Day De-stress Plan
The New Joy of Beauty
The New Ultrahealth
The New Ageless Aging
The New Biogenic Diet
The New Raw Energy (with Susannah Kenton)

Fiction

Ludwig (a spiritual thriller)

Please visit the Hay House Website at: **www.hayhouse.com**

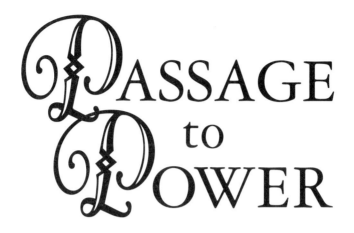

Passage to Power

Natural Menopause Revolution

LESLIE KENTON

Hay House, Inc.
Carlsbad, CA

Published and distributed in the United States by:
Hay House, Inc., P.O. Box 5100, Carlsbad, CA 92018-5100
(800) 654-5126 • (800) 650-5115 (fax)

Edited by: Sarah Wallace and Jill Kramer • *Designed by:* Wendy Lutge

The author of this book does not dispense medical advice or prescribe the use of any technique as a form of treatment for physical or medical problems without the advice of a physician, either directly or indirectly. The intent of the author is only to offer information of a general nature to help you in your quest for emotional and spiritual well-being. In the event you use any of the information in this book for yourself, which is your constitutional right, the author and the publisher assume no responsibility for your actions.

Library of Congress Cataloging-in-Publication Data

Kenton, Leslie.
      Passage to power : natural menopause revolution / Leslie Kenton.
         p. cm.
      Reprint. Previously published: London : Ebury Press, 1995.
      Includes bibliographical references and index.
      ISBN 1-56170-487-3
         1. Menopause—Psychological aspects. 2. Menopause—Complications—
Alternative treatment. 3. Menopause—Popular works. 4. Middle
aged women—Health and hygiene. 5. Progesterone—Therapeutic use.
I. Title.
RG186.K46 1998   98-14278
618.1'75—dc21   CIP

First published in the United Kingdom in 1995 by Ebury Press, Random House,
20 Vauxhall Bridge Rd.
London SWIV 2SA, ENGLAND

ISBN 1-56170-487-3

01 00 99 98 5 4 3 2
First Hardcover Printing, 1995, by Ebury Press
Second Printing (first Hay House Tradepaper Edition), August 1998
Third Printing, September 1998
Printed in the United States of America

*For the hundreds of thousands of women
who courageously seek ways and means of living
their full potential for health, creativity, and freedom,
each in her own way. This book is dedicated to you.*

Contents

PART II: THE SCIENCE OF MYTH

PART III: RITES AND RITUALS

APPENDIX

Acknowledgments

There are so very many people who have either helped me learn what I needed to know in order to write this book, or have painstakingly read the manuscript and have given me their comments and suggestions, that it would be impossible to list them all. There are a few, however, who must be thanked by name: Dr. John Lee, Dr. Robert Jacobs, the late Dr. Dagmar Leichti von Brasch, Dr. Michael Harner, Dr. Barry Durrant-Peatfield, Dr. Shamim Daya, Dr. John Howard, Dr. Ellen Grant, Dr. Peter Mansfield, Dr. Gordon Latto, Willa Shaffer, Celia Wright, Sandra Ingerman, Sandra Coney, Barbara Sommers, and Rhodri Thomas. I am also enormously grateful to my assistant, Yvette Brown—The Fox—for her tenacity in seeing me through the task of researching and writing; and to Sarah Wallace, who has, with such care and skill, edited the book.

— Leslie Kenton
Pembrokeshire, England 1995

Author's Note

The content of this book is intended for informational purposes only. I am only a reporter. None of the suggestions or information is meant in any way to be prescriptive. Any attempt to treat a medical condition should always come under the direction of a competent physician—preferably one knowledgeable about nutrition and natural methods of healing. Neither the publishers nor the author can accept responsibility for injuries or illness arising out of a failure by a reader to take medical advice.

I want to make it clear that I have no commercial interest in any product, treatment, or organization mentioned in this book. However, I have long sought to learn more about whatever can help us to live at a high level of energy, intelligence, and creativity, for it is my belief that the more each one of us is able to reestablish harmony within ourselves and with our environment, the better equipped we shall be to wrestle with the challenges now facing our planet.

PART I

THE MYTHS OF SCIENCE

CHAPTER ONE

BLOODLESS REVOLUTION
The Rise of Natural Menopause

ower, energy, and freedom. These are meant to be the rewards of menopause. This is a book about how we, as women, can bring them into being. It is *not* about how to cope with the "horrors of the change of life." *Passage to Power* explores the transformation in a woman's life that takes place between the ages of 35 and 60 as a journey toward individual freedom. Along the way, the book takes a cold, hard look at Hormone Replacement Therapy (HRT), exposes the common misconception that menopause is an "estrogen deficiency disease," and scrutinizes the rampant misinformation surrounding the use of prescription hormones—sadly, even among many otherwise competent doctors who use them too often because they simply don't know what else to do. It also gathers together diverse information about simple yet effective actions an informed woman can take to improve her physical health and appearance, as well as to maximize her energy and to enhance the quality of her life—whatever her age. In addition, it probes the spiritual nature of the menopause passage that must be experienced through myth and ritual, archetypes and dreams.

For ten years, people have been saying to me, "Write a book on menopause." I have always refused. "I can't until I've experienced it," I used to say. When, finally, menopause arrived, I was unprepared for it. Despite my knowledge of health, I did not know what to expect. Neither had I any idea of the freedom that is available to us on the other side of the menopause passage. The freedom of which I speak is not the "freedom" that advertisers would have us believe comes with owning a pair of Levi 501's or popping in a tampon so that we can swim during a period. It is a freedom of body and soul that enables each woman to experience unfettered her full potential for aliveness. Only by doing so can we call forth our greatest gifts—both for our own personal fulfillment, and to share with our culture and the planet.

Freedom to Be

Despite demands for equal rights at work and our desire to take control of our lives, such freedom too often still eludes us. On a physical level, the proliferation of poisonous chemicals in our environment and the widespread use of chemically grown convenience foods depleted of essential minerals and trace elements have dangerously eroded our freedom to be healthy—so much so that we now experience a Pandora's box of ailments, from infertility and premenstrual syndrome (PMS), to cancers of the womb and breasts—with a frequency and intensity unprecedented in history.

Meanwhile, driven by a desire to exploit the largest commercial market in the world, drug manufacturers spend a fortune each year in an attempt to convince governments, doctors, and the public that using their products is the only choice available to women for contraception and to treat the problems that arise as menopause approaches. Faced with the prospect of a menopause portrayed increasingly as dangerous to body and psyche—an event that, it is intimated, can turn an attractive woman into an old hag—women can become frightened into complying, sometimes to their long-term detriment. Rather like the temple guardians (statues of threatening animals placed at the door of sacred buildings to dissuade the faint-hearted from entering), our fears of menopause need to be seen for the paper dragons they are. Only then will we be able to pass through the doorway that menopause opens to us and return with the boons of meaning, purpose, and freedom that have been hidden for too long.

On a psychospiritual level, too, we are still seeking to define ourselves as women—not as beings *equal* or *superior* to men or as *counterparts* to men—but rather as creatures in our own right, capable of making autonomous decisions and of tapping our resources for creativity and joy. The knowledge and power that enables a woman to play an active role in supporting her own hormonal changes can restore a woman's faith in the miraculous ability of her body to rebalance and heal itself. Menopause can reconnect a woman to her core values, helping her rediscover her connections with the earth. A woman who *knows* such connectedness seldom needs to rely on high-tech medical intervention or prescriptions. Such are the goals of natural menopause.

To experience menopause as a passage to power, a woman needs two kinds of knowledge. First, she needs scientific information to help discern fact from fiction, as well as information on self-help techniques and natural products to support the transformation taking place in her body and her life. Second, she needs knowledge of the soul—access to myths, symbols, and rituals that help her reconnect with the deepest levels of intuition and instinct. As I began to explore the rich interactions between mind and body via hormones, I realized that the two are inextricably woven together.

The Myths of Science

In our society, the basic approach to health has tended to separate body, mind, and spirit, and to opt for symptomatic treatment of ailments with little concern for the underlying effects on the person being treated. As a result, we now live in a world where it is easy for a woman's biochemistry to become distorted by declining physical activity, the proliferation of highly processed convenience foods, and the rise of a whole new—as yet largely unrecognized—phenomenon known as *estrogen dominance*. Now, instead of the estrogen playing its essential role within the rich symphony of steroid hormones in a woman's body, it has begun to overshadow the other players, some would say creating biochemical dissonance and undermining our mental and physical health.

Estrogen dominance has developed for many reasons, including the widespread use of estrogen-based oral contraceptives and the exponential spread of chemicals in our environment that are *estrogen mimics*. Their presence in such force undermines the natural estrogen/progesterone balance and synergy in a woman's body—sometimes with devastating consequences. Every woman needs to be aware of the potential dangers of the "sea of estrogen" in which we now live. She also needs to know what steps she can take both personally and politically to help counter it. Sadly, most still remain largely ignorant of its existence. As a result, we continue to place responsibility for our lives in the hands of others—doctors, drug companies, and government agencies—who we are told will fix things for us. Too often, instead of making use of these agencies to serve our needs, we allow them to become our masters. It is a tendency that needs to be overcome.

This has already started to happen. There is mounting dissatisfaction among women who continue to be told that drug-based HRT is the only answer to midlife depression, hot flashes, loss of sexual appetite, and early aging, probably because such advice goes strangely against our deepest intuition. For many who have followed it, the use of hormonal drugs has ultimately created more problems than it has solved.

There is also a growing sense among women that osteoporosis—the female plague of the late 20th century—*is* stoppable and that we as women need only to understand what is causing this galloping consumption of our bones and take effective action to stop it. How we do this is another question that this book addresses.

At the same time, more and more women in midlife instinctively feel that it should not be necessary to fill their bodies with drugs to keep them from falling apart, nor should they have to plaster their faces with pricey cosmetics to keep their skin from looking like an alligator's rear end. Although scientific information and simple do-it-yourself techniques for natural menopause are readily available, seldom are they drawn together for easy access and use. Neither are they promoted simply because most are not commercial—there is little money to be made from them.

Among so many women, there exists a deep dissatisfaction with the negative image of the postmenopausal woman and the loss of respect for the female that Western society promulgates. Finally, there is a mounting insistence by women worldwide that we will not only find a way to dream our dreams but, as our childbearing years come to an end, turn our dreams into reality.

The Science of Myth

The loss of respect for the female in our world is paralleled by a lack of respect for the earth. We keep looking for solutions to the ecological crisis on the planet, in the same way that we keep reading books about redefining what it means to be female, yet neither brings us much closer to being able to regenerate the earth or ourselves. Perhaps we have been looking in the wrong place. Maybe we need to abandon the language of science for a time and turn to myth. Mythological symbols and rituals on which women can draw are readily available. They explore the nature of what it is to be female and the meaning implicit in our life changes, yet we have mostly forgotten them. Symbols and myths no longer play an important part in the linear, left-brain education we receive. Together, as women, we now need to move beyond science and explore the archetypal processes involved in the transformations that take place as we move out of our childbearing years and toward the years of the crone.

Crone is a much maligned word. It tends to be used to describe the postmenopausal woman only in her negative aspect—the crone as hag, an ugly old woman. When we fall prey to the false notion that hormone drugs hold all the answers to a menopausal woman's worries, then the medical-industrial complex continues to feed our fear of the crone as a negative archetype and blinds us to her wisdom and beauty. An important part of every woman's menopausal journey is meeting the crone face to face in *all* her mythological aspects—from dark witch to gloriously ripe, wise woman. When you befriend the crone, she shares her power with you. She can help a woman to forge a new, more authentic life for herself, as well as create rich new bonds with other women and with the planet; for *crone* is a word that carries great beauty and power hidden within its original meaning, which can help a woman connect with her own infinite female wisdom. The crone can help us dream our dreams afresh. Embracing her wholeheartedly gives each of us access to new energies and healing abilities that not only benefit ourselves, but can also help us to guide others.

Call to Revolution

In recent years, we have witnessed a revolution in pregnancy and natural childbirth. Where women were once dazzled by high-tech medical intervention at birth, and all too willingly surrendered their bodies to epidurals, episiotomies, and fetal monitoring equipment, in the last 20 years this has changed. We have witnessed a demand for natural childbirth, breast-feeding, and good mother-child bonding. And there has developed a growing willingness by hospitals and government agencies to provide the environment for them. It is women themselves, led by a handful of visionary doctors and thinkers, such as Frédéric Leboyer, Michel Odent, and Pierre Vellay, who have helped to make the world aware of the importance of natural childbirth and who have encouraged us to insist upon it for the physical and spiritual welfare of ourselves and our children.

Now we are poised at the brink of a new revolution. This time it is a revolution in women's natural health care that focuses on the years just before, during, and after menopause. This gentle yet persistent uprising takes its impetus from two sources: first, from an urgent demand among women for profound change; and second, from a group of pioneers who present us with the means for bringing it about. A growing number of scientists and doctors now seriously challenge the wisdom of established medical practice—the doling out of potent drug-based hormones from puberty onwards, and the widespread propaganda that accompanies it. Such practices, they insist, are seriously undermining the long-term health and fertility of women, as well as poisoning the environment. These scientists and experts are not trying to damn HRT, but rather to put it in perspective. They insist that, while it may be useful for short periods in the small number of women who actually *need* extra estrogen, the use of drug-based hormones for most women is costly in financial and physical terms. At the grass roots level, more and more women's voices rise up against the use of estrogen and progestogen drugs in the "treatment" of menopause because they have been shown to carry side effects.

The reason for protest is simple. It is *our* bodies that have to bear the consequences. We sense that whatever menopause may be, it most certainly is not a disease in need of urgent treatment. The guidance we need as women to accomplish our ends both spiritually and physically is already available so long as we are willing to look for it, and so long as we adamantly refuse to buy into the fear-mongering world that would make every menopausal woman a "patient" for the rest of her life. While researching this book, I became aware that the whole idea of menopause as a disease to be treated has largely been concocted by multinational pharmaceutical companies in need of a new market for their drugs. Books such as Sandra Coney's *The Menopause Industry* should be read by any woman wanting to understand the ins and outs of the medical-industrial complex and how it functions. Once you have the facts, the question becomes: What then *is* menopause all about? How do we—each one of us—make our own passage to power? These are some of the issues that this book attempts to address.

Male and Female—Dry and Moist

The male-oriented Western world in which we live is linear and hierarchical. The world of the female is cyclical. The female is moist; the male is dry. The female, like the ancient goddess in whose image she is made, is infinitely generous. Her generosity takes many forms. When Christianity came to Ireland, the Irish hung on to their goddess, carving her into the walls of their churches. Sometimes she is depicted sitting on a pig; sometimes she has a huge vagina that she holds open with her hands. In the 18th and 19th centuries, most of these figures were removed, for what most terrifies the male is the absolute licentiousness of female generosity. It is a power that is completely free, that cannot be bought or sold, manipulated or exploited, and that is continually fueled by the seasons, nature, our friendship with each other, and our bonds to the earth. No wonder our materialistic world has devised ingenious ways of trying to contain women's wildness. Control a woman's hormones, and you may for a time be able to contain her wildness. Yet locked within the wildness of woman is her only true experience of freedom and meaning, as well as her sense of connection to the planet. No woman can live without these things for long. It is my belief that the time has come for the wild female energies to be set free.

The pioneers behind the bloodless revolution have already done much of the groundwork that can help us accomplish this feat. These men and women come from many disciplines. They are scientists and thinkers, psychologists, doctors, herbalists, healers, and shamans. In the next decade, a few are likely to be household names, but chances are that you will not have heard of most of them; for the pioneers of the bloodless revolution belong to no great corporation. Their work, much of which you will find described in the pages that follow (together with references at the back of the book so it can be examined further), helps point the way to orchestrating positive changes in our lives. The responsibility for making practical use of what they have to offer is our own.

Pioneers for Change

Mythologists Demetra George and Joseph Campbell, and storyteller Clarissa Pinkola Estés have uncovered many of the myths and archetypes we can draw on to help us come fully into our spiritual power. New Zealand health educator Sandra Coney, biologist Renate Klein, and her medical scientist colleague Lynette Dumble in Australia have all painstakingly amassed information about menopause, the menopausal woman, and the undermining effect that the medical-industrial complex and its insistence on the widespread use of HRT is having on women. Then there are the *wise women*—such as author Susun Weed and midwife Willa Shaffer—who have spent decades resurrecting long-forgotten female secrets about how to use readily available plants for fertility and the treatment of women troubles—even for natural birth control. Another pioneer in the bloodless revolution is Sandra Ingerman. A practicing shaman, Ingerman has devoted her life to teaching a simple technique that can help people retrieve aspects of their own soul from which they have become separated. Soul retrieval, however it comes, is at the crux of a woman's passage to power.

On the scientific side, biochemist Dr. Ray Peat has shared with all willing to listen his research into steroid hormones. It has led to a profound understanding of the mechanisms by which many of women's illnesses—both mental and physical—develop and may be healed *naturally*. In Canada, endocrinologist Dr. Jerilynn Prior at the University of British Columbia claims to have uncovered the real reasons behind the plague of osteoporosis and infertility that we in the industrial world are now experiencing. At the University of Cambridge, professor of clinical gerontology Kay-Tee Khaw investigates how lifestyle and diet can influence a woman's experience of menopause, drawing upon new knowledge in biochemistry and nutrition. A handful of courageous British physicians such as Dr. Shirley Bond, Dr. Shamim Daya, Dr. Patrick Kingsley, Dr. Barry Durrant-Peatfield, and Dr. Yehudi Gordon are already helping individual women find their way. Meanwhile, an expert in natural hormones and brain chemistry, and a researcher in 21st-century energy medicine, Dr. Robert Jacobs heads charitable trusts in Britain and the United States, where the lives of seriously ill people are transformed from sickness into health. The charities also focus on helping people who are well to maximize their energies to become super-healthy. Jacobs and his wife, body therapist Beth Jacobs, use leading-edge techniques to regenerate and rejuvenate women, enabling them to experience better health, greater clarity, and more control over their destiny. Finally—and in many ways the most important pioneer of all in the bloodless revolution—there is American physician Dr. John Lee.

Let There Be Light

Lee is a family doctor who has spent the last 15 years exploring the actions of a *natural* plant-derived form of progesterone available to women in most countries without prescription. Together with a good diet and lifestyle changes, he has found that this natural hormone is capable of eliminating much of the suffering associated with both PMS and menopause. Thousands of women in the Western world now use natural progesterone—generally in the form of a nonprescription cream that you rub on the body—and claim they have not only relief from female symptoms, but experience increased vitality, better skin tone, and renewed emotional balance. Many who have been through the transformations that natural progesterone can bring consider them little short of miraculous. Contrary to traditional medical thinking, Dr. Lee believes that the use of natural progesterone together with dietary and lifestyle change can not only stop osteoporosis, but actually *reverse* it—even in women aged 70 or more. Lee, who discovered this, now spends his life researching, lecturing, and giving help to doctors, scientists, and women who want to find their way out of the labyrinth of suffering—yet he adamantly refuses to accept any money for his work. He is determined to maintain his own autonomy and to return the power for well-being where he believes it belongs—firmly in the hands of the individual woman.

Without the painstaking devotion of these pioneers for change, there would be no bloodless revolution. However, just as so-called common people have created the basis for every popular movement for change in the past, it is only we women who can bring the revolution that has now been seeded into full flower. This is how change has always happened throughout history, whether the revolutionaries have been seeking democratic representation or the end of slavery. Sometimes history books give the impression that successful movements come about solely because of their leaders—that it was only Nelson Mandela and Martin Luther King who brought about the civil rights movement. But these men were not the civil rights movement. Their names appear in history books because many people whose names you never know or whose names are long forgotten were working for change. So it is with the bloodless revolution. When you have enough women devoting themselves to change, then pathfinders such as Jerilynn Prior, John Lee, Sandra Coney, and Demetra George become well known. But that is only because, at the grass roots level, individuals—in this case we women ourselves—are doing the work.

This process has already begun. Groups of women in Canada, the United States, Britain, Australia, South Africa, and New Zealand are already demanding *another way*. They want to know about herbs and homeopathic remedies. They are rediscovering alternatives based on long traditions of use in natural medicine, hard-core scientific findings, and current clinical use. They are also exploring how natural hormones such as progesterone, and leading-edge substances such as melatonin, DMAE, and L-pyroglutamic acid can be used to balance brain and mood, to heighten immunity, and to slow down aging. Such women want to *experience* how various natural substances act upon their bodies. They are demanding methods of self-care that take into account how spirit and body interact and support each other, and they are not content with palliative symptomatic treatments that carry the threat of dangerous side effects. The time has come, they insist, for us to stop thinking of ourselves as victims—victims of cancer, of PMS, of menopausal trauma, or anything else. When you see yourself in the role of a victim, nothing can help you. Only when we let go of the victim role can we begin to take an active part in our own transformation.

Call to Adventure

The radical and fundamental changes that take place in a woman's life around the time of menopause are not signs of decay or pathology, but rather a *call to adventure* signaling the beginning of each woman's archetypal *hero's journey* to her core. When a woman makes such a journey, she discovers that menopause is not only a time for grieving over past mistakes and irredeemable losses, but that it is also a time for rejoicing. It is a time to regenerate and rejuvenate our bodies using a combination of ancient principles and leading-edge science. Most of all, menopause is a time to celebrate that our creativity is no longer bound to our obligations as a member of the human race to propagate the species. Often for the first time in a woman's life, her creativity can be set free for use in whatever way the whispers of her soul dictate.

To me there is little more exciting than being present at the beginning of the bloodless revolution—a quiet moment that promises to bring better health and greater autonomy in its wake. This is where we now stand. This book is designed to serve as a traveler's companion—a guide to both the scientific and the mythological aspects of the menopausal journey. In many ways, it is rather like a collection of rudimentary maps to which a woman can turn in the course of planning and carrying out her own hero's journey. The book is divided into three parts: The Myths of Science, The Science of Myth, and a practical section called Rites and Rituals. As a whole, the book explores the experience of menopause from its spiritual and psychological roots to its hormonal interactions. It draws together the work of trailblazers from a great variety of fields and presents it in a way that hopefully can help a woman wanting to take control of her own life to do so with relative ease. It addresses the knowledge that the pioneers have unearthed and some of the visions held for women—not only around the time of menopause itself, but during the eight to ten years that precede it—as well as the many years afterwards. PMS and osteoporosis, like all the other manifestations of hormonal imbalances, are easiest to prevent by taking action long before menopause arrives. However, no matter what your age or condition, it is never too late to benefit from the newly acquired knowledge.

Each woman is biochemically and spiritually unique. So is the hero's journey that she must undertake if she is to succeed in her quest for wholeness. Although there are useful allies to be found every step of the way, such as birth and death, a woman's menopause passage is one that, by its very nature, she must make alone. After all, when King Arthur's knights set out on their search for the Holy Grail, each entered the woods alone at the place where it was darkest, never dreaming to walk a path that another had walked before him. To do so would have dishonored the quest. Such journeys cannot be codified. They are not package holidays where you pay your money and know exactly what to expect. These are journeys of the soul.

CHAPTER TWO

CRY FREEDOM
Will the Real Menopause Please Stand Up

Nobody ever prepares you for menopause. Nobody tells you that if you are going to have hot flashes or emotional instability, they are likely to be far worse *before* you stop menstruating than afterwards. Nor does anybody explain that waking regularly at two or three in the morning and lying in bed filled with sadness or fear or anger is likely to be not some aberration of nature but a messenger announcing that menopause is near. Because we are told so little, few women in our culture are prepared for the third movement of the hormonal symphony—menopause—nor for the next phase of their life. They seldom expect the intensity of emotion—both pain and pleasure—that can accompany the end of the childbearing years.

Perils of Pathology

Too many women in the Western world first come upon menopause as a result of some pathological event for which they feel forced to seek medical advice: endometriosis, fibroid tumors, depression, loss of libido, vaginal discomfort during intercourse, or the kind of persistent excessive bleeding that can make a woman weak with anemia and weary of the struggle. Such symptoms sometimes result in the loss of a womb. It can be easier for doctors to take out something they are not sure how to handle than to struggle with their own frustration and sense of inadequacy while in search of another way. If surgery is not seen to be the answer, then often a woman is led to believe that Hormone Replacement Therapy (HRT) is. After all, taking estrogen is supposed to halt osteoporosis. "Quite frankly, my dear, I think it would be *dangerous* to try to live without it," one leading gynecologist intimated to me recently. "Be sure to take plenty of calcium pills and drink lots of milk." The so-called experts often add that HRT is important in preventing early aging. "You don't want your skin to go all wrinkled and saggy, do you? You don't want your vagina to dry up! And you *do* want to remain *feminine* and *desirable*, don't you? Well, don't you?"

Just about everybody who is anybody these days will tell you that menopause is an estrogen deficiency disease and that you need to take more estrogen as you approach midlife. What may surprise you is this: Not only is most of such commonly given advice on menopause wrong, but a great deal of it can be positively dangerous. Nevertheless, such is the introduction to menopause for almost half of the women in the industrialized world today. It ignores the freedom waiting to be claimed now that the childbearing years have ended—freedom to surrender to passionate love-making without fear of pregnancy, or to refuse sex altogether if we choose and to channel our libido in other directions. Menopause also brings freedom from the emotional ups and downs that commonly accompany the moon cycles of menstruating women, as well as the freedom to feel radiantly well. For, now, you no longer need to be bound into whatever your role has been. Anthropologist Margaret Mead always insisted that passing through menopause brought a woman the gift of "postmenopausal zest."

Sadly, the menopausal horror stories we hear today have become so far removed from the positive experiences reported by women in the past and still reported by women in other parts of the world, that it is easy to wonder who is lying. Women have begun to ask themselves just what is going on. Is menopause a cosmic joke—an aberration of evolution? Did nature foul up when she made us this way? Are we *meant* to be over the hill at the age of 50? Is the doctor right? If we don't take HRT, are we going to end up as crumpled old bags in ten years—or, even worse, dead after having broken both hips falling down the stairs? If any of this sounds exaggerated, then you have not spent as much time as I have talking with menopausal women in Britain, North America, Australia, New Zealand, and South Africa. For these are very much the fears and exhortations to which women are now subjected. It is not easy for a woman to know what to make of it all until she has a good understanding of what takes place when menopause—the second big initiation—arrives and the third stage of her life begins. Each woman needs to become familiar with what lies behind the various pathologies (illnesses and abnormalities) commonly associated with menopause in the Western world, as well as how relatively easy it can be to counter them if she chooses, often without having to resort to serious medical intervention of any kind.

What Is Menopause?

The first challenge menopause presents a woman is the task of identifying exactly what it is. Apart from those cheerful little booklets on the subject in doctors' offices that are thinly disguised vehicles for the sale of Hormone Replacement Therapy (HRT), information is often not readily available. Even most well-written articles in women's magazines and in newspapers closely follow the "catechism." In recent decades, backed by major pharmaceutical money, an obsession with HRT has developed. As a result, in the past 30 years, very little objective research into other aspects of menopause and the hormonal changes associated with it has even been carried out. Few doctors are as yet aware of what does exist.

When you examine the studies that have been conducted with respect to menopause, you realize that many of the so-called symptoms of menopause have nothing particularly to do with it. They are instead symptoms of aging or of physiological imbalances that have developed out of lifestyles that do not give real support to the proper functioning of mind and body, or symptoms of frustration at the very deepest levels of the soul when a woman is trying to live everybody else's life rather than her own. Such *false* menopausal symptoms can include aches and pains, fatigue, digestive disturbances, and anxiety—all of which develop when a woman's metabolic processes are no longer functioning as they should be. They may be the result of years of eating convenience foods depleted of essential minerals and trace elements yet replete with trans-fatty acids or junk fats (see chapter 11, "Order Out of Chaos"). They can also develop out of having wrestled with the long-term stress of a marriage that isn't working or a career that demands everything of you yet brings you little satisfaction in return. Around the time of midlife, all of these things get thrown together and wrongly labeled "the symptoms of menopause." To treat them as such by papering over the cracks with tranquilizers or hormone drugs (other than temporarily if absolutely necessary) can mean interfering with the power that comes with the menopause journey. It is a journey that, when taken with your eyes open, promises to take you to the very source of your strength and creativity and helps you to make positive changes in your life. This can bring about not just palliative and temporary relief from symptoms, but long-term improved health and the discovery of new spiritual freedom and power.

Will the Real Menopause Please Stand Up

Back in 1973, two epidemiologists at Oxford, John and Sonja McKinlay, set out to survey the research that had been carried out on menopause. They discovered that there had been very little research, and that most of what had been done suffered from serious holes in its methodology. Many studies did not discriminate between women who had undergone a *surgical menopause* resulting from the removal of their womb or ovaries, and women who had experienced a natural menopause. Even much of the research into HRT that examines the use of estrogen in relation to osteoporosis is seriously flawed. Certain that estrogen was the prime factor in preventing osteoporosis, for years researchers paid little attention to whether or not women taking part in various studies had been given anything else as well. Yet when you go back and examine many of the studies frequently cited as "proof" that estrogen counters osteoporosis, you find that the women studied had also been given a progestogen or progesterone. Still, too few stop to ask the question: "Is it really estrogen that is the prime factor in preventing osteoporosis, or might it be something else?" Since the McKinlay research, by far the most revealing investigations into the nature of menopause have been carried out not by medical researchers, but by anthropologists, psychologists, sociologists, and epidemiologists. As a result, despite all the books and articles on the subject and all the leaflets handed out, surprisingly little objective medical information is available about the menopausal woman. The people who know most about natural menopause are the women themselves who have passed through it.

To some women, even a hint that menopause may be on its way seems confirmation that they are "past it," or "it's all downhill from here." At some point in midlife, every woman in our society comes to feel the sadness and frustration that arises because our society links physical aging to a loss of sexual attractiveness and self-esteem. So when menopause arrives, it can seem to be an unwelcome visitor. Women who have long been at home may find that home and family no longer hold the fascination that they once did, nor do they seem to be good sources from which to draw a sense of personal identity any longer. Women who have worked for years in the world, on the other hand, can come to feel that although they may have achieved the success they once yearned for, something fundamental is missing. They ask themselves if life is not passing them by.

As marketing folk worth their salt know full well, the easiest way to sell anything to a woman is to convince her that she is inadequate and in desperate need of whatever is being offered. This is exactly what has happened with HRT. A woman nearing the passage of menopause is particularly vulnerable to such suggestions. If she is told that menopause is a deficiency disease or an inevitable source of struggle, pain, and grief, undermining her sexual attractiveness and pushing her over the hill, she is likely to face her future burdened with these notions. Once a woman, even unconsciously, swallows the negative stereotypes that our culture has created about the older woman, she opens herself up to the idea that she needs "treatment." But take heart. There *is* another way.

Early Start

Strictly speaking, just as the word *menarche* means a woman's first menstrual period, *menopause* means the last period she will ever have. *Meno* comes from the Greek, meaning "month"; and *pause* from *pausis,* meaning "halt." In common usage, however, when most people speak of menopause, they are talking about the entirety of the period a woman goes through—often for years before and after her last menstruation—during which the production of the estrogens and progesterone slow down, her periods may become irregular, and she begins to experience other signs of body change from sudden fluctuations in temperature to alterations in sleep patterns. This total transition from childbearing to post-childbearing is properly known as the *climacteric*. And because each woman is a biochemical and physiological individual, it can last from a few months to as long as 15 years.

The climacteric is usually divided into three parts: *perimenopause* to indicate the time when hormonal shifts have already begun but a woman is still menstruating; *menopause*, the time at which the last period occurs; and *postmenopause*, which among wise women was traditionally considered to have begun on the 14th moon after a woman's last menstruation, since by then her reproductive capacity had most definitely finished. The end of a woman's reproductive life seldom coincides with the time of her last period, in fact. It can either precede the moment of menopause or come afterwards. This is the main reason why it is important to continue to use some sort of contraception for the first year to 18 months after your last period if you don't want another child.

The physiological cause of menopause is simple. It is not a woman's age that brings it about, but rather the "burning out" of her ovaries when the finite number of eggs she has carried since birth are all used up. Since puberty, the ovaries have allowed maybe 400 follicles to ripen while thousands more unneeded and unused eggs have at the same time partly ripened then degenerated and been resorbed into her body. So by the time a woman reaches the age of 45, very few follicles are left waiting to be triggered into action. As the number grows smaller and smaller, follicles begin to mature irregularly. Around the same time, the secretion of estrogens by a woman's ovaries decreases, as does the production of progesterone. Then somewhere between the ages of 40 and 50 (although it can happen earlier or later), a woman's sexual cycles often become irregular because ovulation no longer takes place during some of her cycles—even though she may appear to be menstruating as usual. Gradually, this *anovulatory* menstruation begins to occur more often. Anovulatory menstruation is a menstrual period in which, although you bleed as expected—often more heavily than expected—no mature follicle is released from your ovary, so you are not capable of becoming pregnant. It is common in women in the years preceding menopause and is the major reason why fertility drops greatly as women get older. When ovulation does not take place, progesterone levels take a nose dive since no corpus luteum (glandular mass in the ovary formed after ovulation) has been formed to produce the hormone. Very few people—doctors and women alike—are as yet aware of the implications of anovulatory menstruation or that it can exert powerful negative effects on a woman's body and psyche. Neither do they know how widespread it has become in our society, nor how great a role it is playing in the rise of infertility in the industrialized world—not to mention in the increasing number of women developing negative symptoms, from PMS to menstrual flooding.

Egg-Free Menstruation

Canadian researcher Jerilynn Prior, chief endocrinologist at the University of British Columbia in Vancouver, has done more than any other scientist to bring to light the significance of anovulatory menstruation. Prior and her colleagues made the important discovery that a substantial proportion of menstruating women, long before menopause, are no longer ovulating. Their finding came out of some original work with women athletes whose periods had stopped as a result of heavy training. After studying female athletes in depth, Prior published a paper describing how it is that women in training for marathon running develop osteoporosis. At that time, the medical profession widely believed that this occurs because female athletes are simply not making enough estrogen. (Most of the medical profession still believes this.) Prior meticulously measured estrogen levels in these women and discovered that they were normal. In the process, Prior and her researchers measured a lot of other things, too—including the level of progesterone in their subjects. She and her team discovered that it is the progesterone, not the estrogen, in these young athletes that becomes depleted. In fact, their progesterone levels are not just low, they can be lower than that of a man's. Although the women Prior studied were still menstruating, they were not ovulating; therefore, they were not producing progesterone.

So out of Prior's work, an important discovery emerged. The osteoporosis that occurs in women runners is due not to lack of estrogen as was believed, but rather to lack of progesterone. Now this was hot stuff. When Prior's paper was published in a respectable scientific journal, it should by rights have tossed a bombshell into the medical world, especially since almost every doctor was giving estrogen for osteoporosis. Yet nobody seemed to take much notice.

Female Epidemic

Prior then became intrigued to see what was happening to the hormones of ordinary women. Her next paper, which appeared two or three years later, reported on a similar study carried out on nonathletic women, in which she discovered that the same thing was happening to them. Many women reaching their mid-30s have their periods as usual, yet become anovulatory and are therefore deficient in progesterone. When it comes to female athletes, the theory has always been that since they train so hard and keep their body fat so low, the body thinks that it is not able to have a baby, so does not make the estrogen needed, and periods cease. This was believed by scientists to be some kind of reflex that happened as a result of a lack of cholesterol—the molecule from which the steroids are made, including progesterone and the estrogens.

But Prior's second group of women were not doing extra exercise, and their body fat levels were normal, so something else had to be going on. Whatever it was, unbeknownst to the medical world, it had grown to epidemic proportions. Prior and her colleagues discovered that anovulation and a short luteal phase cycle now occurs in up to 50 percent of North American women's menstrual cycles during the final reproductive years. Just what is it that is causing this epidemic of 35-year-old progesterone-depleted women who are *not* ovulating but *are* developing osteoporosis long before menopause?

It has taken the work of environmental scientists of the caliber of Niels Skakkebaek, researcher at the Rigshopital in Copenhagen, and Richard M. Sharpe of the British Medical Council's Center for Reproductive Biology in Edinburgh to point the way toward an answer. We in the industrialized world, they tell us, now live immersed in a rising sea of petrochemical derivatives. They are in our air, our foods, and our water. These chemicals include pesticides and herbicides, as well as various plastics that all have a phenol ring in common as part of their chemical structure. This means they are capable of mimicking the action of estrogen in an animal's body and that they can also burn out a woman's ovaries, using up her follicles long before their time. When this happens, anovulatory menstruation occurs so that progesterone production decreases or even stops altogether—with potentially devastating consequences for some women.

Chemical Seas

The estrogen-mimicking chemicals that have come to pollute our environment do not break down and disappear. Sprayed on our grain and vegetables, including the corn that is fed to the animals whose meat we eat, these petroleum by-products are fat soluble. They have to be. For only if they are fat-based will they dissolve the insect cuticle so that insects feeding on these plants will be killed. However, these chemicals don't just cease to exist once they have done their insect-killing job. They remain in our foodstuffs. The meat we consume from feed-lot fed animals is full of fat in which these chemicals are stored. The fat we see can always be trimmed off, but most fat in meat is marbled into the muscle and cannot be removed.

Such highly polluting petroleum derivatives have by now been spread all over the industrialized world. Thousands of miles from where they were used to spray crops, they can be found in quantity in the fat of Arctic seals. Gradually, over the years, we accumulate these toxins in the fat of our own bodies. Research shows that they are found in particularly high quantities in women who develop breast cancer. There is an argument raging in medicine at the moment: It centers on the relationship between a high-fat intake and the incidence of breast cancer. In the West, we now consume almost half of our calories in the form of fat, and breast cancer incidence continues to rise. Scientists have known for some time that the incidence of breast cancer can be directly correlated with the levels of fat a woman has in her diet. Now, however, a growing number of experts aware of the rise in estrogen-mimicking chemicals are beginning to suspect that it is not so much the *fat* that predisposes a woman to breast cancer, but the *toxins* that have accumulated in the fat and which then build up in her body.

The leitmotif running through almost all of the "menopausal horrors" for which women are put on HRT—and filled full of yet *more* estrogen—is estrogen dominance—that is, high estrogen or estrogenlike chemicals in the presence of a relative insufficiency of progesterone in the woman's body. You find the same hormonal pattern in anovulatory cycles, breast cancer, mood swings, night sweats, and fibroids, as well as many other illnesses associated with menstruation and menopause. The incidence of fibrocystic breast disease, uterine fibroids, endometriosis, PMS, breast cancer, and cancer of the womb has in recent years become alarmingly high and continues to mount in industrialized countries. Yet these conditions used to be rare. They are still virtually unknown in nonindustrialized areas of the world where women live mostly on a simple diet of compost-grown local foods.

Egg or No Egg?

It can be hard for a woman to know for sure if her cycles are anovulatory or not. Sometimes periods become irregular, heavier, or of longer duration. Sometimes she will have PMS or depression. In many women, their periods can seem quite normal. The only way to know for sure is to have a laboratory test done for low serum progesterone (that is, low levels of progesterone in the blood) between days 18 and 26 of your menstrual cycle. Most laboratories say day 21 is best. A normal serum progesterone level after ovulation is in the range of 7 to 28 picograms. If a woman does not ovulate that month, then the level tends to be around 0.3 picograms. This is a test that your doctor can order.

Where estrogen dominance does exist, the only way to correct it is to reestablish a good balance between estrogen and progesterone. This, too, can be easier said than done, especially if your doctor, like many, has been steeped in the dogma of HRT. Adding one of the progestogens that are now frequently used together with estrogen as part of HRT won't do it. What these synthetics do is to help protect against cancer of the womb if you are on extra estrogen drugs. But, because all the progestogens are end-molecules, your body cannot use them to make the other steroids it needs for hormonal balance, energy, emotional stability, and protection from stress. Only natural progesterone can offer these things. And because the progestogens take up progesterone receptor sites, using them in HRT or contraception further reduces the levels of natural progesterone in your body and can therefore interfere with your body's ability to make more.

Low progesterone levels in a woman experiencing anovulatory menstruation increase estrogen dominance in her body even further as she gets closer and closer to menopause and the complex hormonal feedback mechanisms between the central control station—the hypothalamus—and its first officer, the pituitary, come into play. This can cause disturbances in the feedback mechanisms involving important hormones such as GnRh, LH, and FSH. This creates mood swings, hot flashes, and depression, not to mention disruptions in the thyroid and in the functions of the many other organs and systems that the hypothalamus oversees—all common experiences of perimenopausal women in the industrialized world. Dr. Barry Durrant-Peatfield, one of Britain's pioneers in the menopause revolution, says of estrogen dominance: "Water retention and bloating; increasing enlargement of the bust, mastitis and cystic disease of the breast, weight gain, loss of energy and libido, increased risks of breast and endometrial [womb] cancer and the start of osteoporosis...progesterone will stop all of these problems." He continues: "This situation is really the start of menopause, and the use of progesterone is obviously what is required while the use of estrogen in this situation, as with HRT, may be quite disastrous."

Eventually menopause arrives. Estrogen levels finally fall at the time in a woman's life when they are meant to—usually somewhere between the ages of 45 and 52. Periods become erratic or lighter or irregular in the quantity of blood lost. Eventually they stop altogether, since there is now not enough estrogen to stimulate the proliferation of the endometrium. All of this should take place without much difficulty. Thankfully it still does for most women throughout the world. But in Western industrialized society, more than half of the female population are now thrown into confusion and forced to suffer the negative symptoms of menopause in no uncertain terms—night sweats, hot flashes, emotional ups and downs, even hirsutism (the appearance of hair in quantity on the face and body).

Estrogen Deficient—No Way

Just about everyone these days still leaps to the conclusion that menopausal women *need* estrogen. Many women still believe, and so do their doctors for that matter, that when menstruation finally ceases, a woman's estrogen production falls to nothing. They also think that it is estrogen that keeps skin young looking and sexuality glowing—both of which are patently untrue. A woman's estrogen production does not cease at menopause. Only estrogen production in her ovaries stops so that the monthly buildup of the womb lining in preparation for pregnancy doesn't happen. This is why menstruation no longer takes place. However, provided a woman's body is in good balance and she is healthy, the estrogen she makes now in her fat cells, in her liver, and in her adrenals is all she will ever need.

What does cease, however—or pretty nearly ceases—as soon as menopause arrives, if not earlier, is the production of progesterone. It can fall to near zero. In an estrogen-dominant woman, this produces some of the symptoms commonly associated with menopause, many of which the average doctor is still trying to "treat" by giving a woman more estrogen. In a few women, low or no progesterone can lead to hirsutism, as well as to male-pattern baldness often associated with old age. This is because their bodies, in the absence of progesterone, turn toward DHEA (dehydroepiandrostenediol) and the male hormones, such as androstenediol and androstenedione, as the only metabolic pathway left open to the production of the estrogens.

Other Side Effects

Because progesterone is a precursor to so many other steroid hormones, when the body's production of it ceases or when estrogen dominance gets out of hand, other hormones are not produced adequately either. Some progesterone-derived hormones (hormones to which progesterone is a precursor) are brain chemicals that influence the way you think and feel. Others are needed by the body to protect against inflammation and early aging or to sustain libido. The absence of sufficient quantities of these steroids can produce aches and pains in the joints, chronic fatigue, as well as depression, hot flashes, and anxiety. It can also be a prime cause of the emotional upsets that many women experience in midlife, where a woman is often urged to "pull herself together" or is branded "emotionally ill." Such experiences are most assuredly *not* a natural part of growing older. They are signs that a woman's hormonal balance needs help.

Too often these days, the help that is offered comes automatically in the form of drug-based HRT. The new menopause revolutionaries insist that this is usually not the best way to go. It can be far more helpful to a woman and far more protective of her long-term health to look first to her lifestyle and help her make adjustments in the way she eats, the kind of nutritional supplements she uses, and introduce her to the remarkable healing and balancing properties of natural plant substances. Often this alone will be enough to restore a high level of balance and well-being. Then, if hormones are needed, they claim, it is far better to consider making use of the natural hormones—those that are chemically identical to the hormones her own body produces.

The pioneers are also aware, to a degree that few of their less informed colleagues are, that certain of the natural estrogens such as estriol are far safer than others, such as estrone or estradiol if for a time a woman needs a little extra estrogen to protect against vaginal thinning or help her through a rough-and-tumble period of hot flashes. What is so exciting about the new approach is the way in which its advocates take a genuinely holistic view of women. They know about the dangers of estrogen dominance, and they look for ways to not only help a woman counter it but at the same time enhance her mental clarity and emotional balance so that menopause becomes a true passage to power for each woman. We will be examining closely how they do this in later chapters. First let's take a closer look at the sea of environmental estrogens in which we now live, and examine just how widespread are its potential consequences—not only to the lives of women, but to men and children as well as animal life on the planet.

SLEEPING WITH THE ENEMY

Our Greatest Environmental Menace: The Xenoestrogens

ne of the great ironies at the turn of the millennium is that for almost half a century, women have been encouraged to use estrogens. They have been sold both as a means of birth control and for counteracting negative symptoms experienced at menopause. Yet it turns out that excessive estrogen may well be the greatest enemy any woman in the industrialized world ever faces. It is a silent enemy present day-in-day-out as we eat, as we work, and as we sleep.

20th-Century Plague

Of the thousands of estrogens and estrogenlike chemicals that appear to be responsible for the mounting incidence of estrogen dominance in our culture, none appear quite as sinister as *xenoestrogens*—sometimes called xenobiotics. The word *xeno* means "strange" or "foreign." Xenoestrogen is the name given to environmental pollutants and chemicals now widespread in our foods, our air, and our water that are capable of disrupting biological processes. They mimic the effects of a woman's own natural estrogens, and interfere with the balance of estrogens and progesterone in her body. Because xenoestrogens are taken up by estrogen receptor sites in the body and because the hormones in the body interact with its organs and systems as well as with each other in highly complex and interdependent ways, they can disrupt the workings of the body as a whole. This group of environmental toxins includes hundreds of bedrock chemicals now widespread in our postindustrial society—from the polycarbonated plastics found in our baby bottles and water jugs, the polychlorinated biphenyls (PCBs) used in the manufacture of electronics, to highly poisonous pesticides such as DDT and its even more toxic cousin DDE. It also includes dieldrin, toxaphene, mirex, heptachlor, and kepone, as well as hundreds of other herbicides and pesticides, all of which have an ability to mimic natural estrogen. Even the breakdown products from many common detergents can do this, as can the chlorine compounds now used to bleach paper.

All steroid hormones are derived from cholesterol. However, the estrogen molecule is unique among the steroids—it has a phenol in what chemists call its "A-ring" in the basic cholesterol framework. So whether estrogens are made in the body or come in the form of chemical sprays, all estrogens are what is chemically called *phenolated*. None of the other steroid molecules, such as testosterone, progesterone, or corticosterone have a phenolated A-ring in their molecular structure. A phenolated A-ring is also common among petrochemical by-products, such as the organochlorines and pesticides that get into the food chain. They concentrate in the fat of the animals that we eat and eventually in our own fat. Vegetarians are generally better off than meat eaters in terms of the quantity of xenoestrogens they absorb simply because plants tend to have less fat than animals, and what there is tends to be confined to the germ of a grain. Meat, however, is 50 percent fat or even more, so the great mass of the estrogenic pollutants in our environment finds its way into our bodies—most easily by way of animal fats.

The xenoestrogens resemble other estrogens in some of the effects they exert on the body. Some resemble them molecularly; others can look quite different. All these chemicals and their breakdown products can enter our bodies. Hormones used in birth control and in hormone replacement are other forms of estrogens foreign to the human system. Most forms of estrogens, natural or chemical, are capable of bringing about biochemical changes in the body. Sometimes they are able to attach themselves to receptor sites within the body's cells and prevent the natural hormonal response. Other times they may even stimulate a hormone receptor. Unfortunately, estrogen receptor sites are not particularly choosy. Fraudulent estrogens in pesticides and other chemicals can just as easily hook to them as the real thing.

Locks and Keys

Cell receptor sites normally trigger genetic activity when a hormone or a vitamin is keyed into them, functioning rather like a key that opens a lock. For a long time, scientists believed that each lock would only open when presented with the exact molecular key intended for it. They thought that only the perfect key would turn its "tumblers" to release the gene action as in the estrogen-modulated biology of breast growth, for instance. Recently, however, they have discovered that many foreign chemicals are also capable of opening up estrogen receptors. These estrogen mimics can then fool the body into turning off certain biochemical pathways with the sort of consequences that include the development of cancers of the breast and womb, endometriosis, infertility, and cause changes in the reproductive and hormone systems—not only of adults, but also of unborn children. This happens in several different ways. Some estrogen molecules fit into the receptor keyholes but won't fully unlock them, so they don't trigger normal activity on a cellular level. Others behave like poorly cut keys—sometimes they will turn the lock and sometimes they won't. A third group act like skeleton keys and appear to fit perfectly into a receptor and fully unlock its gene action, yet can still bring devastating effects in their wake.

Reproductive Devastation

One of the most infamous of these estrogen mimics is the drug diethylstilbestrol (DES). Between 1948 and 1971, as many as six million women in Europe and the United States took this synthetic form of estrogen that was enthusiastically touted for its ability to prevent miscarriage. Around the same time—according to John A. McLachlan, a tall, slim, handsome man with a fine sense of humor, who organized the recent world conference sponsored by the National Institute of Environmental Health Sciences (NIEHS) in the United States—some 60,000 pounds of DES were also given to cattle as a "growth promoter." Years down the road, the incidence of abnormalities in the offspring of women treated with DES is still being tallied. Female offspring of women who took it have a high level of T-shaped wombs and other structural abnormalities in their organs, predisposing them to sterility. Many male offspring show similar structural abnormalities, including a high incidence of undescended testicles and deformed urethras, as well as a lowered sperm count. Both males and females show a much higher incidence of certain forms of cancer—from the rare Clear-Cell Vaginal Adenocarcinoma in women, to testicular and prostate cancer in men. McLachlan, who is also chief of NIEHS's laboratory on reproductive and developmental toxicology, looks upon the effects of DES on the off-spring of mothers given the drug as a model for the kinds of effect xeno-estrogens may be having today. DES is the only estrogenic substance so far known to trigger the body's estrogen receptor activity even more efficient-ly than the body's natural estrogens.

At a recent conference in California called "Environmental Estrogens: Pathway to Extinction," McLachlan pointed out that screening chemicals using traditional toxicology for their hormonal effects is virtually impossi-ble since these may not show up until the next generation is born. We can-not, he points out, judge a chemical's hormonal activity by any specific attribute of its molecular structure. He therefore suggests that we turn to what he calls "functional toxicology" when chemicals are defined not by their chemical structure but by how they act on an organism. Chemicals could be tested, for instance, for their ability to occupy, activate, or turn off cell receptors. This information could be included with chemical informa-tion such as molecular weight, melting point, and solubility to help us bet-ter anticipate chemical dangers where they are present. So far, we are a gen-eration away from doing this. Meanwhile, we keep taking more and more xenoestrogens into our bodies.

Secrets of Estrogen

In order to grasp how xenoestrogens affect the body, it is important to know how the natural estrogens work. There are three major kinds of estro-gens made in the human body: estradiol (the most common and the most potent), estriol, and estrone. These estrogens are produced mainly in the ovaries, although small quantities are secreted from the adrenal glands, the placenta during pregnancy, and in fat cells. The estrogen production in a woman's body begins when she is still a fetus, reaches its peak after puber-ty, and then declines at menopause. While you were in the womb, estrogens stimulated the development of your ovaries and uterus and ensured that you developed properly into a female child. Men, too, produce estrogen, but in much smaller quantities than we do. High estrogen levels in a male fetus prevent the full development of masculine characteristics needed for a boy, even if its genes are programmed to produce a male child. When puberty arrives, estrogens in a girl encourage the development of breasts and the expansion of the uterus. After that, they help regulate the menstrual cycle and play other important roles, such as helping to maintain bone mass and keeping blood cholesterol levels in check. When excessive quantities of estrogen, regardless of source, are present in a young woman's body, they will burn out her ovaries and undermine fertility. It is this phenomenon that many eco-scientists believe to be largely responsible for the rapidly decreasing fertility in Western women.

Each year, evidence mounts further that women in industrialized countries are suffering from an overexposure to estrogen mimics. In 1960, the chances of a woman developing breast cancer were only one in 20. Today, one in nine women are statistically destined to get the disease. Only about 30 percent of women who get breast cancer now are in what are considered high-risk groups—women who have an early menses, don't breast-feed or breast-fed for a limited period, come from a family with a history of breast cancer, or who have their first pregnancy late in life. A number of studies have recently demonstrated that women exposed to polycyclic aromatic hydrocarbons (PAHs) and polychlorinated biphenyls (PCBs) have a significantly higher rate of breast cancer than women not exposed. Devra Lee Davis at the U.S. Department of Health and Human Services is one of the scientists who has closely examined the issue of breast cancer. She points out that many studies have shown elevated breast cancer rates in women who have worked in the chemical industry and who have been exposed to PCBs or PAHs in drinking water, or who have breast tissue that contains high concentrations of DDT.

Good-Guy Estrogen

To make things even more complicated, not all estrogens or estrogen-like substances exert the *negative* effect on the body that estrogen drugs and xenoestrogens can. In the same way that medicine now recognizes that there is a good-guy cholesterol and a bad-guy cholesterol in relation to protecting the body from heart disease, so are there "good" estrogens and "bad" estrogens. According to Herman Aldercreutz, nutritional chemist at the University of Helsinki, and others, a number of weaker natural estrogenlike ingredients in foods actually help protect us against cancer of the breast and reproductive system by binding with estrogen receptor sites so that dangerously strong estrogenic compounds are not so readily taken up. Many of the best protective foods contain estrogenlike compounds called isoflavoids. They are found in many of the soya-based foods eaten daily in the Orient, such as tofu, tempeh, and miso, as well as in rye bread and in legumes, such as lentils. A number of other edible plants, including pomegranates and French beans, contain phyto-estrogens of a different kind that also boast protective properties. At the Children's Hospital Medical Center in Washington, D.C., when Kenneth Setchell fed rodents on soya protein, he discovered that his animals developed far fewer tumors than animals fed on a soy-free diet. This, plus the fact that Japanese women also eat a great variety of land and sea plants that continually help to detoxify the body, may explain why Asians still have very low rates of breast cancer and few menopause-related problems compared to Europeans and North Americans. However, when Japanese women move to the United States and take up a Western diet, they rapidly develop the same diseases we have.

Not Created Equal

Devra Lee Davis at the United States Department of Health and Human Services is one of the researchers delving into the way in which estrogens are not all created equal. She says that when the body produces estradiol, this estrogen can be broken down via two different metabolic pathways. One turns into a form of estrogen called 16-hydroxy estrone, which can damage DNA—the cell's genetic material. It is the kind of bad-guy estrogen implicated in triggering breast and testicular cancers. The other metabolic pathway breaks down estradiol to a form of estrogen called 2-hydroxy estrone that is not only harmless but is beginning to be hailed by scientists as beneficial and protective against cancer.

In Germany and the United Kingdom, doctors working with natural methods for treating hot flashes and vaginal dryness prescribe phyto-estrogens in tablet or capsule form or as herbal tinctures or extracts, and claim to get excellent results from them. When beneficial phyto-estrogens bind to estrogen receptor sites, they can not only supply an alternative form of natural estrogen where needed, but, by taking up her estrogen receptor sites, they may protect the woman from the xenoestrogens in her environment that are continually trying to key into them.

Poisoned Consensus

Less than a year ago, some 300 scientists from all over the world gathered at a conference in Washington D.C., sponsored by the NIEHS. The intention was to share specific information on the effects that environmental chemicals are now exerting on human and animal health. It was only the third such conference ever held. Mary S. Wolff of New York City's Mount Sinai School of Medicine also reported that DDT and DDE are likely to be playing an important role in the huge rise in breast cancer incidence we are witnessing in the Western world. Wolff and her colleagues compared levels of DDE in 58 women with breast cancer with those of 170 women who were cancer free. All the women were carefully screened so that they matched in age, socioeconomic status, and every known risk factor. They discovered that the risk of breast cancer was four times greater in the women with the highest levels of DDE than in those with the lowest. The general consensus among conservative scientists investigating the link between environmental chemicals and breast cancer is that as much as a third of breast cancer now developing is directly related to the use of xenoestrogen chemicals in our environment, but many experts insist this is far too low an estimate.

As far as cancer of the womb is concerned, estrogen dominance in the body is the *only* known cause of this illness. Meanwhile, the whole business of exposure to excessive estrogenic compounds becomes an increasing worry when you consider that estrogens are also the hormones most commonly prescribed for women—not only for birth control, but also for HRT. Exposure to xenoestrogens and environmental pollutants over a period of time, say experts, is exacerbated by estrogens prescribed as drugs to women and may be producing breast cancer by disrupting the normal processes of cell regulation in breast tissue.

Dr. Ana Soto, an endocrinologist at Tufts University, discovered for herself quite by accident just how powerful an effect a xenoestrogen can exert on breast tissue. She and her colleagues had been experimenting with cancer cells taken from the breast, then cultured. They found the cells would only grow if they were fed estrogens. In fact, the technique Soto was using—bathing the cells with specific chemicals and then recording whether or not the cells proliferate—may one day prove to be an excellent test for whether or not a specific chemical exhibits an estrogenic effect.

One day the tests simply stopped working. The cancer cells continued to grow even when no estrogens were fed to them. This had been going on for four months when Soto realized that the manufacturers who made the disposable flasks in which she had been culturing her cells had started to use a different plastic—one that, when it becomes warm, releases minute quantities of the estrogenlike compound nonylphenol. Her tissue samples were being continually contaminated by these leaking estrogens. Once Soto determined the cause and changed to glass flasks, she found that she could carry on with the experiments as usual, but the experience stunned her. It has since made her voice extreme concern about the effect that plastics we use day to day may be exerting upon our health.

The Perils of Plastic

Our world is full of plastics—containers that we use every day to store leftovers in the refrigerator or to cook food in the microwave, cups that we drink coffee from, and bottles that our mineral water comes in. Most companies who manufacture plastics are not even aware themselves of whether or not their products slough off estrogenlike molecules. The use of a number of PCBs may have been restricted in many industrialized countries but, like DDT and a few pesticides known to be highly toxic, the products of their breakdown persist in the environment for decades. As endocrinologist David Feldman from Stanford University says: "It is very possible—and it is frightening—that we may be drowning in a sea of estrogens." The xenoestrogens that occur in highest concentrations in many of our effluents are the nonylphenols and octylphenols. These are the break-down products of surfactants in our detergents and common household products, and in spermicides.

While examining fish populations, John P. Sumpter of the Department of Biology and Biochemistry at Brunel University in Uxbridge, England, discovered that powerful estrogenic chemicals are being discharged from sewage treatment plants into rivers. More than 70 percent of the wastewater he and his colleagues sampled contained between 0.1 and 5 micrograms per liter of dissolved nonylphenol. He, like most scientists investigating the rising estrogenic sea, voices great concern for the implications of xenoestrogens in our rivers on human health and on the health of fish and other animals. As far back as the late 1960s, discharges of almost two million kilograms of DDT into the coastal waters of Southern California brought about the collapse of the brown pelican and double-crested cormorant populations. Since then, with the introduction of restrictions on DDT, populations have recovered. However, DDT has a very long half-life. Even were it to be banned worldwide, it would continue to poison the earth for many generations to come. But it is still used in many countries today. DDT is part of a group of xenochemicals that travel easily in the environment and that have been shown capable of inducing and promoting mammary cancers in laboratory animals.

DDE-Sexed Alligators

Not long ago in Lake Apopka in Florida, wildlife biologists discovered that strange things were happening to the alligators living there. Lake Apopka is a large body of water not far from Disneyworld, with a southern channel on which lies a petrochemical factory making pesticides. A toxic spill took place in 1980, but it was forgotten and was unknown to scientists who were called in five years later to investigate a decline in the numbers of alligators. The population of alligators in 1980 had been 30 per square mile. By 1987 it had dropped to a mere three per square mile. It was discovered that in those eggs that hatched, the male alligators that emerged from the eggs had abnormally small penises. They were 75 percent shorter than average. Almost certainly, said scientists investigating the phenomenon, this was the result of residual concentrations of DDE from a lakeside spill of the chemical dicofol and DDT that took place many years before. Following up this hypothesis, Louis J. Guillette, wildlife endocrinologist at the University of Florida, experimented with these xenoestrogens. He discovered that painting alligator eggs with the same doses of DDE that are now present in concentrations in the lake (such low doses that they can only be measured in parts per billion) brings about the same reproductive problems in laboratory animals. Only 10 percent of the treated eggs hatch, and most of these animals turn out to be female.

Alligators are not the only beasts being affected by the "feminization" of the environment. Wildlife biologist Michael Fry, a bird physiologist from the University of California at Davis, has examined birds in areas where concentrations of PCBs are high and found that female gulls are producing extra egg-laying organs, while males have a mixture of female and male reproductive structures. At the University of Texas, David Crews works with turtle eggs. He reports that even very low doses of estrogen-mimicking chemicals applied to the shells of turtle eggs can cause ovary formation in otherwise male turtles. Meanwhile, in Europe and North America, a group of studies have been carried out to investigate the decline of certain species including gulls, turtles, frogs, deer, and alligators. Different animal experts report the same apparent causes— the females of these species have enlarged ovaries. Like consistently anovulatory women, their egg follicles have been burned out and are simply gone.

The old saying: "These days a man is only half his grandfather" may no longer be hyperbole. Speaking at an international conference held last year, Danish endocrinologist Niels Skakkebaek, a researcher at the Rigshopital in Copenhagen; and Richard M. Sharpe of the British Medical Research Council Center for Reproductive Biology in Edinburgh, presented strong evidence that the increased incidence of male birth defects, testicular cancer, and prostate cancer is likely to be the result of exposure to environmental xenoestrogens begun while the male fetus is still in the womb. After carrying out a 21-country study of semen quality that analyzed records from 50 years starting in 1938, Skakkebaek and his colleagues reported in 1992 that there has been a 50 percent drop in sperm counts worldwide. During this same period, the incidence of testicular cancer has tripled in many countries, while that of prostate cancer has doubled. Meanwhile in Germany, researchers have recently discovered that women with endometriosis (the condition that very commonly occurs in women over the age of 40 where the secretory lining of the womb painfully proliferates) have significantly higher levels of PCBs in their bodies than women without the disease. Seventy years ago, only 21 cases of endometriosis had been reported in the world. Now, there are over five million cases in the United States alone.

Plague of Plagues

What appears to be happening is that a strange and potentially highly dangerous marriage is taking place between the proliferation of estrogen-mimicking chemicals in the environment and the rise in various estrogens prescribed medically to women. It is out of this union that estrogen dominance has probably developed. The estrogens and progesterone in a woman's body must balance each other for a woman to remain healthy. In many of us, they are becoming more and more out of kilter. As a result, we are now seeing a widespread rise in many diseases and discomforts for which—with a strange irony—doctors are prescribing more estrogen.

Go to the Source

So potentially dangerous is estrogen dominance that it is essential that we communicate information about it both to other women of all ages and to our doctors. It is also important that we put pressure on our politicians and government leaders to increase control over what chemicals are allowed to be used in the world around us. Scientists throughout the Western world are working to identify as many specific agents responsible for the increase in xenoestrogens in our environment as they can. However, we are constantly exposed to so many chemicals that exhibit an estrogenic characteristic that it may turn out to be a task as complicated as finding the proverbial needle in the haystack. Some researchers suspect that ethynylestradiol (EE)—the primary estrogenic compound in birth control pills (the Pill)—plays a big role as well.

EE in the urine of women on the Pill is able to pass through water treatment plants so it ends up in our drinking water. EE is a much more potent estrogenic compound than estradiol. To test the effect of EE and other estrogens on wildlife, researchers incubated fish in aquariums that had dilute concentrations of either EE or estradiol, the primary estrogen in the whole of the animal kingdom. They found that even concentrations of EE as low as 0.1 nanograms per liter of water exert significant effects. Researchers concluded that EE is one of the most potent biologically active molecules. Since then, at the Fish and Wildlife Services in Atlanta, Georgia, scientists have issued a prohibition on the use of estrogenic chemicals, including pesticides, in more than a hundred wildlife refuges managed by the federal government.

As yet, little of the information about the mounting effects of xenoestrogens and estrogen dominance in women has even *begun* to filter down to the general public. Neither has it been made easily available to the busy doctors to whom the women suffering from PMS or menopause-related symptoms turn to for help. For any woman eager to take control of her own reproductive destiny in terms of fertility, PMS, menopause, and beyond, it is essential that she be aware of just how widespread the challenges of environmental chemicals have become.

Magnetic Powers

It may not be only chemicals in our environment that are capable of unbalancing hormones and undermining health and reproductive capabilities either. For many years, there has been a recognition that the presence of certain electric energies, radio waves, and electromagnetic fields seems to increase susceptibility to breast cancer. There are indications that they may also alter the development of male fetuses. Researchers have discovered, for instance, that prenatal exposure of animals to low frequency fields

(15 hertz) can demasculinize males so that they do not mark their scent in the way normal mature males do. More than 20 years ago, researchers at the University of Manitoba in Winnipeg exposed male rats to chronically magnetic fields, either while in the womb or just after birth, and then monitored the results. Scientists discovered that when the rats were prenatally exposed, they developed larger testicles, whereas if they exposed the animals as adults, testicle size decreased. Like the good-guy estrogens and the bad-guy estrogens, some magnetic fields appear to be beneficial and some detrimental. So does exposure to light itself. Studies show that both can influence the secretion of a brain chemical that among its many other properties helps to regulate estrogen concentrations in the animal's body. For the past quarter of a century, researchers have wrestled with epidemiological data that tie together electromagnetic fields and cancer. They have had a tough time making sense of their findings since most low-frequency fields (associated with household electric currents, microwaves, and radio waves) appear to be too weak to break the chemical bonds that would bring about the genetic changes typically associated with the production of cancer cells.

Then, in the April 1987 issue of *The American Journal of Epidemiology*, Richard G. Stephens of the Pacific Northwest Laboratory in Richland, Washington, published an interesting theory that scientists concerned about environmental influences on human health now take very seriously indeed. It goes something like this:

During the hours of darkness, the pineal gland in the center of the brain secretes a hormone called melatonin in direct response to the amount of sunlight that we are exposed to during the previous hours of light. It is a deficiency in melatonin production that produces the now widely publicized Seasonal Affective Disorder, or SAD, where some people become depressed during long, dark winters. Melatonin is also largely responsible for the experience of jet lag when we cross time zones. And, taken as a nutritional supplement, melatonin has shown itself useful in counteracting jet lag. Among its other attributes, melatonin inhibits the body's production of both estrogen and prolactin, the hormone that stimulates milk production. However, animal studies have shown that exposure either to electromagnetic fields or to light during the night hours can suppress the secretion of melatonin from the pineal. Stephens's work suggests that the chronic exposure to artificial lights that most of us in the industrialized world continually live with may be increasing our cumulative lifetime dose of estrogen and also be increasing our risk of developing breast cancer.

Not long after Stephens published his theory, two researchers at the University of Arizona in Tucson announced another important discovery that supports it. David E. Blask and Stephen M. Hill found that giving melatonin can directly inhibit the proliferation of human breast cancer cells in a culture. Even more important, the quantity of melatonin needed to do this is extremely small, comparable to the amount present in human blood at night. Blask believes that melatonin may have the ability to increase the levels of naturally occurring antioxidants in breast cancer cells that not only help protect against the development of cancer, but heart disease, too. Melatonin may even be capable of reducing the number of estrogen receptor sites on breast cancer cells. Since it is estrogen that feeds the growth of hormone-responsive breast tumors, increased melatonin may help decrease tumor growth. Meanwhile, at the University of California at Berkeley, scientists such as Robert Liburdy have shown that some magnetic fields can limit or block melatonin's ability to inhibit the proliferation of human breast cancer cells in a culture. Other researchers speculate that it may be the suppression of melatonin by electromagnetic fields and light that tends to promote cancer, especially breast cancer.

The whole melatonin issue is a particularly important one for menopausal women. First, the production of melatonin tends to drop as the body gets older. Many age researchers now believe that supplements of melatonin have anti-aging properties. One of the things menopausal women commonly tend to suffer from is wakefulness at night. It is a strange kind of wakefulness not treatable by ordinary natural tranquilizers such as valerian or passiflora. For such women, taking 15 milligrams of melatonin before bed can often make the difference between a night spent half awake and hours of blissful sleep. (See chapter 24 for more information about melatonin.)

We shall probably be well into the 21st century before the devastating effects of the 20th-century postindustrial environment can even begin to be tallied. Our wildlife was the first to send signals that something is seriously wrong. However, in the face of economic pressures from manufacturers of chemical products, governments may never be able to pass laws adequate to control the addition of new poisons to the rising sea of estrogens around us. But there is a great deal that a woman who feels respect for the wisdom of nature and for her own body can do to protect herself now, as well as to protect the world around her.

SEARCH FOR THE GRAIL
Probing the Mysteries of Progesterone

hink of menopause, and chances are you think of estrogen. For menopause, they tell us, is simply an estrogen-deficiency state. We are also led to believe that problems that arrive at menopause—from hot flashes to weird emotions—are the result of this estrogen deficiency and are therefore fixable either by "estrogen replacement" or HRT. So deeply ingrained have such notions become in the industrialized world that to challenge them seems sacrilege. Yet challenge them we must if we are to tap into the power of the bloodless revolution.

Two main sex hormones dominate a woman's reproductive life—estrogen and progesterone. To be healthy emotionally and physically so that menopause becomes a voyage of discovery instead of a living hell, they need to be balanced. In recent years, we have been bombarded with information—and misinformation—about estrogen, but little has been said about the equally important role progesterone plays in female well-being. It is time to redress the balance, time we delved into the mysteries of estrogen's silent partner. This is a task easier said than done, for the role of progesterone has been both neglected and misunderstood even by the so-called experts. The mysterious progesterone holds many secrets. Some are brand new, some long forgotten. They are secrets that can empower women.

Forgotten Hormone

An understanding of what progesterone is and how it works is central to the revolution in natural menopause. Among this hormone's many attributes is an ability to do what most medical science still considers impossible—*reverse* osteoporosis. Exciting as all this may sound, progesterone is not some miracle substance nor is it a new-fangled alternative to HRT. It is simply a forgotten piece of the menopause puzzle. As such, the story of how progesterone's role in women's health has been discovered is an ideal jumping-off point for our journey into natural menopause.

For the past 15 years, while the high-powered medical world has been extolling the virtues of estrogen drugs and HRT, John Lee, a country doctor in northern California, has been diligently researching the actions of natural progesterone. When he began to apply his knowledge of this remarkable hormone, Lee discovered that women who use it are able to eliminate a myriad of menstrual and premenstrual problems, as well as banish a litany of menopausal complaints for which conventional medical science still has no answers. In some cases, natural progesterone has even shown itself useful in making barren women fertile. Lee and many other physicians and health practitioners in several countries of the world who use and recommend progesterone have watched it transform the lives of first hundreds, then thousands, of women.

A tall, soft-spoken man of Norwegian descent, John Lee retired from a busy practice as a country doctor five years ago to create more time for writing and research. Before that he had for many years been gravely concerned about the widespread phenomenon that scientists in the field of ecology are now reporting evidence of throughout the industrialized world. Chemical after chemical in our environment is capable of exerting an *estrogenic* effect on the human body, thereby upsetting the delicate balance of hormones and exerting a detrimental effect on human health and fertility.

Bad News, Good News

It was Lee who a few years ago coined the phrase *estrogen dominance*. He used it to describe a biological state in which the finely tuned balance between estrogen and progesterone in a woman's body has been disturbed, often as a result of high levels of these mock estrogens. So far, estrogen dominance is something about which the majority of doctors throughout the world remain ignorant. That is the bad news. Happily, there is good news too: Estrogen dominance is relatively easy to correct once you know how. And correcting it when it has occurred in the body brings enormous benefits to a woman's overall health.

Here are a few of the ways in which estrogen dominance can manifest itself:

- When estrogen is not balanced by progesterone, it can produce weight gain, headaches, bad temper, chronic fatigue, and loss of interest in sex—all of which are part of the clinically recognized premenstrual syndrome, or PMS.

- Not only has it been well established that estrogen dominance encourages the development of breast cancer, thanks to estrogen's proliferative actions, it also stimulates breast tissue and can in time trigger fibrocystic breast disease—a condition that wanes when natural progesterone is introduced to balance the estrogen.

- By definition, excess estrogen implies a progesterone deficiency. This, in turn, leads to a decrease in the rate of new bone formation in a woman's body by the osteoblasts—the cells responsible for doing this job. Although most doctors are not yet aware of it, this is the prime cause of osteoporosis.

- Estrogen dominance increases the risk of fibroids. One of the interesting facts about fibroids—often remarked upon by doctors—is that, regardless of their size, fibroids commonly atrophy once menopause arrives and a woman's ovaries are no longer making estrogen. Doctors who commonly use progesterone with their patients have discovered that giving a woman natural progesterone will also cause fibroids to atrophy.

- In estrogen-dominant menstruating women where progesterone is not peaking and falling in a normal way each month, the ordered shedding of the womb lining doesn't take place. Menstruation cycles become irregular. This condition can usually be corrected by making lifestyle changes and using a natural progesterone product, and is easy to diagnose by having the doctor measure the level of progesterone in your blood at certain times of the month.

- Endometrial cancer (cancer of the womb) develops only where there is estrogen dominance or unopposed estrogen. This too can be prevented by the use of natural progesterone. Some of the artificial progestogens may also help prevent it, which is why a growing number of doctors no longer give estrogen without combining it with a progestogen drug during HRT.

- Waterlogging of the cells and an increase in intercellular sodium, which predisposes a woman to high blood pressure or hypertension, frequently occurs with estrogen dominance. This can also be a side effect of taking a progestogen. Progesterone usually clears it up.

- The risk of stroke and heart disease is increased dramatically when a woman is estrogen dominant.

Like British scientist James Lovelock, father of the Gaia theory that views the earth as a living organism, John Lee is an *independent* scientist. He does not work for anyone. He is not a consultant to any drug manufacturer, cosmetic manufacturer, or health-food company. Lee takes no money for the talks he gives to doctors, scientists, and women's groups throughout the world, and he has nothing whatever to sell. Blessed with down-to-earth common sense and a brilliant inquiring mind, Lee has spent decades searching for simple answers to complex questions. His area of greatest knowledge and expertise with regard to women's health is the use of plant-derived progesterone—a molecule that is chemically *identical* to the progesterone produced by a woman's body. As such, natural progesterone is very different in its actions and effects from the drug-based hormones now prescribed for contraception or HRT.

Mysteries of Mistletoe

John Lee's first encounter with plant-derived progesterone came about almost by accident. In the late 1960s, he was the editor of a bulletin for his local medical society. Obliged to produce an editorial each month, he was always on the lookout for interesting subjects to tackle. Stuck for copy for the December issue one year, and conscious that his deadline was approaching, Lee came across two interesting articles. One had appeared in the *Harvard Alumni Journal*. It concerned the origins of the Christmas custom of kissing under the mistletoe. This mysterious ritual, the article said, originated with the Celts, although reasons for it remained unknown. The second article had appeared in the *Journal of The American Medical Association*. It was about a retired doctor who, on returning to his birthplace in Texas, met an old gypsy, a woman much celebrated in the community for her "morning after" cures for pregnancy. The gypsy had told the doctor that her success came from the use of European mistletoe berries. Curious, the retired physician had gone to the trouble of having the European mistletoe berry analyzed. He discovered that European mistletoe contains high levels of progesterone, together with some other steroid hormones and glycosides, including digitalis.

Lee became fascinated by the mystery. He knew that most of the information that we have about the Celts and their practices comes from the Roman historian Pliny, so he went in search of what Pliny had to say. Pliny recorded the respect that the Celts had for the medicinal properties of the mistletoe plant. Lee discovered that the name *mistletoe* translates to "all heal" and that the Celts believed the plant to be sacred. Each year at the time of winter solstice, their Druids would hold a week-long ritual in worship of the sun, importuning it to be reborn instead of dying, with a promise that spring will return. At this time of year, they would give gifts to one another, feast, and drink deeply of hot mead laced with the holy mistletoe, which had been carefully gathered in a white cloth that was never allowed to touch the ground. Then, with the usual restrictions on sexual behavior lifted, they would party long and hard.

Sexy Progesterone

One of the major characteristics of progesterone is its ability to stimulate libido. Another is that when the level of progesterone in a woman's body has been relatively high and then falls abruptly (as happens naturally around day 26 to 28 of her menstrual cycle), this drop in the hormone triggers a flow of menstrual blood, causing the lining of the womb to be shed. Lee reasoned that this was probably what happened with the Druids' mistletoe rituals. After a week of sacred orgying on progesterone-tinged alcohol, any fertilized ovum was likely to be eliminated with the subsequent menstrual flow that would take place after the feast was over and all the progesterone-laced mead had been drunk. No one would get pregnant. No wonder the Celts looked on the plant as a gift of the gods. Now all that remains of their winter solstice ritual is our Christmas tradition that a man can still kiss a woman with impunity under the mistletoe.

Learning about the Celtic ritual and the mistletoe gave John Lee just the material he needed to write an amusing editorial for the Christmas issue. This he did, then promptly forgot about it all. After his editorial was published, he received some interesting letters. From them he learned that mistletoe is not the only plant that contains phytohormones (plant-derived hormones) capable of producing shifts in female hormonal balance. There are over 5,000 known plants that boast either precursors to progesterone or estrogens (precursors are chemicals that can easily be converted by the body) or hormones themselves. In fact, it is from such plants that wise women's traditional healing repertoires for female complaints have been fashioned throughout history. Both the hormone progesterone and its plant source origins now began to intrigue John Lee. He wanted to know more, but he had little time as a busy country doctor to pursue his curiosity. Time passed until, almost before he knew it, his 40-year-old patients had become 60-year-old patients, and by the mid 1970s, Lee found himself faced with more and more women in his practice who were suffering from osteoporosis. Their spines were crumbling and their bones kept fracturing, but he did not know what to do to help them.

Darkness at Noon

In 1976—the heyday of estrogen replacement in the United States—a general consensus conference was held at the world-famous Mayo Clinic. Doctors from around the world gathered there to decide that estrogen—then the only hormone given for osteoporosis and menopause-related symptoms—should no longer be given on its own since more and more of the women on estrogen replacement were developing cancer of the uterus (womb). Like many other physicians, Lee found himself faced with a dilemma. The medical profession and drug manufacturers claimed that extra estrogen was necessary to protect a woman from crumbling bones. But if this were true, then to stop osteoporosis and prevent fractured hips, Lee would either have to give estrogen replacement and tell a woman that she might end up with cancer of the uterus as a result, or he would need to add one of the progestogens to the treatment. (Progestogens are drugs now commonly used with estrogen as part of the HRT package.) But progestogens, Lee believed, carry a range of pretty ghastly potential side effects of their own, including possibly an increased risk of breast cancer. It was a dilemma that nobody in medicine had ever been able to solve to the satisfaction of conscientious doctors wanting to do their best for women patients yet dissatisfied with current thinking on hormonal treatments. But let's pause a moment for a couple of important definitions before we continue with Lee's tale.

Initial Principles

Surrounding the word *progesterone,* you will find many misunderstandings in both the medical and the lay world that take a bit of sorting out. For starters, the word *progesterone* tends to be used erroneously and collectively by doctors, researchers, and the media alike to describe not the natural hormone itself (which Lee and others have now investigated), but rather one or more of the *progestogens*—these synthetic progesterone-analogues such as the widely used drugs Medroxyprogesterone acetate (Provera), Dydrogesterone (Duphaston), and Norethisterone (Primulut). Together with one or more forms of estrogen, progestogens—also called *progestins* or *gestins*—are incorporated into contraceptive pills and HRT. You will often hear doctors say that "progesterone does this or that." When you actually pin them down and get them to clarify exactly what they are talking about, 99 times out of 100 you find that the word is being used not to describe the natural hormone progesterone, but rather one of these synthetic analogues.

The effects of natural and synthetic hormones on the body differ enormously. The synthetics do not match the body's chemistry, so the body is not equipped to metabolize them properly. Taking a progestogen can inhibit ovulation in a menstruating woman—and can produce abortion—which progesterone protects against. It can also suppress her body's production of its own natural progesterone and trigger other negative side effects. You will find them listed at length in the manual your doctor refers to when prescribing drugs. Progesterone itself, on the other hand, has none of these. The use of synthetic progestogen in HRT can all too often aggravate some of the problems a doctor is trying to treat by making a woman moody, irritable, and ill-tempered. Natural progesterone, by contrast, tends to make women feel calm and stable. A growing number of doctors and women who have used it in Europe and North America report that progesterone also banishes hot flashes, reestablishes fertility, eliminates PMS, and reverses osteoporosis. But, since the natural hormone and the various progestogens so often get lumped together in common medical parlance, progesterone frequently gets blamed for negative effects that it doesn't cause. Meanwhile, doctors and women alike remain ignorant of the natural hormone's potential for good.

The Proliferator

And it is not only progesterone about which confusion abounds. Estrogen, too, needs clarification. Although people commonly refer to estrogen in the singular, this hormone is not a single compound like progesterone. It is a group of many different compounds, each with different characteristics and actions. Estrogen is the *collective* name used to describe all natural and artificial chemicals that are able to trigger estrus—the release of an egg in a woman. Estrogen is secreted primarily by the ovarian follicles of menstruating women. During pregnancy, it is also secreted by the placenta. To be absolutely accurate, there is no such thing as estrogen, but the word is used to describe many compounds—found in nature, in our foods, and in our bodies, as well as made synthetically either in the form of hormone drugs or petrochemical derivatives—which exert an estrogenic effect on the body.

The estrogens are also responsible for the development of a woman's secondary sex characteristics. After puberty, together with progesterone and a few other steroid hormones, estrogen, or more properly stated, *the estrogens* help regulate menstrual cycles, building up the endometrium or womb lining during the first half of each cycle. Many women have been taught that after menopause, a woman's body stops making estrogen. This common error ultimately leads to an even greater untruth—that menopause is an "estrogen deficiency disease." The truth is that even after menopause, estrogen is still made in a woman's body, only in smaller quantities.

The Protector

The antagonist to the collective "estrogen," progesterone is the name for a *single* steroid female hormone—one specific molecule—made by the corpus luteum. The corpus luteum is the yellow granular mass in the ovary formed each month after an egg has been released. Where estrogen is the major female reproductive hormone during the first half of a woman's menstrual cycle while the endometrium is proliferating, progesterone is the most important hormone during the second half. Not only does progesterone help make other hormones, it is important for countering stress and immunity and is concerned almost entirely with holding on to the endometrium in final preparation of the lining of the womb for pregnancy.

Progesterone does this by promoting changes in the womb lining that make the uterus ready for implantation by a fertilized egg. When a woman is pregnant, the placenta takes over her body's production of progesterone, which now increases 10- or 20-fold—sometimes more—above the level of progesterone produced before. Progesterone during pregnancy helps the womb hold the fetus safely until a baby is ready to be born. Women who habitually miscarry often do so because their bodies do not produce enough progesterone—especially during the early stages of pregnancy. Progesterone, and plants containing other chemicals from which the body can make this hormone, have been used throughout history to arrest threatened miscarriages. Midwives and wise women have relied on wild yam and other botanicals, which are rich in phytochemical precursors to progesterone, in the treatment of pregnant women who are experiencing breakthrough bleeding. It is also the high level of progesterone synthesized during pregnancy that makes many women feel and look so well during the last few months before birth—often better than at any other time in their lives.

By the time of the Mayo conference in 1976, it had been well established that giving excess estrogen as "estrogen replacement" to women with a history of breast cancer was highly dangerous, because in some women the proliferative character of estrogen reactivated cancerous growth. Progesterone, on the other hand, has no known negative side effects. Progesterone is an important compound in the body for another reason, too: From it the body derives more than a dozen other important hormones—including the estrogens themselves. More about this in a moment, but for now let's go back to Lee's story.

Mission Impossible

John Lee had a number of osteoporosis patients with a history of breast cancer. He believed that for them, estrogen was absolutely contraindicated since it could stir up metastases, causing the cancer to recur. There seemed to be no way out. Treating their osteoporosis the accepted way by giving estrogen meant exposing these women to the possibility of more disease—something he did not feel right in doing. Then, in 1979, while he was wrestling with these issues, John Lee heard a talk given by another of the trailblazers in the menopause revolution: Dr. Ray Peat.

An outspoken and tireless investigative biochemist at Black College in Oregon, Peat had spent years studying the effects of progesterone on the human body. His research had taken him back to studies carried out half a century earlier—long before the Pill and HRT became big business and the investigation of the natural hormone had been replaced by studies into its drug-based analogues. In the lecture, Peat pointed out that the medical profession had virtually forgotten that natural progesterone exists. He said that progesterone is easy to obtain without a prescription and that it can be derived from many plants. Unlike the progestogens, progesterone has no negative side effects, said Peat. It is even included in the formulas of certain cosmetics because it is so good for the skin. It was time, insisted Peat, for doctors to include progesterone in their thinking about how to manage the treatment of women patients. Peat's words rang bells for John Lee. Lee contacted the biochemist and asked for all his research references. Later, ploughing through scientific papers, Lee discovered that Peat was right. There had indeed been masses of research into the uses of natural progesterone right from the early 1900s up to around 1960. After that, with the development of the synthetic progestogens, little further research or clinical work was carried out with the natural hormone—except in Britain.

British Breakthrough

Back in the 1950s, pioneering British gynecologist Dr. Katherina Dalton first identified premenstrual syndrome (PMS) and coined the phrase. In fact, she was herself a victim of it. Having suffered terrible migraines associated with her menstrual cycle, Dalton discovered that many of the symptoms associated with PMS could be alleviated when progesterone was given by injection. She chose to experiment with progesterone because she noticed that her migraines disappeared during the final months of her own pregnancy when progesterone levels in the body soar. Dalton published her first reports as far back as 1953. Although she had to fight hard to have PMS accepted as a genuine condition requiring medical attention, she was able to treat some women successfully with natural progesterone.

Progesterone is not always easy to take. Dalton's methods involved regular injections of relatively large amounts of the hormone. This can be costly and inconvenient, and in a few cases, according to Peat, can lead to a serious reaction at the injection site in part because the solvents used for the injectable progesterone are unfriendly to the body. So a few doctors experimenting with the use of the hormone changed to using progesterone suppositories. But they too can be cumbersome and frequently do not absorb easily, yielding at times as little as 5 percent of the hormone present. Progesterone can also be taken orally. After all, mother's milk contains significant quantities of progesterone. This is an important ingredient in breast milk, for progesterone makes a considerable contribution to the health of a baby's developing endocrine system. Later on, a few doctors began to use an oral pill filled with powdered micropulverized progesterone, but some were disappointed with the results. They claimed that progesterone, in oral form, tends to be converted into a water-soluble metabolite that is mostly excreted.

However, most progesterone given by mouth is first digested in the small intestines then passed through to the liver. One of the liver's tasks is to filter out and dispose of excess hormones and, once there, oral progesterone is converted into a water-soluble form and put back into the digestive tract. Here it blends with other chemicals, and much of what remains of the hormone can be excreted instead of absorbed. To overcome this "first-pass" phenomenon in the liver, oral progesterone has to be carefully "packaged." Even so, it can be hard to give small doses of the hormone by mouth and be sure about absorption, although some doctors still use larger quantities of progesterone in this form with good results. (It is worth remembering that the major success of the contraceptive Pill only happened because scientists developed a form of hormones that would be absorbed by the digestive system without being destroyed in the process.)

After much experimentation with various forms of the hormone, the most successful and now the most widely used has turned out to be *transdermal* progesterone. Progesterone in a cream is applied to the skin, which readily absorbs it, and it is then distributed throughout the body. This form of the hormone can be derived from plants—most commonly from the wild yam.

Down in the Valley

The first progesterone that scientists experimented with had been derived from animal sources—mostly pig. It was, therefore, expensive.

However, the exact same molecule you find in a woman's body can easily be made from plant sources. Plant-based hormone can be derived from *steroidal saponins*—compounds that are found in some foods—such as beans or yams—as well as in many other herbs and wild plants. Many saponins resemble cholesterol, cortisone, estrogen, progesterone, and vitamin D. As such, they are capable of acting as *exogenous* steroids (meaning from a source outside the body); helping to regulate the body's steroid hormonal actions, as well as to protect it from the negative effects of stress. Some plants that boast hormone-regulating abilities are also *adaptogens*. This means that they are capable of strengthening an organism's "nonspecific resistance" to aging, illness, and fatigue. These include many "rejuvenating" plants such as ginseng, damiana, and sarsaparilla—all of which are capable of enhancing the body's ability to adapt itself to all forms of stress, while at the same time normalizing its biochemical activities. There are also literally thousands of plants that contain phytohormones or precursors to the body's natural hormones. They include licorice, black cohosh, blue cohosh, squaw vine, false unicorn root, fenugreek, and wild yam. One of the most important plants of all for women's health is the wild yam. One might call it the mother of progesterone, and among progesterone's many beneficial properties is an ability to balance excess estrogen in the body, thereby helping to protect against its side effects, including cancer of the womb. Perhaps progesterone, reasoned Lee, would offer his osteoporosis patients on estrogen replacement the protection they needed without the side effects implicit in giving a synthetic progestogen.

Leap in the Dark

John Lee had spent some time gathering Ray Peat's references. He had also discovered many new ones, too. He found that everything Peat had said about progesterone seemed to be true. It has hardly any side effects, and as far as its benefits were concerned, they turned out to be far more than Lee had ever imagined. Progesterone helps the thyroid hormone do its job properly, for instance. It protects against the edema that excess estrogen can cause, and against the retention of sodium that results in water logging. It also helps keep cell membranes intact so they are not easily damaged by viruses or toxic substances from the air we breathe, the water we drink, and the food we eat. Progesterone even exerts anti-aging effects on skin. It is a natural antidepressant and can restore lost libido. All of this sounded pretty good to Lee, so he suggested to his women patients who suffered from osteoporosis—whether or not they were taking estrogen replacement—that they go to their pharmacy or their health food store, buy a jar of progesterone cream, and try it for themselves.

At about that time, a new technique for measuring bone mineral density called photon absorptiometry had been developed. Photon beams pass through skin and soft tissues but are reflected back by bone. The number of reflected photons can be counted as an indication of the density of bone mineral. The new technique enabled a technician to measure the bone mineral density of any woman to within 96 to 98 percent of absolute accuracy. It was a real breakthrough. Methods in use before the 1980s were highly inaccurate. X-rays, for instance, besides subjecting women to doses of radiation, are not able to show a radiologist the degree of bone loss until it exceeds 30 percent. And if a woman has a 30 percent bone loss, she already has a terrible risk of fracture.

Lee not only wanted to see what effect topically applied (that is, on the surface of the skin) progesterone would have on women, he wanted accurate objective measurements of how progesterone, used regularly, would affect osteoporosis. So he persuaded his women patients to have bone mineral density tests done in this new way. He took measurements of bone mineral density before they began using progesterone cream and then again at intervals afterwards, and he kept extensive records of changes observed. All a woman had to do, in addition to taking a few vitamins and minerals, watching her diet, and getting a bit of exercise, was to rub a little of the progesterone cream onto her skin once or twice a day. To Lee's amazement, six months to a year later, not only had progesterone been able to protect these women from further bone mineral loss, it had actually *improved* the state of their bones.

Lee's discoveries about the reversal of osteoporosis using progesterone are rapidly changing the whole face of women's natural health care, for such improvement had never in medical history been recorded before. What had been already established was that estrogen supplementation could *slow* bone loss to some degree by preventing some of the breakdown of old bone. But estrogen can do nothing to create new bone once mineral loss has taken place. Progesterone can. John Lee's discovery took place more than ten years ago. Since then, information about Lee's clinical studies using progesterone has been published in *The Lancet, International Clinical Nutritional Review*, and *Medical Hypothesis*, as well as in many other journals, magazines, and even in a few books. Still, however, John Lee's findings remain virtually unknown in the mainstream medical community. As yet, too, far too few women know enough about it all to be able to put progesterone to work to improve their own lives.

The Color of Money

One of the closest molecular relatives to progesterone is the plant saponin, known as diosgenin—well supplied by nature in the wild yam root. In a laboratory, this phytochemical is easily converted into progesterone—the exact same molecule you will find in your body. By further conversions, it can also be changed into any number of other molecules, both into those that are molecularly identical to the body's own hormones, and also into synthetic unique molecules that can be sold as drugs. In fact, diosgenin is used by many pharmaceutical manufacturers to synthesize their hormone drugs. Drug companies have access to thousands of acres of wild yams from which they make their products. But why, John Lee asked himself, would pharmaceutical manufacturers forgo a perfectly natural hormone like progesterone, which is chemically identical to the body's own hormone and which offers all these benefits with no problems of safety and no negative side effects, choosing instead to market products that are synthetic and that, because they are foreign to the body, carry potentially serious side effects?

One reason comes to mind. Progesterone cannot be patented. Patent law lies behind the continuing insistence from the medical-industrial complex that drug-based HRT is the treatment of choice for just about every perimenopausal, menopausal, and postmenopausal complaint you can imagine. Once you have synthesized a compound in the laboratory—once you have created a unique molecule—one which is not found in nature, you have a new *drug*. You can put a patent on it and you can *own* it. As soon as a company patents such a compound, they can control its sales and its prices so nobody can undersell them. In fact, nobody else can sell it at all for a number of years. This is what the pharmaceutical business is all about. And a very big business it is, with enormous profits.

Selling drugs is a very different kettle of fish compared to selling herbs, nutritional supplements, or a generic hormone such as progesterone. With a generic therapeutic substance such as vitamin C, vitamin D, or natural progesterone, a company can sell it, but it will never be able to acquire a patent on it since these are all compounds obtainable from nature, and anybody else can sell them, too. To do further medical research on a new use for a compound such as progesterone would cost in the hundreds of thousands—as much as the research into a new drug does. If any pharmaceutical manufacturer were to undertake such research and spend the huge sums of money necessary to establish that progesterone is beneficial, the money they invested would be largely wasted, because their competitors could then produce the same product and reap all the financial benefits without ever having spent a penny. So, naturally, pharmaceutical companies who manufacture contraceptives and HRT drugs choose instead to grow massive quantities of the Mexican wild yam, extract its diosgenin, turn it first into progesterone, then, by altering the molecule further, produce a unique and patentable synthetic drug. In fact, the seven most common progestogens used in the Pill and HRT are all synthesized either from the 21-carbon nucleus of progesterone or from the 19-carbon nucleus of the male hormone nortestosterone. Meanwhile, natural progesterone never has been produced in a major way by a large drug company because it will never be a patentable commodity from which a pharmaceutical manufacturer can derive big profits.

Pale Mimics

Although progesterone and the synthetic progestogens can both be made out of diosgenin taken from the Mexican wild yam, they have little in common in most of the actions they exert on the body. Both can sustain the lining of the womb—the secretory endometrium. Both also appear to offer some protection against cancer of the womb to a woman being given estrogen-replacement drugs. Beyond that, the synthetics differ as dramatically from the real thing as night from day. Where the natural hormone given during pregnancy protects the development of the fetus and is used to guard against miscarriage, medroxyprogesterone—a commonly used progestogen—carries a warning that its use during pregnancy may increase the risk of early abortion as well as birth defects. Dosages of synthetic hormones when they are given as HRT need to be carefully controlled since, unlike natural progesterone, they become more toxic the more you take. By contrast, progesterone is safe regardless of dose. Although by now, thousands of women have used natural progesterone for many years, doctors with expertise in its use have not found it to be toxic at any levels. Ray Peat confirms these findings from animal studies: "Animals are generally more sensitive to progesterone than humans are," he says, "and in animals no toxic level has been found, except that in the highest doses it is anaesthetic. In humans, even this effect has never been reported in the medical literature, and it is clearly anti-toxic in nature. Besides preventing acute poisoning of many kinds, it also reduces the incidence of birth defects and cancer."

Yet, due to the confusion over the definition of progesterone, and the fact that the word is so frequently misused, even many doctors learning about the side effects of the progestogens wrongly assume that they also apply to progesterone. You can still hear so-called experts in women's health claim that natural progesterone is dangerous—that it causes dangerous irregular bleeding or migraine, depression, weight gain, painful breasts and leg cramps—when in fact not one of these things is true. Even many of the library and computer references to research and clinical studies refer to the dangers of "progesterone." However, when you go back to the papers themselves and look carefully to see what researchers were actually using, without exception you find that what in the references has been called "progesterone" turns out not to have been the natural hormone at all, but one of the synthetic progestogens. This is a major reason why the majority of doctors remain ignorant of progesterone's power.

Women using a progesterone product consistently report a sense of increased energy and well-being both mentally and physically. However, the official product information on Provera, issued to doctors by its manufacturer, Upjohn, contains a list of contraindications and adverse reaction warnings wide-ranging enough that were prospective women users to read it while sitting in their general practitioner's waiting room, many, I suspect, would have some very searching questions for their doctor.

From the Horse's Mouth

Since his first successes with the natural hormone, John Lee has recommended progesterone in cream form to hundreds of doctors and thousands of women. But it is primarily the women themselves who pass on the good news to one another by word of mouth. It is also they who have reported back to Lee and other professionals on the hormone's remarkable effects. Like the French surgeon Michel Odent, who claims he learned about childbirth by watching women give birth and listening to what they could tell him about their experience, Lee has learned most of what he knows about progesterone from women themselves. Many using the cream have found their hypothyroidism disappeared as their bone densities went up. Aches and pains in the body also often vanish. Women report they feel calmer and stronger and their skin improves. It was also from women using progesterone cream that Lee learned about a phenomenon called *estrogen rebound.*

When you first use a progesterone cream, it can make you temporarily more sensitive to the estrogens in your body, so for a short time symptoms such as breast tenderness can get worse. This is because estrogen and progesterone, while antagonistic in some actions, are synergistic in others. Alter the level of one, and you affect the actions of the other. This means that some women get temporary breast swelling, tenderness, or other signs of excess estrogens right at the beginning of using progesterone. These symptoms soon pass as the estrogen dominance disappears and the system rebalances itself. Lee also discovered from working with his patients that the presence of adequate progesterone in a woman's body means that her need for estrogen is automatically reduced. So, Lee believes, if a doctor decides to give progesterone to a woman on estrogen replacement, he will need to cut her dose of estrogen in half or more. She will then get all the benefits of estrogen replacement—but in a much lower (and much *safer*) dose. Most women taking progesterone, however, find that they need no extra estrogen at all, since progesterone can be converted into estrogen by the body.

Lee observed that a simple progesterone cream rubbed on a woman's body eliminated the excess facial hair that some women develop as they get older and the weakened nails and loss of hair from the head that others experience postmenopausally. Many of his women patients reported that after using the cream, the hair on their heads grew thicker. He learned, too, that women who had previously relied on diuretics to prevent water retention usually didn't need them anymore, as progesterone is a natural diuretic. He frequently found that women with high blood pressure no longer needed to take their hypertension medication. Many women on thyroid medication no longer need treatment either since progesterone makes the body's use of its own thyroid much more efficient.

The Champions

Now that John Lee has retired, he continues to learn more and more about progesterone from doctors, biochemists, and—most important of all—the women who use it. They come to him for information, for help, and to share knowledge about diet, lifestyle changes, and other factors that can help revolutionize the lives of menstruating women, as well as their menopausal and postmenopausal sisters. Lee frequently receives letters and phone calls from medical colleagues who, coming upon the wonders of natural progesterone for the first time, are astounded. "My God, it works!" reported one doctor from New York City. She had pooh-poohed the whole idea of using a progesterone cream when a patient first told her about it. "First of all, you can't absorb hormones through the skin," her doctor had argued. Then she said, "Anyway, you can't get proper hormones from a wild yam." Her patient pointed out that this is exactly where many major pharmaceutical companies get theirs—by growing wild yams from which they derive progesterone, which they then sell to other pharmaceutical manufacturers for use in making synthetic progestogens. "Well, I just don't think it will work," insisted the doctor. "Do you mind if I try it for three months?" asked her patient, a woman who had fibrocystic breast disease, ovarian cysts, and endometrial thickening, together with fibroid tumors. The doctor agreed, "Okay, you can do it for three months. But if the tests show any positive results, I will personally eat the report."

The patient used the progesterone for three months. Her fibrocystic breast disease vanished. The ovarian cysts went away, and the fibroids shrank by 18 percent—all of which showed up clearly on sonograms and mammograms. Delighted, the woman rang John Lee to report her success and to tell him everything that had been said. Lee asked, "What are you going to do?" The woman replied, "I'm just on my way to my doctor's office. I am going to sit there until she eats the medical reports."

Living in Time

It is in many ways not surprising that most of the medical profession remains ignorant about the powers of progesterone. In the last half of the 20th century, scientific and medical knowledge is changing so rapidly that it is almost impossible for anyone to keep up with what is taking place. John Lee recalls that, when he attended the 20th class reunion of his medical school, the university dean told the doctors in attendance that the half-life of what is now taught in medical schools is only about ten or fifteen years—that is, ten or fifteen years after a doctor leaves medical school, half of what he has been taught will be found to be wrong in one way or another. The dean said he had known at the time they graduated from medical school that half of the things that they had been taught would turn out to be wrong. The problem was nobody could tell which half. "Next year, when I attend my 40th class reunion," muses Lee, "I suspect he will say that the half-life of medical information is down to six or seven years because of the accelerated rate at which things now change."

So when you ask your doctor what he thinks of natural progesterone, don't be surprised if he doesn't know what you're talking about, or if he makes the mistake of confusing the natural hormone with synthetic progestogens, or if he lumps them all together as "progesterone." And reporters in the media and writers of books on women's health can sometimes be as uninformed as scientists and doctors. For instance, after wrestling with the whole question of progesterone and its synthetic analogues, Gail Sheehy, author of the well-known book on menopause, *The Silent Passage*, admitted to being so confused about names that she decided to call all of them "progesterone" throughout the book—even though most of what she has written refers not to progesterone but to the synthetic progestogens.

Given progesterone's ability to enhance women's health, it might be easy to fall into the trap of believing it to be some kind of miracle cure-all that will solve your problems while you go on living a stressful life that doesn't feed your soul, swigging back the gin, smoking like a chimney, and going on and off crash diets. It most certainly will not. Although it is central to the bloodless revolution, progesterone is but one important piece in the natural menopause puzzle. For this natural hormone to yield up the finest it has to offer a woman in terms of enhanced health and emotional well-being, it needs to be joined together with all the other pieces as well— specific nutrients that facilitate progesterone working in the body fully, and the use of specific herbs, plants, and brain-enhancing metabolites, as well as the best that leading-edge energy medicine can bring. Finally, it needs to be placed within a much larger context that examines not only an individual woman's health, but her relationship to her own deepest values, to the environment in which she lives, and to the health of the planet. All of these things must work together to help women make menopause a true passage to power. Nonetheless, given all that natural progesterone has to offer a woman, one big question arises: Why should any woman need progesterone anyway? In search of an answer, first we need to examine the whole process of hormone cycles in a woman's body, going back to long before menopause arrives.

CYCLES OF THE MOON

Menstruation, Hormones, Magic, and Madness

ike the moon's waxing and waning, or the snake that sheds its skin to be born anew, woman is a cyclical creature. Both the fecundity of the moon and the snake's bondage to the changes of life through time are endemic to her nature. They are, in fact, so much a part of our make-up that seldom do we stop to think about them. Yet both depend upon the almost infinitely complex multiple interactions of hormones within our bodies. In short, hormones matter a lot. An awareness of the profound influence they exert on a woman's health and emotions is essential to making menopause a passage to power rather than a source of misery. So complicated are the interactions between hormones in the human body that many are still not understood by science. But bear with me while we explore the basics. Some of what follows may sound a bit like one of those children's manuals on sex, but it really is important to understand how the main steroid hormones in your body act and interact if you are to maximize your health and make menopause an adventure instead of a catalogue of miseries.

Spiritual Interface

So central are hormonal events to how women think and feel that it would be no exaggeration to say that the female endocrine system is an interface between body and spirit. Even our hopes and dreams are echoed in surges of hormones and in their shifting patterns—much as chords and rhythms develop into the themes and movements of a symphony. Changes in hormonal balance from day to day—even from moment to moment—can not only alter the way you feel emotionally, they can even affect your view of reality. Whether you see life as a challenge to be met or a source of constant misery and disappointment can also be reflected in hormone shifts. This is why hormonal imbalances create such emotional and spiritual agonies in women, such as those associated with PMS or menopausal symptoms.

The psychic and spiritual aspects of a woman's hormonal interactions are all too often forgotten, living within the confines of the mechanistic thinking that rules our society. Instead of recognizing the changes in mood and personality as natural to any cyclical creature, we tend to think we should always be the same—always rational, reliable, reasonable, and steady. Meanwhile, synthetic hormones continue to be doled out to us from puberty onwards, with no respect for a woman's cyclical nature and little concern for the long-term consequences these chemicals can have on our health and emotions. There is, I believe, far too little awareness of the way in which the use of one or two artificial hormones year after year may not only undermine our long-term health, but can also affect a woman's ability to fulfill her potential—perhaps even impeding her spiritual development.

I Excite

The word *hormone* comes from a Greek word, *hormao*, which means "I excite," and this is exactly what hormones do. They are messenger chemicals made in minute quantities in the brain, or in special endocrine glands such as the thyroid, adrenals, pancreas, and ovaries—sometimes even in fat cells. They are then carried by the bloodstream to distant parts of the body, where they control, activate, and direct the ever-changing system and organ functions, urges, and feelings that *are* you. Your body is continually creating new hormones out of amino acids, peptides, and cholesterol in the presence of certain vitamins and minerals—all in response to its specific needs. Hormones are also continually being destroyed—that is, metabolized and removed from your system—as your need for one or another of them changes. All this happens in much the same way that a theme or cadence in a piece of music gives way to the next. So rapidly can hormonal shifts take place and so closely interwoven is the endocrine system with your thoughts, feelings, and external events, that measurements of estrogen or progesterone levels can differ drastically when taken only an hour apart.

Hormones perform many tasks. Some help produce or store energy, some trigger growth or balance blood sugar, some affect your water balance, others your metabolic rate. Still others regulate respiration, cell metabolism, or neural activity. It is the task of the steroids affecting brain and mood that we are mostly concerned with here. They are nature's servants for regulating sex and reproduction, as well as for balancing brain chemistry and helping the body handle stress without succumbing to illness. Although they are only produced in small doses, steroids pack a big wallop. Each is highly specific in its actions. Each hormone will only excite the particular cells it is designed to affect.

A molecule of a certain hormone—take progesterone or DHEA—has a unique shape. It will be ignored by all receptor molecules (key-holes on the cells) as it travels through your body until it is at last recognized by the particular receptor molecule with which it is meant to connect. Into this receptor site in cells, and into it alone, the hormone molecule fits perfectly, just the way a key does in its lock. So powerful are a hormone's actions that your body only needs to make minute quantities of each as they are required. For instance, at any moment, there may be as little as one molecule of a particular hormone to every fifty thousand million other molecules in your bloodstream. This is how powerful hormones can be and why giving relatively large quantities of synthetic hormones can be so potentially damaging to the body. The body's production of hormones and the way in which the relationship between them is continuously adjusted relies on complex interactions involving your pituitary (a tiny gland at the base of your brain) and your hypothalamus, often called the master gland, as well as other glands such as the adrenals.

Let's look at the hormonal symphony that is played between the major sex hormones estrogen and progesterone—not in your 40s or 50s when you are most likely to be faced with symptoms that can cause you grief, but long before. For it is how you live during the menstrual years—the way you eat, how you use your body, and the decisions you make about what medications you take or don't take—that sets the stage for a trouble-free natural menopause.

Moon Cycles and Ovarian Rites

Only since the late 19th century have women's menstrual cycles—the *menses*—been investigated scientifically. The name *menses* also comes from a Greek word meaning "month." It, in turn, is derived from an even older word meaning "moon." Quite literally, the menses is the period of waxing and waning between one new moon and the next. Once menstruation begins at puberty, which is a woman's first rite of passage, the ebbs and flows that her body goes through each month are the stuff of which the second movement in her life's hormonal symphony is made. This part of her life has one principal goal—childbearing. And its success depends greatly upon the two major steroids—the estrogens and progesterone—working in close communication with her body's chief control centers, the pituitary and hypothalamus.

The hypothalamus is the control center. It balances and oversees biochemical and energetic changes throughout the body. The limbic system in which it sits is the most primitive part of the brain. It is the part that deals with emotions and with our sense of smell, with our passions and with all the unconscious interfaces that take place between mind and body. The actions of the limbic system lie beneath the level of the thinking mind. This is one of the reasons that the hypothalamus is often referred to as the "seat of emotions." When excited, the hypothalamus triggers desire—for food, for water, for adventure, and for sex. Its actions can also be influenced by inhibitory thought patterns. In a woman frightened of becoming pregnant, for instance, the fear itself—via the hypothalamus—can dampen sexual desire or even disrupt menstrual cycles so she remains barren.

The hypothalamus even reacts to bodily changes that take place as a result of meditation. Its activities are influenced by spiritual practices, which is a major reason why women who meditate regularly tend to develop greater emotional balance, as well as why repeated experiences of joy or stillness can dramatically improve various female complaints such as PMS and hot flashes in both menstruating and menopausal women.

Sacred Cycles

There are three main branches of the female endocrine system involved in menstruation. The first is the control center, the hypothalamus. It releases hormones with complicated names that you certainly don't need to remember, including gonadotrophic hormone (GnRH). The second branch is the anterior pituitary, which releases follicle-stimulating hormone (FSH) and luteinizing hormone (LH)—both of which are secreted in response to GnRH from the hypothalamus. The third branch is made up of the estrogens and progesterone which, during a woman's nonpregnant childbearing years, are secreted by the ovaries in response to FSH and LH. What is important to understand is just how complex and interlaced the actions of these hormones are.

All the hormones released during a menstrual cycle are secreted not in a constant, steady way, but at dramatically different rates during different parts of the 28-day period, a cycle which, like everything else in the natural world, involves birth, maturation, and death, only to lead to new birth again—in this case, the egg a woman's body produces. Menstruation itself is simply the elimination of the thickened blood and blood-filled endometrium in the womb—the lining developed in preparation for a possible pregnancy. When a pregnancy does not occur, this lining is shed at monthly intervals under the control of estrogen and progesterone, with a little help from their friends GnRH, FSH, and LH. When ovaries are not stimulated by the gonadotrophic hormones from the pituitary, they remain asleep, as they were during childhood and as they become again after menopause.

For the first eight to eleven days of the menstrual cycle, a woman's ovaries make lots of estrogen. It is estrogen that prepares the follicle (a small excretory sac or gland) for the release of one of the eggs. The word *estrogen*, like the hormones produced in a woman's body that belong to this family—estrone, estradiol and estriol—comes from *estrus*, a Greek word meaning "frenzy," "heat," or "fertility." It is estrogen that proliferates the changes that take place at puberty—the growth of breasts, the development of a girl's reproductive system, and the reshaping of a woman's body.

Each girl baby is born with all the primary follicles she will ever need. At the time of puberty, a girl's ovaries contain about 300,000 of these follicles. And while each woman only produces one or two fully developed eggs each month, somewhere between 100 and 300 follicles have to start developing in order for one to become fully grown. This is why a woman can lose between 100 and 300 follicles a month. However, since she started with 300,000, she will have enough to last all her reproductive life.

On day one of each monthly cycle—that is the day of the onset of menstruation—hormones trigger a group of ovarian follicles, causing accelerated growth in the cells surrounding them. As cells around the eggs grow, they secrete fluid that contains a high concentration of the estrogen estradiol to bring about many other changes, developing the potential of the egg so that it becomes capable of being fertilized by the male sperm.

It is not only the estradiol secreted by the follicle that brings about the maturation of the egg. The interaction of this hormone with other reproductive hormones helps the process along for a week or more, until one of the follicles outgrows all the rest. This is the one that will become the female egg ready for impregnation, and so the final follicular growth can be completed and *ovulation* can occur—that is, the release of the egg into the fallopian tubes for its journey down into the uterus. Ovulation takes place, usually around the 14th day, in the middle of your cycle.

Enter Progesterone

The rate of estrogen secretion begins to fall on about day 13, one day before ovulation occurs. As small amounts of progesterone begin to be secreted, very rapid growth of the follicle takes place. Beginning with this secretion of progesterone, ovulation occurs, too. During the first few hours after the ovum has been expelled from the follicle, more and more rapid physical and chemical changes take place to the egg, in a process called luteinization. At this stage—known as the *luteal stage* of a woman's cycle—the follicle becomes known as the *corpus luteum,* or yellow body. The cells around the follicle begin to secrete larger quantities of progesterone as the level of estrogen decreases. Some of the cells around the follicle become much enlarged. They develop inclusions of lipids or fats, which give them their distinctive yellow color. From now on, development becomes rapid, until seven or eight days after ovulation when it peaks.

Ovulation changes the whole ball game. No longer is there a need for further buildup of the womb lining. The challenge now is to hold on to the secretory endometrium and to render it capable of nurturing a fertilized egg long enough for it to grow into a baby. That is progesterone's task—and remember that progesterone is only secreted when you ovulate.

The corpus luteum that forms each month is a tiny organ with a huge capacity for hormone production. It releases large quantities of progesterone, plus some estrogen that causes a feedback decrease in the secretion of pituitary hormone so that no new follicles begin to grow. But as soon as the corpus luteum degenerates at the end of its 12-day life—which is about the 26th day of the female sexual cycle—this lack of feedback triggers the anterior pituitary gland to secrete several times as much FSH, followed a few days later by more LH as well. This, in turn, stimulates the growth of new follicles to begin the next ovarian cycle. And at the same time, a fall in progesterone and estrogen secretion triggers menstruation.

Peaks and Valleys

From day one until about day thirteen of a woman's menstrual cycle, the level of progesterone in her body is very, very low. Yet at the point at which a follicle is released, it continues to rise dramatically until day 21 to 23, when it begins to fall again to its lowest level as menstruation begins around day 28. In addition to maintaining the endometrium and shifting down activity in the other ovary, the progesterone provided each month travels to other parts of a woman's body to fulfill other roles. It protects her from the many negative effects of estrogen dominance by balancing the estrogen in her body. Progesterone also brings surges of libido. You still hear a few experts say that estrogen increases libido. But think about it. Which hormone would you rely on for sex drive—estrogen, which is present *before* the egg is made, or progesterone, which comes *after* the egg is released and is ready for fertilization? Libido increases with progesterone surges.

When this rhythmic cycling of estrogen and progesterone during each lunar month gets out of sync (and many things in modern life can cause this), then all sorts of things can go wrong—from infertility to PMS, depression, bloating, endometriosis, and fibroids. For the estrogens and progesterone each have their characteristic roles to play, and for a woman to be healthy, they must balance each other.

The Last and the First

So do all the other steroids. This group of hormones to which cortisol, aldosterone, progesterone, DHEA, testosterone, and the estrogens belong is intimately involved in how you feel both physically and emotionally, as well as how rapidly your body ages. Steroids have a characteristic molecular structure that resembles cholesterol, from which they are all ultimately derived. Cholesterol is the vital fatty substance that has had such bad press in recent years, but which is absolutely essential to life. Out of each steroid hormone made from cholesterol, yet another and another can be made in a knock-off effect. For instance, pregnenolone is the steroid manufactured directly from cholesterol. It, in turn, becomes a precursor to progesterone, as well as to many other hormones (see diagram that follows).

Steroidogenesis pathways

Every hormone in the shaded area can be made by your body from proges-terone. If you don't have enough progesterone, then you may not be able to produce enough of the anti-inflammatory hormones such as cortisol, as well as other hormones that affect brain and mood. (From *Natural Progesterone*, by John Lee M.D., BLL Publishing, 1993.)

Natural steroid hormones such as progesterone made by biosynthesis in your own body have a remarkable capability to act as precursors. In other words, they are capable of being turned into other hormones further down the pathways as your body needs them. Progesterone is the mother of many other hormones. It can eventually be turned not only into various estrogens, but also into cortisol (the anti-inflammatory hormone) and into other steroids such as corticosterone or aldosterone with equally important jobs to do. All of these conversions happen through slight alterations in the shape of a molecule, thanks to the actions of enzymes, each of which carries out a specific task. But these conversions can only take place if the molecules on which the enzyme is acting "fit" precisely. All of these changes that take place through the magic of enzymes occur in the presence of vitamin and mineral co-factors such as magnesium, zinc, and B6, which catalyze each enzyme reaction. Like the menstrual cycle, they too are carefully modulated by elaborate feedback mechanisms. The names and chemical transformations from one steroid to another are not important to remember. Again, what is important is that you get some sense of just how complex hormone synthesis and interactions can be and how important it is to have sufficient co-factors, as well as "primary" hormones such as pregnenolone and progesterone to be able to synthesize others. A rich hormonal symphony? Immeasurably. Yet all this still does not take into account the myriad pathways by which these steroid hormones interact with other hormones. Neither does it take into account how they master central mechanisms within the hypothalamus and pituitary or psychoneuroimmunological pathways, through which hormones affect our emotions, and emotions our hormones.

Sabotage

It is in coming face to face with the rich textures of such hormonal symphonies that the synthetic progestogen drugs can be confusing. When you look at the structures of their molecules, you find that although they resemble the body's homemade hormones, their shapes have been altered slightly by adding extra atoms here or there at unusual positions. It is this that has enabled them to qualify as patentable drugs.

However, unlike the natural hormones (which they attempt to mimic and which not only fulfill their own functions by binding with their own receptor sites, but also act as precursors for a myriad of other hormones with other important jobs to do), the progestogens are *end-product molecules*. They are also completely foreign to the living body. Unlike nature's own steroids, they cannot be augmented or diminished as necessary to maintain balance and to keep the body's hormonal symphony flowing smoothly. They also cannot easily be eliminated when their levels get too high. Like the xenoestrogens in our environment, although the synthetics can still bind with the receptor sites of the hormones they are made to mimic, they don't fit as well as the homemade steroids do into the enzymes meant to act upon them. This means that they are not under the watchful eye and control of these enzymes, nor of the body's self-regulating capacities. This is why drug-based estrogens and progestogens in contraceptives and HRT cocktails can significantly disrupt a woman's normal hormonal cycles by introducing foreign elements into her body. They also virtually wipe out the moon cycles to which a woman's natural fertility and spiritual balance are inexorably bound from puberty onward. So, although in the short term they may do a job such as provide birth control or quell heavy bleeding or hot flashes in a menopausal woman, in the long run they only sabotage hormone balance.

Friends and Lovers

Quite apart from their biochemical actions, rather like people, hormones have characters with highly individual personalities. To the biochemist, the "personalities" of the estrogens and progesterone will always remain a mystery. The biochemist is interested in nothing beyond their molecular configurations. But many women come to know these personalities well—by allowing intuition and instinct to be their teachers. When progesterone is surging through the body, a woman can feel high. Provided her body is producing enough of this steroid, she is likely to feel great. Your senses are keen when progesterone is running. Smells smell sweeter—or more horrible. Touching, sensing, tasting, and hearing are all richer experiences than usual. In the presence of progesterone, women have a desire to *do* something, to create something, to work in the garden, to dance or sing a song, or make love. Sometimes progesterone surges can feel like falling in love. This can happen during the luteal phase of the menstrual cycle after ovulation when the follicle turns into the yellow body or corpus luteum, but it becomes far more intense when you are pregnant. It is a high level of progesterone that makes a woman feel on top of the world during the last months of pregnancy. At this time, the placenta churns out an amazing 300 to 400 milligrams per day of the steroid. During the luteal phase of your menstrual cycle, it will have only been producing 20 milligrams or so a day.

I suspect that among those women who seem to get pregnant over and over and who so love the whole experience, you are likely to find high progesterone levels. You also find them in women who have trouble-free menstruation. Sadly, the opposite is true, too. When progesterone is low— as it is in a growing number of women who have become estrogen dominant—women never seem to feel well even during pregnancy. Many have all sorts of trouble with their female organs and cycles, including PMS— sometimes from puberty right through to death.

When Estrogens Flow

The estrogens have quite a different character. When estrogens peak in the menstrual cycle just before the "fall" of ovulation, a woman feels less independent. She is more willing to adjust herself to the needs of others. When the estrogens are running, women like to attract a mate, not so much to draw him into her body, as to comfort, admire, and care for her. Her ovaries seem to be smiling—"Whatever you want, I'm happy to give," they seem to say. A few women who by nature are high estrogen producers feel quite dependent on others for approval, and for the definition of their being. While such an experience can be lovely and make a woman feel highly "feminine," it can also go too far. However, in these women, when menopause finally arrives and estrogen levels drop dramatically, often they find to their surprise and delight that for the first time in their lives, they feel complete in themselves—as though they don't need anybody else to validate their lives. Provided they are otherwise well, menopause can be sheer joy in the sense of the freedom it brings to these women, once they get over the shock of being such a "different person."

From a biological point of view, there are many important actions that progesterone and estrogen exert upon the body and psyche. Since these are little known among women and doctors alike, it is worth looking at a few (see next page).

Effects of Progesterone	**Effects of Estrogen**
Increases libido	Decreases libido
Prevents cancer of the womb	Increases risk of womb cancer
Protects against fibrocystic breast disease	Stimulates breast cell activity
Helps protect against breast cancer	Increases risk of breast cancer
Maintains the lining of the uterus	Proliferates the lining of the uterus
Stimulates the building of new bone	Slows down the resorption of old bone
Strengthens skin	Thins skin
Is a natural diuretic	Encourages salt and water retention
Antidepressant	Can produce headaches and depression
Encourages fat burning and the use of stored energy	Lays down fat stores
Normalizes blood clotting	Increases blood clotting
Concerned with procreation and survival of the fetus	Concerned with the development and release of the egg
Precursor to important stress hormones	End-molecule steroids

The reproductive hormonal menstrual cycle of a woman between puberty and the menarche is a superbly ordered natural work of art. It becomes so much a part of our lives that unless we have some particular difficulties with PMS or fertility, we hardly give it any thought. Not, that is, until things begin to alter. Once they do—in most women sometime between the age of 40 and 50—they usually change gradually until finally a woman senses that something deep in her being has shifted. Such feelings herald the coming of menopause—the third phase of a woman's life.

CRAZED WOMAN

Hormone Replacement Therapy (HRT):
False Promises and Real Truths

here are many bizarre ironies surrounding HRT. For example, despite all the glossy pamphlets and pro-HRT articles in newspapers and women's magazines, most women—including those who actually take HRT—are enormously ill informed about what it is and why they are taking it. In one national opinion survey of over 1,000 women on the treatment, most claimed that they were taking it in order to help them stay young and sexually attractive, something that it most decidedly does not do. Only 3 percent of the women polled were the least concerned that it might reduce the risk of a heart attack (the reason why it is currently being aggressively marketed), while two-thirds did not even know the cause of menopause. No wonder there are so many crazed women trying to make sense of it. Let's look at HRT, how it came into being, and what is being claimed for it by whom.

Just what is HRT, anyway? Based on the assumption that menopause is not a natural occurrence in which hormonal changes take place in a woman's body, but an estrogen deficiency disease—much as hypothyroidism is a thyroid deficiency disease—HRT is an attempt to restore hormonal "normality" by *replacing* the hormone or hormones that are deemed to be missing in perimenopausal, menopausal, and postmenopausal women.

HRT comes in four presentations—tablets, implants, creams, and patches. Tablets are most commonly used in three- or four-week packs.

Creams are sometimes prescribed for women whose main difficulty is either vaginal itching or dryness or inflammations of the urinary system. Patches are put on like plasters, generally to the lower abdomen, and then changed every three or four days. HRT also comes in four main forms:

- giving estrogen alone, which is called *unopposed estrogen;*
- *opposed sequential therapy,* where estrogen is given for a period, followed by a shorter period where a progestogen is given;
- *opposed continuous combined therapy,* where both estrogen and a progestogen are given at the same time; and
- giving a *progestogen alone.*

Within each category, there are numerous drugs in different combinations that a doctor can choose from. For an unopposed estrogen regime, for instance, he might use conjugated equine estrogen in doses of between 0.3 to 1.25 mg a day, or estradiol valerate in a dose of 1 to 2 mg a day, or an implant of micronized estradiol, or some form of transdermal estrogen. If he decides to give opposed sequential therapy, he might choose transdermal estradiol together with norethisterone acetate, or conjugated equine estrogen together with medroxyprogesterone acetate, or estradiol with norethisterone acetate, and so on. The possibilities are many. Each drug company promotes its own packages, and each doctor has his or her favorite treatment program.

Hobson's Choice

Because there are many unpleasant as well as dangerous side effects to the hormones used in HRT, and because such problems as the development of endometrial cancer have been shown to be directly related to the levels of estrogen a woman is given, most doctors try to use as little of the drugs as possible to get results. After all, there would seem little purpose in putting a woman on estrogen for 20 years in an attempt to protect her from osteoporosis if she ends up developing cancer of the womb in the process. But any doctor prescribing HRT is faced with a delicate balancing act in which there are many unknowns, for each drug used in any of these combinations of treatments will affect different women in different ways, and each drug has its own list of characteristic possible side effects.

In Britain, as in many industrialized countries of the world, the popularity of HRT is still growing. In a recent four-year period, the number of

British women choosing to take hormones more than doubled. In 1990 only 9 percent of postmenopausal women took HRT, but by 1993, 18 percent did. By the millennium, pharmaceutical companies hope to have more than 50 percent of menopausal women in Britain on HRT. Many doctors insist that HRT is likely to be "the most important advance in preventative medicine in the Western world for half a century." They proselytize that it is through taking hormone drugs that postmenopausal women are going to be able to safeguard their bones and hearts. So powerful is the HRT rhetoric and so widespread has this message become that, as American physician Christiane Northrup, author of *Women's Bodies, Women's Wisdom*, says:

> By combining so-called medical fact with fear, an entirely new generation of women is being brainwashed that ERT [Estrogen Replacement Therapy] is the gold standard—"Don't leave menopause without it" The current "medicalization" of menopause has been so successful that most women's own menopausal wisdom and trust in their bodies to remain healthy during this natural life-stage is almost nonexistent....The rare woman who wants to get through menopause *without* estrogen replacement now has to fear that she may not be making the right choice. She doesn't get the cultural seal of approval that she would get if she were on ERT.

Despite the impression created that HRT is both a miracle of modern science and an essential treatment for menopausal women, there is much evidence that once the immediate flush of excitement over a new treatment and all the promises it carries is over, women's experience of HRT does not back up these assertions. A recent Swedish survey of the university town Linkoping has shown that there, as in other countries such as New Zealand, 49 percent of the women who go on HRT stop taking the drugs within a year. Many starting on HRT initially experience a kind of euphoria, primarily because the one thing that estrogen replacement gets rid of almost immediately is the hot flashes that may have been disturbing sleep and contributing to exhaustion. Many women report that a few months later, their experience of HRT has worsened dramatically because of side effects such as mood swings, decreased control over the bladder, fatigue, and headaches. The most common side effects that women complain of are migraines, depression, bleeding, water retention, increased blood pressure, weight gain, thrush, breast problems, varicose veins, and chest pains.

Some researchers believe that the depression that frequently follows in the wake of HRT may to some extent be a result of disappointment at its not having lived up to expectations. According to a British study, among women's reasons for giving up HRT are these: About half stop taking it because of side effects, about one-fifth because they are advised to do so by their doctors, and about one-third either because they are afraid of long-term consequences such as cancer or because HRT has shown itself to be ineffective in helping them.

Chemical Addictions

For some women, addiction is the worst problem that arises when on HRT. Researchers S. Bewley and T. H. Bewley recently reported in *The Lancet* that estrogen, like other drugs that are potentially addictive and abusive, have the potential to cause symptoms of both tolerance and withdrawal. Advocates of HRT strongly deny that this is so. Other researchers have established that the use of estrogen implants can result in a buildup of what is called *supraphysiological* estrogen in the body of a woman receiving HRT, and lead to a diminished responsiveness (known as *tachyphylaxis*) to increasing amounts of physiologically active substances. It is a phenomenon that hormone drugs appear to share with other drugs already known to be addictive.

There is another issue in relation to the use of Premarin—whose name gives a clear indication where it is derived from (PREgnant MARes urINe—pregnant mares' urine)—that women and animal rights groups object to. They are troubled by the conditions under which the horses used to collect the hormone are held. In a recent editorial in *Townsend Letter for Doctors*, American physician Alan R. Gaby, M.D., writes that "the way the horses are treated in the production process is anything but 'natural.' To produce the drug, horses are impregnated, then fitted with a rubber collection device so that all of their urine can be collected...The mares are then forced to stand on concrete floors in stalls measuring just 8 feet long and 3½ feet wide for most of their 11-month pregnancies. This is because allowing the mares to roam about in the pasture might result in the loss of precious urine, which is worth $17 a gallon to Wyeth-Ayerst Laboratories, the makers of Premarin." The horses' physical confinement makes it virtually impossible for them to turn around or even to lie down properly, according to the American animal rights organization PETA—People for the Ethical Treatment of Animals. This, they claim, results in some of the mares becoming crippled, while occasionally an animal dies. Soon after giving birth, say PETA, the foals are taken from their mothers, who are impregnated yet again. Some of the foals, they say, are killed immediately, while others are fattened and slaughtered or retained to replace the burnt-out mares from which they came.

Risk-Benefit Assessments

It is very hard to sort out the benefits that are quoted by HRT support-ers from the risks. Proselytizers for HRT often refer to follow-up studies done on American postmenopausal women who took estrogen a decade or more ago. They are all studies that are highly prone to bias, since the women studied tended to come from a higher socioeconomic group, and as such, were likely to be healthier in the first place than women from the lower socioeconomic groups. When it comes to looking at the effects of hormone treatments, it has always been difficult to do randomized stud-ies—that is, studies in which women enter a trial without knowing whether or not they will be put into the group that will take HRT, or the control group that will not. Women just won't go for it. When it comes to examin-ing the results of studies that have been carried out, it is important to remember that the hormonal mixtures being prescribed now differ tremen-dously from the formulations that were used in the 1960s, 1970s, and 1980s. We really have no way of quantifying what the long-term effects of HRT are on women's health.

Nonetheless, medical and commercial apostles for HRT continue to back up their assertions by referring to all sorts of follow-up studies of American postmenopausal women on estrogen. One major thing that they claim now is that HRT can decrease a woman's risk of suffering a heart attack or stroke by 50 percent, as well as reduce the chance of fractures from osteoporosis. Before going any further, it is important to take a look at what they are claiming. Fifty percent sounds like a lot and makes you think that 50 out of 100 women are going to be safer if they take HRT. This is not the case. What is really being claimed does not amount to much. Sta-tistics show that, in general, women between the ages of 65 and 75 in indus-trialized countries have a 6 percent relative risk of heart disease. Translated into real people, this means that 6 out of every 100 women are at risk of having heart problems at some time in their lives. A 50 percent reduction in the number of women at risk would mean that instead of 6 women out of every 100 running the risk of heart problems, this figure is reduced to 3 women per 100—a long way from the 50 out of 100 women that is commonly perceived when 50 percent reductions in risk are talked about.

The force of the assertions about the ability of various forms of HRT to give a woman long-term protection against degenerative diseases, the complacent manner in which they are made, and the way they are attributed to numerous frequently cited studies, often bear little relationship to the facts stated when you closely scrutinize the studies quoted and the overall conclusions drawn from them. For instance, the study most often cited to back up the assertion that HRT protects against heart disease was carried out in the United States on 48,470 nurses and reported in 1971. It mentions a decreased risk of major or fatal heart disease in estrogen users. When you look closely at the coronary risk factors of the study, you realize that the decreased cardiovascular disease among HRT users is likely to have little to do with the HRT these women were taking, but a great deal to do with the fact that they came from a self-selected group of healthy women with less severe vascular risk to begin with, and that the women studied, unlike the general population, all had a continued commitment to preventative medicine in general.

Carol Ann Rinzler, author of *Estrogen and Breast Cancer: A Warning to Women*, describes this phenomenon well when she says: "It might look as though estrogen kept a woman healthy when in fact it was just the other way around: Healthy women took estrogen." Meanwhile, the believers in estrogen drugs seem occasionally to behave like ostriches—burying their heads in the ground and ignoring the fact that estrogen in the contraceptive pill has already been credited with thrombosis in women who smoke or already have heart disease. So the effects, if any, of HRT on coronary heart disease and its prevention remain uncertain. Meanwhile, there is also conflicting evidence about the relative risk of stroke in women being given HRT.

As far as the role of hormone drugs in relation to osteoporosis is concerned, data from a number of randomized trials have shown that estrogen drugs can indeed reduce the rate of decline in bone density after menopause. This is a result of the fact that estrogen slows down the rate of bone resorption. However, unlike natural progesterone, estrogen can do nothing to build new bone, and the small benefits that it can confer are only maintained as long as the HRT is continued. Once HRT is discontinued, then bone density is lost at a similar rate to that which happens in women on a Western diet without adequate exercise or adequate progesterone during menopause.

Most important of all, after all the studies are cited and all the positions aggressively defended, it is essential to remember that what is most frequently obscured by the medical-industrial complex in their claims for HRT is that a woman's lifestyle is far more important in protecting her from cardiovascular disease and osteoporosis than giving hormone drugs could ever be. The discrepancy is wide between what is claimed for HRT and what it delivers, not only in these two areas, but in many others. It is an excellent example of just how irrational the so-called rational assessments of HRT have become. There is also something ironic in such inconsistencies, especially considering the way in which women themselves have for many years been accused of being irrational by the male-dominated medical profession. But then the history of drug-based hormone treatments is full of inconsistencies.

History Speaks

As far back as the 1930s, scientists knew that estrogen would produce abortion even when given in small doses. When given early enough, it will also prevent implantation of fertilized embryos. It was also known that estrogen could cause various forms of cancer in animals. And as early as the 1940s, scientists were aware that progesterone was capable of protecting against many of estrogen's toxic effects, including its abortifacient actions. But until the mid-1940s, chemists assumed that progesterone's activity was very narrow. In the words of Carl Dyerassi, who reported on "The Making of the Pill" in *Science*, they believed "that progesterone's biological activity was extremely specific and that almost any alteration of the molecule would diminish or abolish its activity." As a result, any interest drug companies might have had in progesterone was overridden by commercial interests, since it is only possible to profit from patentable substances, and you can only patent something that has been chemically modified to produce a unique molecule.

In the 1950s, the search was on for chemicals that would prevent ovulation and that could be used for birth control. Chemists discovered that there are many chemicals that have estrogenic actions. Out of this discovery the contraceptive pill was born. It created a gigantic market. Ten years later, having developed the technology of using estrogen in contraceptives, it was only logical for pharmaceutical manufacturers to look toward wider markets for their applications. New Zealand health educator Sandra Coney describes the way in which it all happens:

> Medicine can create diseases to provide a market for new products developed by the pharmaceutical industry. There are two alternate scenar-

ios in the development of drugs: Biomedical scientists can go looking for a cure for a known illness, such as cancer; but new compounds are sometimes synthesized in the laboratory without anyone being initially clear what purpose they can be put to. The end result is a drug in need of a disease. The more broadly the disease can then be defined, the greater the treatable population and the greater the potential sales. Well people and others experiencing social problems are obvious targets.

Once estrogen drugs and delivery systems had been developed as contraceptives, the next logical step for drug manufacturers was to find a new use for them. The menopausal woman, standing poised at the threshold of profound changes in physical and spiritual life, was ideal.

Hidden Persuaders

Until the 1960s, medicine was not much interested in menopause. It was something that women patients were told they would simply have to put up with. Then as the *psychotropic* (mind-altering) drugs began to hit the market, medical journals became littered with advertisements for Librium and Valium as treatments for "women's complaints"—crying jags, lethargy, anxiety, insomnia, and depression. These drugs were then touted as "cures" for the "symptoms" of menopause, and doctors began to write prescriptions for them. It was not long before the use of estrogen followed suit, thanks largely to three forces: first, a book called *Feminine Forever,* by New York gynecologist Robert A. Wilson, M.D., which made estrogen drugs sound like the best thing ever; second, women's magazines, which carried articles on this newly discovered magic bullet treatment that was to keep women young forever; and third, massive promotions and advertising by pharmaceutical companies.

Wilson's book represented "estrogen replacement" as a kind of youth pill that would save poor fading women from the horrors of age. The crusade that he launched almost single-handedly to rescue women from what he termed the "living decay" of menopause has all the hallmarks of a fundamentalist religion. He spoke of the "tragedy of menopause," which often "destroys her character as well as her health." Wilson's message is clear—that menopause is a hideous disease with disastrous consequences. And only estrogen carried by the noble White Knight of medicine is able to save her from its clutches. Wilson's paternalistic desire to prevent the aging woman from becoming "redundant" by making her "feminine forever" has echoes of the very worst of cosmetic marketing about it. "The unpalatable truth must be faced," says the good doctor, "that all postmenopausal women are castrates..." Wilson obviously felt it was his mission to identify the "serious consequences" of the loss of estrogen that happens to a woman at menopause.

According to Wilson, they include heart attacks, osteoporosis, tough, dry, scaly, and inelastic skin, "atrophic" breasts, and shriveled genitals. As Sandra Coney says, "There is something unpleasantly voyeuristic about his desire to ensure that all women are walking around with plump, juicy genitals. Wilson's views as a man determined his clinical judgment. He was the Hugh Hefner of Menopause." A lot of Wilson's rhetoric reads like something out of Monty Python. By now, it has lost whatever Pythonesque humor it may once have had. After 30 years of propaganda based on such nonsense, it now reads more like a blueprint for fear, which we are still being sold.

In 1963, Wilson founded a private trust known as The Wilson Foundation for the sole purpose of promoting the use of estrogen drugs. Its funding of $1.3 million came from the pharmaceutical industry. Each year, Wilson received money from pharmaceutical companies including Searle, Wyeth-Ayerst Laboratories, and Upjohn, all of which made hormone products that he claimed were effective in *treating* and even in *preventing* menopause. Since then, Wilson's foundation has become very much the prototype for similar organizations in industrialized countries that continue to further the sale of HRT, usually under the banner of saving women from postmenopausal agonies. Then it was more loss of femininity, neurosis, and haggard, shriveled skin that was threatened. Now it tends to be osteoporosis, stroke, and coronary heart disease. The words may change, but the message remains constant: Midlife women need hormone drugs to rescue them from the horrors of menopause.

Comedy of Errors

Now, more than 30 years later, things have changed. In the 1970s, it became known that estrogen used in the way Wilson had pioneered it—*unopposed*—had led to a tenfold increase in cancer of the womb. First, warnings about HRT were substantiated by two articles published in the *New England Journal of Medicine,* followed by a third that appeared in 1976. An editorial in *The Lancet*, "Dangers of Eternal Youth," made the bizarre makeshift suggestion that women who wanted to continue on HRT should have hysterectomies, since no woman could get cancer of the womb if her womb had been surgically excised. Other scientific articles around the same time linked estrogen replacement with gall bladder disease, with the increased development of fibroids, and increased frequency of breast and ovarian cancer.

Overnight, estrogen replacement lost its glamour with both doctors and the patients who had been using it. The United States Food and Drug Administration (FDA) demanded that all estrogen medications carry a package insert warning of its dangers, as well as back-pedaling their sale as a "youth pill." But with the backing of the American Medical Association—which is *supposed* to be an independent body—United States drug manufacturers went to court in an attempt to resist printing the package inserts. Their main argument was that such information would unnecessarily "frighten women." Before long, the first studies indicating that estrogen replacement is associated with reduced fractures from osteoporosis brought hope to drug manufacturers who were trying to pick up the pieces left by the cancer scares. Yet, many doctors were afraid to use unopposed estrogen due to the link with uterine cancer.

So in 1976, Wyeth-Ayerst Pharmaceuticals hired a top American public relations firm to help refocus their marketing of Premarin, taking it away from the eternal youth image and toward a product used for the prevention of osteoporosis and heart disease. Their advertising was altered. The pharmaceutical companies as a whole also came to the rescue by altering the "product" they were selling—unopposed estrogen. By adding one of the newly developed progestogens such as Provera, they were able to come up with a new "product"—a cocktail of hormone drugs that (they insisted) would reduce the risk of estrogen's overstimulating the womb lining and causing cancer. Some also started referring to hormone treatments not so much as ERT (Estrogen Replacement Therapy), but as HRT. A new product. A new name. A new image. Over the next 15 years, hormone manufacturers funded study after study and publicized the findings to doctors and the press in an attempt to demonstrate the benefits of HRT.

Sweet Talk

To some extent, the relaunch of HRT has been a successful project. Some women are reassured by the calm, rational voice of books such as the British publication *The Amarant Book of Hormone Replacement Therapy*, offspring of the Amarant Trust, which relates that "There was a scare in 1975 that HRT 'caused' cancer, but at that time estrogen was used by itself, without the added progesterone...What doctors had not realized then was that progesterone was needed as well to induce the womb to shed the lining and so prevent the buildup." Its authors, Gorman and Whitehead, go on to explain that the new "opposed therapy" produces a monthly bleed that they define as a safe, "normal period." They reassure their readers that so successful has the campaign to promote HRT been in some countries that certain gynecologists now claim that *all* postmenopausal women need HRT in order to reach their health potential. To other women, however, such rhetoric seems reminiscent of TV advertising for dishwashing detergents. The same book also speaks of "long-suffering husbands" as a result of their wives "letting themselves go," wives "looking hot and bothered," and wives who have "gone off sex." It concludes that men should encourage their wives to see a doctor since "it may save your marriage," and insist that for over a third of a woman's life, she is living in a state of estrogen deficiency. "HRT is the greatest treasure of a middle-aged woman's life," claim its authors. With HRT, they promise, a woman can have "reached fifty but feel like twenty."

Meanwhile, doctors unaware of how lifestyle alterations, the use of botanicals, and natural progesterone can transform the health and energy of women in midlife, are beginning routinely to warn women of the dangers of *not* using HRT. And journalists, fed information by supposedly independent organizations, which are in fact largely funded by pharmaceutical manufacturers, conclude in articles published in such papers as *The Guardian* that: "Once the only cure for menopause was said to be death...now there are other options."

Cancer Scares

According to recent research, what women seem to worry about most in relation to HRT is that it may increase their risk of cancer, especially endometrial cancer, but breast cancer, too. There is much evidence that hormone supplementation does indeed increase the risk of some cancers. As far back as the mid 1970s, epidemiologists remarked that endometrial cancers were rising at an alarming rate. The culprit was identified as unopposed estrogen, which encourages the proliferation of the womb lining. This is why most doctors today add a progestogen to their estrogen replacement.

However, it is not even known whether or not adding a progestogen to the HRT cocktail may be wiping out any postulated benefit that estrogen replacement may offer as a protection from heart disease. This is an example of how incomplete the highly vocalized research into the supposed benefits of HRT may be. As far as the effect of taking estrogen on the development of breast cancer in postmenopausal women is concerned, Elizabeth Barrett-Connor of the University of California at San Diego concluded, as have others, that taking estrogen for five years or more increased the risk of breast cancer by as much as 50 percent. Meanwhile, many other scientists, including Kay-Tee Khaw, professor of gerontology at the University of Cambridge and editor of the scholarly book *Hormone Replacement Therapy*, suggest that adding a progestogen may actually compound the risk.

Forgotten Estrogen

Amidst all the arguments, confusion, and disagreement over HRT, there are two benefits that it undeniably brings to the few women who are genuinely very low in estrogen after menopause and who can therefore benefit from supplementary estrogen. These lie in the ability of this important female hormone to relieve vaginal dryness and to stop hot flashes.

What is usually forgotten is that estrogen is not the only way of eliminating either symptom. Neither is it necessarily the best way for most women. For the majority of women, who in the Western world tend to be estrogen dominant, adding more estrogen drugs only serves to mask the underlying hormonal fluctuations taking place in their bodies that involve the hypothalamus—triggering hot flashes while further increasing estrogen dominance. And although hot flashes do not usually respond to the use of natural alternatives as rapidly as they do to estrogen drugs, they do respond well, frequently bringing permanent relief with no side effects. Similarly, a natural progesterone cream or oil used regularly both on the body and in the area of the vulva and inside the vagina itself is usually enough to clear vaginal dryness, itching, irritation, and the thinning of vaginal tissue, in the vast majority of cases within a few weeks. For that matter, a good cream based on comfrey is usually enough to do the trick for most women. For the very small number of women to whom such actions don't bring relief, a small amount of estrogen used for a while will bring relief. But what kind of estrogen?

All estrogens are not created equal. Estrogen (E1) and estradiol (E2) are highly stimulating to breast tissue, and, like the artificial estrogen used in

HRT and the xenoestrogens in our environment, have been implicated in breast cancer. By contrast, the third estrogen that the body makes, estriol (E3), being a weak estrogen, has actually been shown to inhibit the development of cancer in animals and may help protect from it in women. At the beginning of HRT, there were few alternatives to artificial estrogen drugs. Now, less carcinogenic forms of estrogen, such as estriol itself, or what is known among doctors who favor natural methods of helping women deal with menopausal difficulties as *triple estrogen*, are available. An invention of American physician Jonathan Wright, triple estrogen is made up of 80 percent estriol with 10 percent each of estrone and estradiol. It is available in the United States through pharmacies and can be ordered by doctors outside the United States by prescription. So can excellent vaginal creams containing high levels of the safer estrogen—estrogen that is chemically identical to the hormones secreted by a woman's ovaries. In the rare cases when small amounts of estrogen are needed temporarily as part of a woman's bloodless revolution, such products have become the treatments of choice by doctors who take a natural approach to the treatment of menstrual and menopausal problems.

As far as getting off HRT, if you are already on it and dissatisfied, this is not a difficult thing to do. It should be done slowly, and it is best carried out with the help of a physician or health practitioner knowledgeable about the techniques and products that form a part of the natural menopause revolution.

In Praise of Straight Talk

The one thing on which almost everyone seems to agree is that women should have the right to make an informed choice about whether or not to use HRT. However, becoming informed enough to make that choice is another matter. Most "educational" materials readily available to women on HRT that purport to present objective information are in truth a travesty of objectivity. Under the guise of rational language, these publications lay out all the supposed benefits HRT offers, sometimes in rather patronizing language. The average woman wanting to inform herself about the pros and cons of treatments available to her through her doctor has little access to *real* information and is unlikely even to know where to go to get it.

Some excellent material has been written that does give the facts— books such as Sandra Coney's *The Menopause Industry*, and Gail Vines' *Raging Hormones*, for instance. Often such books have received little publicity, since even much of the press has been indoctrinated into the value of HRT, and books like these challenge it—sometimes in highly technical terms. They also demand an intellectual commitment to the search for information on HRT that many women have neither the time nor the inclination to carry out. There are also some excellent official reports such as "Hormone Replacement Therapy," a report to the National Advisory Committee on Core Health and Disability Support Services in New Zealand, published in 1993, and some well-researched papers produced with the support of women's groups, such as the highly erudite and hard-hitting "Disempowering Midlife Women: The Science and Politics of Hormone Replacement Therapy," by Renate Klein and Lynette J. Dumble from the Women's Studies International Forum in Australia in 1994. But, unlike the slick little booklets available in every doctor's office, the paperback books, and the 2,500-word reassuring articles informing women about the latest benefit of HRT readily available in the general press, few women as yet have access to the other side of the story.

Stepford Wives Revisited

As Klein and Dumble say of HRT, "Given the fact that millions of [peri]menopausal women are advised to use this therapy, we believe that this amounts to nothing less than 'drugging' healthy women and furthermore does this without even informing them of the possibility of addiction." It is a sentiment with which I heartily concur. They continue:

> We reject the view that menopause is a disease and believe it to be extraordinarily unethical to risk drug dependence in healthy women. Midlife women have arrived at an important point in their lives where many of them feel the time has come to focus on their own needs and interests. By medicalizing the menopause and administering addictive drugs, this empowering process of self-determination is threatened...HRT has the potential to *disempower* midlife women...another form of medical violence against women.

One of the interesting issues surrounding the whole question of HRT, and yet another strange irony, lies in the way some feminist groups view it. An important question in the future will be whether or not feminists take the lead in exposing the way in which midlife women are being disempowered or whether they, too, become pawns in the hands of profit-oriented pressure groups. McCrea and Markle investigated the attitudes of feminist groups on both sides of the Atlantic. They came up with some fascinating observations about the differences. In the United States as long ago as the late 1960s, feminists had begun to challenge the notion that menopausal women are suffering from a deficiency disease that needs treatment. They presented menopause as a normal event in a woman's life and in doing so attempted to remove the stigma that has surrounded it ever since Robert A. Wilson first issued his warning that a woman's worth ends in midlife. American feminists pointed out that to take the standard view of menopause is to acquiesce in the belief that menstruation, like menopause itself, is a physical and emotional handicap rendering women incomplete in comparison to men. Out of such thinking, a number of active American, Canadian, Australian, and New Zealand women's health and consumer groups have developed who have become highly vocal in their opposition to the use of hormone drugs. Klein and Dumble say:

> Many long-time feminists are approaching midlife. Will we personally resist HRT and politically expose the extraordinarily paralyzing consequences if millions of women at the prime of their lives and ready to challenge the world instead become the Stepford Wives of the 1990s: rigid in their "happy" state, heterosexually active because they must, running from mammography to bone density test to endometrial biopsy, coping with migraines, hypertension and weight gain; stressed out from surviving the cancer scare which resulted in a breast biopsy—all from a drug for the prevention of osteoporosis and heart attacks which they might never get?

By contrast, in Britain and some other Western countries, with the exception of Germaine Greer who has put together a powerful case against HRT, many feminists have campaigned enthusiastically for hormone treatments. Together with consumer groups, they have tended to view HRT as something they believe British doctors are denying women the right to— too often, they say, by insisting that the problems women have around the time of menopause are figments of an overactive imagination. As Gail Vines, author of *Raging Hormones*, says:

> American feminists have tried to show that differential socialization, not biological difference, accounts for women's inferior social status. In Britain, on the other hand, feminists tend to be more closely aligned with

the socialist movement, and have tended to see the roots of women's oppression in the structure of capitalist societies and so to give the biological debate less priority.

But, as McCrea and Markle point out, "It has been individual feminists and not a whole social movement who have militated for ERT [HRT] in Great Britain." A major problem with all the talk about HRT is that it has stolen the whole women's health agenda by taking attention away from the real issues about women's health. The crux of preventing heart disease and osteoporosis lies not with HRT, but with making lifestyle changes—particularly and especially to diet. Our bone fracture rates in the West have been increasing dramatically so that both men and women have three times more hip fractures now than were experienced in the same age group some 30 years ago. It is important that we don't become so focused on looking for "magic bullets" that we beg the real question of how far-reaching an effect lifestyle change can have on women's lives.

Of major importance in the success of the bloodless revolution and the rate at which it is carried out is the attitude that feminists and women's groups take to it. It is essential that they, like all women, become aware of the work of its trailblazers so that we can make the best possible use of all the information, techniques, and substances now available to us. Important, too, is our finding ways to reconnect with the energies of instinct and deepening our awareness of the powerful and life-enriching archetypes of menopause. All of these things are here to help each one of us. Until HRT or some other "magic bullet" is able to promise that kind of freedom and fulfillment, it is of minor importance.

———✦———

CHAPTER SEVEN

DARK GODS

Is Cancer Preventable?

ancer is probably the most serious disease affecting women. Certainly it is the most terrifying. We are continually being urged by the medical profession to guard ourselves against death from breast, cervical, and womb cancer by getting regular mammograms and Pap smears. We are bombarded with information from the media about the dangers of breast cancer. Yet, instead of equipping us so that we can take action to make cancer's appearance in our own lives less likely, most of the information we receive day to day about the illness fills us with the kind of fear that makes it difficult to sort out the facts from the fantasies. Each woman responds to fear in a different way. For some, fear of cancer has them booking regular appointments at women's clinics. Others hope against hope that the cancer terror will pass them by. Even the words we use to describe someone who has the illness—a cancer *victim*—give to the illness a power that it does not deserve. Meanwhile, the threat of cancer—both real and imagined—continues to disempower us.

The Perils of Protection

Ask most medical experts about what you can do to best protect yourself from dying from some form of female cancer, and they are likely to tell you that early detection is the answer. The theory is that the earlier you detect cancers, the better your chances of survival. Breast cancers are diagnosed through a combination of sonograms, aspiration of lumps, physical examinations, mammograms, and, if necessary, surgical biopsy, where a piece of tissue taken from the breast is removed and examined under the microscope. A mammogram is an x-ray of the breasts that is used to diagnose breast cancer at its earliest appearance—supposedly before it can be felt by a physical examination. It is standard medical procedure in most countries to have mammograms taken of the breasts of women who can afford it every year or two.

Some interesting research came to light as the result of the largest study of its kind ever carried out in Canada. The Canadian National Breast Screening Study followed the fate of 89,836 women between the ages of 40 and 49 for an eight-year period, during which half of them were given mammograms every year to eighteen months, while the other half were only examined physically. To the amazement of the researchers, when all the results were tallied, they discovered that deaths among the women who got regular mammograms were significantly higher than those who had none. When finally the results were published—which incidentally did not happen until a full four years after the study was completed—the National Cancer Institute finally announced that the increase in death from breast cancer was 52 percent. In simple terms, this means that you are half again as likely to die of the disease if you do get regular mammograms than if you do not. Unlike much of the research that appears unheeded by the general public, this report made the headlines. "Breast Scans Boost Risk of Cancer Death," announced the headline in an article that appeared in *The London Times* on June 2, 1991. It then went on to announce that "middle-aged women who have regular mammograms are more likely to die from breast cancer than women who are not screened, according to dramatic new research."

Another common notion about breast cancer is that the earlier it is detected and surgery is performed, the better your chances of survival. This, too, appears to be untrue, as Petr Skrabanek reported in *The Lancet* as far back as 1985: "There is no evidence that early mastectomy affects survival. If the patients knew this, they would mostly likely refuse surgery." At the University of California, Berkeley, Professor Hardin Jones is an expert in the areas of medical physics and physiology. He had reported to the American Cancer Society more than 15 years before that every serious attempt to relate early treatment to survival has been unsuccessful. Jones studied many reports that looked at detection and survival and found that those subjects chosen for treatment for cancer tended to be patients who were considered capable of being cured by operations, while the inoperable or terminal patients tended to be lumped together as part of the untreated control groups. When he had made adjustments in the statistics to take this into account, Jones concluded that "My studies have proven conclusively that untreated cancer victims actually live up to four times longer than treated individuals." That was more than a quarter of a century ago, yet Jones's investigations, like those of other researchers since then, have gone largely unheeded.

Mammogram Miasma

Not only are mammograms not a cure-all for breast cancer, a clean mammogram is no real guarantee that you *do not* have a cancer developing. Mammograms are capable of missing its presence altogether in between 10 and 15 percent of all cancers. They are also open to a great deal of confusion and interpretation, since reading them is not an exact science but an art dependent upon the competence and judgment of human beings.

There is a great deal of fear in women that tends to surround the whole practice. American specialist in internal medicine Dr. H. Gilbert Welch, a senior researcher at the Department of Veterans' Affairs in White River Junction, Vermont, has looked carefully at the difficulties that go with the excessive diagnosis of diseases like breast cancer. He discovered that in women who die from other causes, an amazing 40 percent have had microscopic changes in their breasts. These are common lesions that show up on mammograms, and there is no way that any expert, no matter how skilled or highly experienced, is capable of knowing which of these will remain dormant and which will turn into cancer.

According to recent research, neither does a biopsy after a suspicious mammogram improve survival rates from breast cancer. A biopsy entails cutting through the suspected lump and invading the protective pocket that helps keep a tumor from spreading, and, as a result, this very procedure that is designed to confirm the existence or nonexistence of a cancerous lesion can actually encourage any cancer present to metastasize—to spread to other parts of the body. German researchers who looked at the survival rates of patients with breast cancer discovered that those who'd had biopsies died earlier than those who did not. Even biopsies done with a needle rather than a scalpel do not appear to be safe—quite apart from what the worry over waiting for results and the pain involved in the procedure can do to undermine a woman's immune system. George Crile Jr., M.D., a surgeon emeritus at the Cleveland Clinic in the United States, says, "It gives credence to what our patients already think and tell us—that cutting into cancer spreads it and makes it grow."

The point to consider from all of this is that it is time we stopped falling victim to the pronouncements and procedures of high-tech medical procedures, as well as to cancer itself as a disease, for the answers to its prevention lie mostly in our lifestyle. The answers depend upon things we can do ourselves to change the way we eat and live and think for the better and should not be left in the hands of abstract medical theorizing and the fear-mongering that too often accompanies it. As a recent editorial in *The Lancet* pointed out, "Some readers may be startled to learn that the overall mortality rate from carcinoma of the breast remains static. If one were to believe all the media hype, the triumphalism of the profession in the published research, and the almost weekly miracle breakthrough trumpeted by the cancer charities, one might be surprised that women are dying at all from this cancer."

Precancerous Power

Another common procedure to which women are subjected is the Pap smear for diagnosing cervical abnormalities. Its name comes from a Dr. George Papanicolaou, who developed the procedure almost three-quarters of a century ago. It has since been refined and is now used as a way of identifying abnormal (often called *precancerous*) cells as early as possible. Using a simple instrument inserted into the vagina, a doctor scrapes away a sampling of cells from the squamocolumnar junction of the cervix just inside the cervical opening at the bottom of the womb. These are then fixed on a slide with a chemical preservative and examined under the microscope by a technician or doctor used to reading them. Pap smears are frequently credited with the decline in the death rate for cervical cancer that has occurred in the past couple of decades. They, too, can be highly unreliable and produce a number of both false-positives and false-negatives, and there have been no controlled randomized trials that prove that they actually save lives.

When a trial was carried out in British Columbia where mass screening by Pap smear had been done, deaths from cervical cancer did indeed drop. Not a lot could be deduced from this fact, since they also dropped in the rest of Canada to just the same degree even when mass screening was not conducted. Meanwhile, in Britain, the death rate from cervical cancer has not dropped despite 40 million smears having been conducted. As Dr. E. Robin points out in his fascinating book *Matters of Life and Death: Risks vs. Benefits of Medical Care*, the Pap smear is not only one of the most common and popular laboratory tests, it is also one of the most unreliable. He writes about one study where two Pap smears were taken from the same women at the same time. An amazing two-thirds of the women's two tests showed different results.

Cancer is not, as we have been led to believe, the inevitable curse visited upon innocent victims without warning. In the past five years, a great deal of information has come to light about how the way you eat and live either protects or predisposes you to cancer. Forward-thinking researchers are awakening to hormonal links in the development of breast and womb cancer and finding ways of using natural hormones to protect against it. At the same time, the evidence mounts that all those Pap smears and mammograms we have been putting ourselves through are not only pretty useless in protecting against cancer death, they may even be contributing to its development. Happily, the rest of the news about cancer that is emerging out of the bloodless revolution is all good—especially in terms of what it can do to protect your life and the lives of your daughters.

Cells Gone Wrong

Cancer is defined as a "malignant neoplasm"—a powerful abnormal cellular growth that first invades and then eventually takes over normal tissue. Every cancer begins with an alteration to a single normal cell, which causes an increase in cell division or reproduction, as well as a loss of differentiation. Ordinary healthy human cells reproduce continually in a controlled manner as part of the body's normal growth and repair processes. This remains under the control of the body's normal patterning mechanisms, which differentiate a cell from every other kind of cell in the body in line with the purpose this cell serves. Cancer cells are different. They multiply faster than normal and lose all definition so that newly replicated cancer cells become incapable of carrying out the tasks for which normal cells of a particular kind have been designed. Cancer cells revert to a more primitive form of cellular life, relying on glucose for their metabolism rather than oxygen, and avariciously reproducing, unchallenged by the body's normal control and regulating mechanisms. A woman's immune system, which is superbly designed to handle foreign invaders, finds it almost impossible to oust cancer cells because the membranes of cancer cells resemble closely enough the membranes of normal cells so that it does not recognize how dangerous they are.

No one knows for sure why cells become cancerous. There are two main theories. The oldest is known as the *genetic* theory. It says that a cancer cell is the result of damage to DNA (which holds the body's chromosomal codes for replication within it), which has been brought about by radiation, toxins, or viruses. The genetic theory goes something like this: Damage is always occurring to the chromosomes of cells throughout the body and then being repaired by gene-repair mechanisms. However, more damage can occur than a cell's repair processes can handle. When enough unrepaired damage accumulates, says the theory, cancer develops. A more recent theory about the origins of cancer—more likely according to a rapidly growing number of scientists, as well as practitioners of natural medicine—is known as *epigenetics*. The epigenetic hypothesis insists that it is not time passing, but toxic elements within a cell's cytoplasm, that trigger chromosomal changes that result in the cell's reverting to a more primitive mode of behavior. In effect, cells become cancerous in direct response to the toxic threat.

All this may sound like high-falutin' theorizing by abstract scientists and of little relevance to any woman concerned about the prevention and treatment of cancer of the breast, cervix, or womb, but it is actually great news, because where once a woman was forced to see herself as a helpless victim of the great demon cancer, which struck without apparent warning, we now know that there are specific lifestyle changes we can make and actions we can take that not only help prevent cancer, but at the very least, significantly prolong the life of a woman who has it. These changes include cleaning up our environment and following a diet that is low in fat, high in fresh vegetables, rich in beta-carotene, and that includes taking supplements of the antioxidant nutrients such as vitamin C, selenium, and beta-carotene. Many studies also show that a shift in attitude can both help prevent cancer and extend survival time in someone who already has it. So can the use of certain natural hormones. All of this is particularly welcome news, since what has become blatantly obvious in recent years is that the usual treatments for most types of female cancer—surgery, radiation, and chemotherapy, where toxic chemicals are introduced into the body—have little success in treating most kinds of cancer, for cancer cells can be hard to kill. Preventing cancer is much easier than trying to cure it.

Hormone Links

Both breast cancer and endometrial cancer (cancer of the womb) are related to a woman's hormonal balance. And while endometrial cancer still remains relatively rare, in recent years the incidence of breast cancer has increased manifold in industrialized countries. In the United States, one female in nine between the ages of one and 85 now gets breast cancer, and it is the leading cause of death among women between the ages of 40 and 55. Only 20 years ago, the figure was one woman in 20. Now there are 180,000 new breast cancer cases each year and 46,000 deaths, while another 150,000 women submit to mutilating mastectomies. Worldwide, breast cancer is the most common cancer among women, accounting for 20 percent of all malignancies. Britain has the highest breast cancer mortality rate in the world. In Britain, in 1992, there were 13,663 deaths from breast cancer and 53,000 total or partial breast excisions. Over 20,000 new cases are now discovered each year.

The relationship between the development of breast and endometrial cancer and sex hormones daily becomes more clear. Both breast tissue and endometrial tissue are sensitive to reproductive hormones. Estrogen is well known to stimulate breast tumors in animals. Every published study on breast cancer turns up evidence that estrogen—or, to be more exact, estradiol and estrone, which are the most commonly prescribed estrogens—is somehow related to breast cancer. The now-famous Swedish research carried out by L. Berkgvist and his colleagues at University Hospital in Uppsala, and reported in 1989, showed an increase in breast cancer after only seven years of estrogen use. Several other studies have linked estrogen replacement to increased risk of breast cancer, although not all studies as yet support this finding. Still, many so-called medical experts continue to downplay the risk and insist that even women who have already had breast cancer are putting themselves under no special risk in taking estrogen replacement or HRT, using both estrogen and a progestogen.

When the dangers of estrogen replacement first began to come to light, many doctors expressed the hope that they could minimize the risk of breast cancer by adding a synthetic progestin to the cocktail of hormones being given to women. This was a reasonable assumption, since the progestins had been shown to offer some protection against endometrial cancer in women given estrogen replacement. However, like many stopgap measures taken in medicine, this approach simply has not worked. This is perhaps not surprising when you know that the *Physician's Desk Reference* lists breast malignancies in beagle dogs as one of the side effects of giving them Provera—one of the most commonly prescribed progestins in many countries of the industrialized world. The Berkgvist study showed that taking an estrogen/progestin combination (still commonly prescribed for HRT) quadrupled the breast-cancer risk, compared with women who were not taking it.

Then in 1992, not long after the Berkgvist study was published, an important review of studies was carried out that examined the relationship between HRT and breast cancer, published in *Obstetrics and Gynecology*. It showed a 63 percent increase in breast cancer risk for women on estrogen/progestin-based HRT. Such findings have prompted many experts on breast cancer to set warning bells ringing. Dr. Jonathan S. Berek, Director of Gynecologic Oncology at the UCLA School of Medicine, has said that it "hits at the heart of our philosophy that patients should be on estrogen and progestin. This questions the assumption that it is entirely safe, at least from the standpoint of the breast." Meanwhile, evidence continues to mount that xenoestrogens and other environmental pollutants are also in part responsible for the rising incidence of breast cancer in the industrialized world. Yet more and more estrogen/progestin HRT is doled out every year, and our environment becomes more and more polluted by petrochemically derived estrogen mimics.

Beware Estrogen Dominance

Both breast cancer and endometrial cancer tend to develop during periods of estrogen dominance in a woman's life. Breast cancer occurs most often in menstruating women with either normal estrogen levels or high estrogen levels but low progesterone—a set of circumstances most likely to present itself after the age of 35 when anovulatory menstruation becomes common in Western women. Breast cancer also develops easily after menstrual periods have stopped, when women are being given estrogen replacement either on its own or together with a progestin but *without* natural progesterone.

A study carried out by Dr. Linda Cowan, which was reported in the *American Journal of Epidemiology,* clearly showed the protective benefits of progesterone. Menstruating women with low progesterone levels were found to have almost five and a half times the risk of developing breast cancer. They also experienced ten times the number of deaths from malignant neoplasms, compared with women whose progesterone levels were normal. Anyone willing to take the time to look in depth at what is known about the factors that predispose us to, or protect us from, breast cancer will find two things: First, estrogen—particularly estrogen unopposed by progesterone—lies behind the development of cancer; and second, sufficient progesterone helps to protect from it.

There is a drug called Tamoxifen now commonly given to women who have had breast surgery in an attempt to prevent cancer from recurring. The way Tamoxifen works is simple: As a weak estrogenic substance, it blocks the uptake of estrone and estradiol in breast tissue since it is taken up by estrogen receptor sites on the breast, thereby protecting the breast tissue from the cancer-promoting estrogen present in the body. Unfortunately, the drug has some rather nasty side effects. A growing number of doctors insist that the same results can be achieved by giving natural progesterone. The fact that Tamoxifen works by protecting against estrogen's effect on breast tissue is yet another thing that strongly supports the notion that estrogen at levels that are too high is a major factor in the development of breast cancer. So is the fact that a woman's risk of developing breast cancer is much diminished by full-term pregnancies—particularly those that occur before the age of 18. (You will recall that the progesterone level in a woman soars during pregnancy, apparently conferring protection.) Women who have never had children have a much higher risk of getting breast cancer than mothers.

When men are given estrogen as a treatment for prostatic cancer or after sex-change surgery, this too is accompanied by an increased risk of breast cancer. However, when a woman's ovaries have been removed before the age of 40, her estrogen production decreases dramatically, as does her risk of breast cancer. This protection is lost, of course, if she is given HRT. Recent research shows that, strangely, a woman's chance of survival after breast surgery is even influenced by whether or not her body is in a state of estrogen dominance when it is performed. Menstruating women who have breast surgery carried out during the second half of their menstrual cycle—the luteal phase, when progesterone is high to balance estrogen—survive far longer than do women whose surgery is done early on in their cycle during the estrogen-dominant follicular phase.

It may take 20 years before all of the measurements are in, which will enable scientists to prove unequivocally that excess estrogen in a woman's body allows both cancer of the breast and cancer of the womb to develop. From a commercial point of view, it may be far longer. In the meantime, we need to begin looking upon cancer not as some terrifying disease against which we are helpless, but rather a result of biological and ecological imbalances that each of us is capable of taking action to rectify. For this is the truth of things. It is a truth much obscured by all the "cancer drama" that surrounds us.

The Strong and the Weak

Even some of the weaker natural estrogens themselves can have important roles to play in cancer prevention. You will recall that your body produces three main estrogens or hormones with estrus activity: estrogen (E1), estradiol (E2), and estriol (E3). In common parlance, they are usually lumped together under the "estrogen" banner. Each of these estrogens has unique characteristics. When you are not pregnant, it is primarily estrogen (E1) and estradiol (E2) that are secreted by the ovaries in relatively large quantities (measured in micrograms), while estriol (E3) is only made in minute quantities as a by-product of E1 metabolism. During pregnancy, when the placenta becomes the prime site for estrogen production, this pattern is completely reversed. Now estriol becomes the dominant estrogen and at the same time, progesterone production by the placenta also soars. It is only estrogen (E1) and estradiol (E2), which are highly stimulating to breast tissue, that have been implicated in breast cancer, not estriol. Studies carried out more than 20 years ago showed that estradiol, and to a lesser degree, estrogen, increase a woman's risk of breast cancer, while estriol is actually protective against it, for estriol (E3) is a weak estrogen. Like some of the phyto-estrogens, it appears to occupy receptor sites so that they are protected from the cancer-inducing properties of E1 and E2. So much weaker is E3 that the ratio of activity between estradiol (E2) and estriol (E3) is an amazing 1,000:1.

The Amazing Estrogen Quotient

In animal experiments where both rats and mice were treated with cancer-causing chemicals and then one group was given estriol (E3), researchers discovered that breast cancer was inhibited by this estrogen. Much impressed by the protective effects of estriol on animals, American researcher Dr. Henry Lemon began to investigate how this estrogen behaves in relation to human breast cancer. He developed a fascinating formula that he dubbed the *estrogen quotient*, by which he meant the ratio of the cancer-inhibiting estriol (E3) to the cancer-promoting estrogen (E1) and estradiol (E2) in any woman. If a woman's estrogen quotient is high, then her body is producing a lot of the protective estriol in relation to the other estrogen. He theorized that in these women, the risk of breast cancer would be reduced. If, on the other hand, a woman's estrogen quotient was low, then very little of the protective estriol would be produced relative to the other two, and she would be expected to have a higher risk of cancer.

To test all this out, Lemon measured the various kinds of estrogen both in the urine of healthy women and those with breast cancer. In healthy women, the average estrogen quotient was 1.3 before menopause and 1.2 afterwards. Only 21 percent of the healthy women had estrogen quotients that were below normal. By contrast, in the women with breast cancer who had received no hormonal treatment of any kind, the average estrogen quotients were between 0.5 and 0.8. A surprising 62 percent of these women had values below normal.

Lemon's work strongly suggests that women with breast cancer have low levels of estriol relative to the other two estrogens. It has also been confirmed by epidemiological studies. In countries where there is a low incidence of breast cancer, women tend to have high levels of urinary estriol excretion and low levels in their blood compared with women in countries such as the United States where the incidence of breast cancer is high. Later on Lemon and his co-workers carried out another interesting study on women whose breast cancer had metastasized (spread to other areas of their body). One group was given estriol in doses of between 2.5 and 15 mg a day. The other was not. By the end of the study an amazing 37 percent of women who got the estriol had either had their cancer arrested or experienced a complete remission.

In the light of what is generally expected in women with metastasized breast cancer, such results are nothing short of astounding. Not only is there strong evidence that unopposed estradiol and estrogen are cancer-causing in relation to breasts, both estriol and progesterone—the two hormones that are produced in good quantity during pregnancy—help protect against it. Sadly, the protective properties of natural progesterone remain largely unknown. Meanwhile, to block the side effects of estrogen and estradiol on breast tissue, it is not the safe natural estriol (E3) with virtually no side effects that is regularly used, but rather the drug Tamoxifen—known to increase the incidence of womb cancer when given to women. Why? There are probably several reasons. But without a doubt, one of the most important is that the protective powers of estriol are little known by specialists, let alone the average general practitioner (GP).

Estriol, the dose of which needs to be individualized for each woman, is a natural hormone derived from plant sources. As such, like natural progesterone, it is a generic hormone of little interest to drug companies, since there is no way it can be patented as a drug. It is worth noting that estriol— far and away the safest of all the estrogens—has all sorts of other useful properties. It has the ability to alleviate vaginal and urinary infections in postmenopausal women without causing breakthrough bleeding and eliminates vaginal dryness in the small number of women who need extra estrogen after menopause. Yet estriol (E3) is still rarely used. I suspect that only when women themselves demand it will this change.

Endometrial Help

Endometrial cancer (cancer of the womb) is not only relatively rare, it is much less dangerous than breast cancer. Because it tends to cause abnormal bleeding, it is not so difficult to diagnose early. It also tends to remain isolated for a long time before spreading to other parts of the body. The general treatment for endometrial cancer is hysterectomy. Once a woman who has had it has had her womb removed, she is usually warned to stay away from HRT forever. When it comes to endometrial cancer, the relationship between excess estrogen and its development is even clearer than in the case of breast cancer. As John Lee says, "It is generally acknowledged that the only known cause of endometrial cancer is unopposed estrogen. Here again, estradiol and estrogen are the culprits. When estrogen supplements are given to postmenopausal women for five years, the risk of endometrial cancer increases 6-fold, and longer term use increases it to 14-fold." It is not only postmenopausal women who are at risk either. "In premenopausal women, endometrial cancer is extremely rare except during the 5 to 10 years before menopause when estrogen dominance is common," Lee continues. "The addition of natural progesterone during these years would significantly reduce the incidence of endometrial cancer as well as breast cancer."

John Lee and other doctors working with natural menopause are not only suggesting the use of natural progesterone cream as a preventative measure against both endometrial cancer and breast cancer, but many of them also use progesterone as a way of helping to protect these women from progressive osteoporosis, and from urinary tract infections and vaginal atrophy, which occurs in some women. In fact, it was with these women—those who could not be given the estrogen and progestins of ordinary HRT—that Lee first began his highly successful natural progesterone therapy. It was through his clinical work over many years that Lee discovered that natural progesterone therapy would not only reverse osteoporosis and correct vaginal atrophy, it can also prevent the further development of all sorts of cancer in these women. None of the women Lee originally treated with progesterone who'd had breast cancer have to his knowledge ever had any recurrence of the illness.

Fat Chance

Specific foods and nutrients can also play a vital role in protecting a woman from cancer of the breast or womb—in no small part because certain compounds in food actually help lower a woman's estrogen levels. In a review of data from 12 case-controlled studies that appeared in *The Journal of the National Cancer Institute*, investigators concluded that 25 percent of postmenopausal breast cancers can be prevented by changes in diet alone. Research shows that 60 percent of breast, womb, and ovarian cancers are associated with a diet high in fat, for instance. In another study, where the dietary histories of 455 Italian women with ovarian cancer were compared with the histories of 1,385 normal women, a high-fat diet—especially from meat or butter—elevated the risk, while a diet high in green vegetables, carrots, whole grains, and fish provided the lowest risk.

High levels of most varieties of estrogen are what you want to avoid to protect your body from breast cancer. Eating a high-fat diet rich in animal-based proteins such as meat and milk products increases a woman's concentration of these estrogens dramatically. Estrogens in your bloodstream are filtered through the liver where they become combined with elements that make them difficult to absorb. Then they are sent to the intestines to be eliminated from the body before any excess can cause damage to the body. But if you eat a lot of fat in your foods (and almost half the calories in the typical Western diet come in the form of fats), then the intestinal environment becomes riddled with just the kind of bacteria that are able to break down estrogen compounds so that the estrogen is reabsorbed into the bloodstream. Not only does this increase the level of estrogenlike compounds in the body, but it also tends to prolong what is known as a woman's "menstrual life." Menstrual life is how many years in a woman's life she actually menstruates. When it comes to assessing the risks of breast cancer, women with a long menstrual life are twice as likely to get the illness as women with a short menstrual life.

For example, American women who live on a high-fat diet rich in animal products on average begin to menstruate at around the age of 12 and do not go through menopause until the age of 50. This is considered a long menstrual life. Asian women or young women on a vegetarian diet low in fat and only moderate in protein, on the other hand, begin menstruating later—around the age of 16—and go through menopause earlier—at approximately 46 years old. They have a much smaller risk of ending up with breast cancer, although it is interesting to see that when Japanese women who have been raised on such a low-fat diet move to the United States and eat more of the high-fat Western fare, their risk of getting breast cancer rises significantly.

Alcohol drinking also increases your risk of breast cancer. All but three of the case-control and cohort studies reported recently in the *New England Journal of Medicine,* which have investigated the association between alcohol intake and breast cancer incidence, have shown a 40 to 60 percent increase in risk even with only moderate drinking. Sugar, too, is implicated in cancer development. An epidemiological survey of 21 countries showed that a high-sugar intake is a major risk factor for the development of breast cancer in women over the age of 45.

A Passion for Healthy Foods

Just as certain kinds of diet predispose you to cancer, so others can protect you from it. There are many anti-cancer constituents in common foods. They include methylated flavones, selenium salts, phenols, indoles, aromatic isothyiocyanates, protease inhibitors, and, of course, the important plant sterols. There are also certain foods that have proven anti-cancer properties. Many are soya based, such as tofu, miso, tempeh, and tamari. Made from soya beans, they contain plant sterols or phyto-estrogen that have weak estrogenic activity. Research shows that Asian women who eat a lot of these foods have very little trouble with hot flashes around the time of menopause and afterwards. They also have very little trouble with any other menopausal symptoms, apparently because the weak estrogen that the foods contain bind with estrogen-receptor sites and protect them from the negative effects of circulating estrogen in the body and from xenoestrogens in the environment. There are other foods that in their natural, unprocessed state contain significant levels of plant sterols or phytohormones as well. They include corn, wheat, apples, almonds, cashews, oats, and peanuts. Meanwhile, the cruciferous vegetables, such as cabbage and cauliflower and broccoli, also boast anti–breast cancer elements such as indole-3-carbinol (I3C), which deactivates the estrogen hormones that can encourage breast cancer. At the Foundation of Preventative Oncology in New York City, researchers concluded a study examining the actions of these foods by saying that "dietary I3C may provide the basis for a novel approach for preventing breast cancer...."

Natural fiber also offers protection against cancer. Fiber alters the metabolism of estrogen in the bowel so that more is excreted and less reabsorbed. It has also been well established that optimal quantities of certain nutrients—most of them antioxidant vitamins and minerals, such as vitamin A, C, beta-carotene and the mineral selenium—have a great deal to contribute to cancer prevention. Researchers have discovered while examining 89,000 women nurses who were followed over an eight-year period that those who had an intake of less than 6,630 IU of vitamin A per day also had a 25 percent higher incidence of cancer than women whose daily intake of the vitamin was above this level. The B vitamins, too, are important for immunity and may help prevent cancer. This group of vitamins is very much involved in the metabolism of estrogen in the body, as well as in good bowel function, so that toxic wastes can be efficiently eliminated. Yet most of the B complex vitamins are destroyed or drastically reduced in the milling of flour and the preparation of convenience foods so that many women in the Western world are deficient in them.

The best diet to follow for cancer prevention is low fat, where less than 20 percent of the total calories you consume come from fats—a primarily vegetarian way of eating that rejects highly processed convenience foods, eliminates processed oils, is high in complex carbohydrates, and rich in fiber to help control the body's cycling estrogen. Consider taking extra antioxidant nutrients to boost your levels of these important protectors and fortify your immune system to help protect against cancer as well. We are not powerless to deal with cancer. Banishing fear, losing our reverence for high-tech diagnostic procedures whose effectiveness needs to be questioned, and taking back our responsibility for our own life and health hold the real promise for prevention. Knowing how is the first step, and taking action ourselves with the help of our doctors and health practitioners is the next. Once again, in the bloodless revolution, the power for change lies largely in our own hands.

GREMLINS IN THE ARCHITECTURE
Banishing the Fear of Osteoporosis

steoporosis is a terrible disease. A progressive loss of minerals, bone mass, and bone density, it affects men as well as women; and can result in fractures of the hip, shoulder, ribs, vertebrae, forearm, or wrist. Statistically, bone loss in women begins several years before menopause and then gets worse afterwards, creating an ever-increasing risk of debilitating breakages. In Britain, where the incidence of the illness has increased six times in the past 30 years, one in three women now develop it, and one in eight men. In the United States, statistics are even worse. The illness currently costs the country more than $11 billion a year. Twenty-five percent of women whose hips fracture die within two years—not always directly from the fracture, but from ending up in nursing homes where inactivity, alienation, and loss of control over their lives defeat them. Today, more women in the industrialized world die of fractures related to bone thinning than from cancers of the womb, cervix, and breast put together.

Silent Killer

Osteoporosis is not a simple disorder. And it is most certainly not another so-called estrogen deficiency disease, as some would still have us believe. Neither is it treatable by drinking masses of milk or stuffing yourself with calcium supplements. Surprisingly, both of these actions can actually make the condition worse. Like coronary heart disease, which few people even know they have until a heart attack strikes, osteoporosis is an insidious illness. The *Harvard Medical School Newsletter* recently dubbed it the "silent epidemic." It develops secretly over the years until one day its presence in the body surfaces to devastate a life. It need not. The idea, which is still taught in medical schools, that bone mass decline is a normal consequence of aging is quite simply false. There is nothing normal about bone thinning.

A few facts. Osteoporosis regularly occurs in men who are deficient in testosterone and in women who are deficient in progesterone. Black women have less bone loss than white women, big women less than small women, and fat women less than their skinny sisters. Meat eaters are at a far greater risk of the disease than vegetarians. A high calcium intake is often mentioned as being essential in preventing bone thinning. Yet, people in Third World countries whose daily intake of calcium is less than half our own have a very low incidence of the disease, whereas in our culture its incidence is very high and continues to mount. Users of prescription drugs have more osteoporosis than people who do not take medication, and couch potatoes are far more prone to the condition than women who get regular exercise. To prevent osteoporosis, you need to understand it. The earlier a woman learns why it happens and the sooner she takes action to counter it, the better. Ideally, this should be in her 20s and 30s. However, if those years are already long past, take heart. Despite all the fear-mongering surrounding the disease, the truth is that there are actions you can take not only to halt bone loss if it has begun, but even to *reverse* it—no matter what your age.

Living Bone

Bones may seem like tough, inanimate objects, but they are not. They are actually living support tissue that is constantly changing and growing. Bone is made up of a combination of a flexible noncellular collagen matrix that has been embedded with hard and inflexible mineralized crystals. It is a kind of mineralized cartilage. Without the flexibility of collagen, your bones would be so brittle that they would easily shatter. Without the crystalline hardness of minerals, they would resemble the soft cartilage of a shark. Unless you spent your entire life under water, your skeleton would be unable to support the weight of your body. The combination of both this tensile strength from the minerals and compression strength from the collagen creates just about the finest structural resistance to breakage found anywhere in the living world.

Your bones are constantly being renewed, at a surprising rate. This is what makes it possible for breaks to mend and for a child's body to grow taller. There are two kinds of bone—*cortical* and *trabecular.* The heavy bones of your body, such as the long bones of the legs and arms, are cortical bones. Designed to give great directional strength, they are densely cast in spirals around tiny tubular channels through which cells can travel. Cortical bones renew themselves completely about every ten years. The other kind of bone (trabecular) is found in the vertebrae of your spine and at the ends of the long bones of the legs and arms—in places where you need compression strength. Trabecular bone is more weblike in its structure, and its turnover is even faster than cortical bone, completely renewing itself every two to three years.

When you are born, the growth hormone made by your body stimulates bones to grow at a rate that in general matches the rate at which the rest of your body is growing. Children start life at about 22 to 24 inches long, growing eventually to 64 inches, 69 inches, even 74 inches. The bones, muscles, tendons, and ligaments all keep in touch via a mysterious and beautiful inner harmonic—of which bones are a part—that synchronizes growth rate. One day puberty arrives, and the pineal gland switches on the reproductive hormones of the pituitary. The pituitary, in turn, activates the ovaries; and the ovaries start making estrogen and progesterone. When this happens, women have a growth spurt for a year or so, after which they grow no more in height. Now the hormones of the ovaries take over. It becomes the job of estrogen to slow up or moderate the rate at which old bone is being broken down. Meanwhile, progesterone gets busy encouraging the manufacture of new bone. If the speed of these two processes are in complete harmony—working at the same rate—your skeleton will stay at that particular bone density. When new bone formation exceeds breakdown, then your bones will grow more and more dense and stronger. But if breakdown begins to overtake new bone production, then osteoporosis develops.

Bones can be thought of as similar to the fibers that make a scarf or shawl—fibers that are knitted together with little spaces in between. When osteoporosis occurs, not only have the fibers become finer, you actually have fewer of them. In effect, you have lost a number of bone strands, and each strand that is left has become thinner. Under the microscope, sometimes even with the naked eye, you can see that there are spaces in such bone that make it look spongy and porous. That's where the word *osteoporosis* comes from. Whenever the resorption of bone is faster than the making of new bone, you will have osteoporosis. In fact, osteoporosis can be described as the condition that happens when there is a relative deficiency of osteoblasts resulting in inadequate bone formation.

Personal Pac-man

The ability of bones to break down and re-form depends on a process called *remodeling,* which relies on two very special kinds of cells in the substrate out of which all bone develops. The first are called *osteoclasts.* If you have ever played the video game Pac-man, it is easy to understand how they work. It is the job of the estrogen-modulated osteoclasts to travel through the spirals and weblike structures of your bone tissue like Pac-man, seeking out old, mineralized bone and then to gobble it up or dissolve it away (the proper name is *resorb* it) in order to make way for new bone. The minerals contained in the gobbled bone are released into general circulation and only empty spaces—called lacunae—are left behind. After the osteoclasts have done their Pac-man work, along come the other kind of bone cells—the *osteoblasts.* These cells, whose activity is modulated by progesterone, are drawn to the same sites and make their way into these lacunae. There they get busy creating new bone.

When you are growing up, your pituitary is pumping out growth hormone so the action of your osteoblasts dominates and more bone is created than is destroyed. Around puberty, the activity of osteoclasts and osteoblasts becomes more balanced. Later on, however, the balance can shift in favor of the bone-eating osteoclasts, while osteoblast activity declines. It is now that osteoporosis first takes hold. You get a shrinkage in bone mass, since more bone is being resorbed than being built, and more spaces are appearing than are being filled. If this goes on for a long time, too many minerals can be lost, and bone gets less hard and less dense until at last it becomes finely honeycombed and highly susceptible to breakage.

Stressing Your Body

When any crystal structure, such as bone, is put under stress, there are changes in the voltage of the electric fields around and through it. These electromagnetic changes draw the osteoclasts to the areas of your bones that need replacing, as well as encouraging the production of new bone via the work of the osteoblasts, which form the patterns of arcs and curves that create bone texture—a bit like weaving a scarf. When they are properly formed, these patterns provide resistance to all the day-to-day stresses your bones are put under. In fact, the more you stress your bones through exercise, the better quality will be the electric fields that govern remodeling—provided, of course, you supply your body with all the nutrients it needs to create new bone tissue. All any woman needs to maintain good, strong, dense, well-mineralized bones is a good balance between the activity of her osteoblasts and her osteoclasts. A woman in the Western world living a sedentary life and eating convenience foods will find this virtually impossible.

Secrets from the Grave

Once, osteoporosis was considered a menopausal disease. If it occurred at all—and it was still pretty rare—then it would only happen at menopause or afterwards. A fascinating article appeared in the prestigious British medical journal *The Lancet* not long ago. During the restoration of Christ Church in London, some skeletal material dating from between 1729 and 1852 was unearthed from the crypt. This gave medical researchers the chance to compare the rate of bone loss in the legs of these bone samples with those of present-day women of the same age. Using dual-energy x-ray absorptiometry, investigators discovered that there was significantly less bone loss in these women of 200 years ago compared to modern women—despite our supposedly better diet. Equally surprising, when investigators calibrated bone density with age, they could find no sign of a menopausal change in the unearthed bones. Now, however, unlike our ancestors, more and more women arrive at menopause having already lost between 20 and 30 percent of their bone mass. And this loss begins much earlier than most women realize.

It is during the five to eight years before menopause when, unknown to them, many women are experiencing anovulatory cycles that they are most vulnerable to bone loss. When a woman is not ovulating during a monthly cycle, no corpus luteum produces progesterone even though her periods may seem normal. Insufficient progesterone leads to insufficient osteoblast activity, for without enough progesterone, the osteoblasts are unable to produce new bone properly, so more bone is resorbed than built, and osteoporosis sets in. Statistically, bone mass in healthy women reaches a peak in the early 30s. After that, osteoclast activity tends to increase, while osteoblast activity decreases so that it declines gradually. At menopause, the decline further increases for three to five years, after which it tends to slow again to a rate of between 1 and 0.5 percent a year. Most doctors still believe that this is inevitable. It most certainly is not. To prevent it, to stop it, and to reverse bone loss, you need to do two things: Change your lifestyle, and get your hormone balance right. Let's look at hormones first.

Hormone Connections

Both estrogen and progesterone help protect against osteoporosis. The average doctor knows that estrogen replacement can slow down the rate of bone loss. This it does by regulating the "gobbling" actions of the osteoclasts. What the doctor is probably not aware of, however, is the far more important role that progesterone plays both in protecting against osteoporosis as well as in reversing it. And where estrogen's role is a minor one, progesterone's is a major one.

As far back as the early 1940s, researchers noticed the relationship between the decline in female sex hormones and the development of osteoporosis. Not until the 1970s, however, did they discover that estrogen replacement slightly decreased the rate of bone loss in women on HRT. Around the same time, epidemiological studies indicated that there was a decrease in the number of fractures that occurred in women who had been put on HRT. With reports like this, backed by marketing and public relations money from pharmaceutical manufacturers eager to find new groups of women to sell their drugs to, it did not take long for statements to appear drawing the conclusion that, like menopause itself, osteoporosis is an "estrogen deficiency disease," and then spread the news far and wide that estrogen replacement was the *treatment of choice* against the disease.

Unfortunately, the news that was spread has turned out to be one of those dangerous "half-truths" to which 20th-century medicine is particularly prone. Yet it has continued to spread despite the fact that highly respected researchers and reviewers writing in prestigious medical journals, from the *Journal of the American Medical Association* and *The Lancet*, to every up-to-date standard medical textbook, have long since refuted it.

The early studies on which the estrogen-protection assumption were based had gross scientific defects. Some were carried out on too few participants to be significant. Others made use of imprecise methods for measuring bone density. Later scientific papers (post–1976) praising the value of estrogen in managing osteoporosis failed to take into account that often either progesterone or a progestogen had also been included with the estrogen supplementation. It could well have been that the minor benefits that were reported came not from the estrogen itself, but from the combination of the estrogen and progesterone or estrogen and a progestogen—or even from the progesterone or the progestogen itself. When medroxyprogesterone—a common progestogen—was used on its own without estrogen in postmenopausal women, researchers reported that a small gain in bone mineral density of 5 percent took place. It is not much, but even this small gain is better than what can be achieved using estrogen on its own. However, estrogen continues to be considered as the treatment of choice for osteoporosis.

A Touch of Evil

Unopposed estrogen—that is, estrogen given on its own—carries with it serious long-term health dangers, both minor and major. They range from encouraging the laying down of fat stores in a woman's body and causing water retention to increasing her risk of endometrial cancer, liver disease, and breast cancer. Nonetheless, when hormone replacement began, estrogen was given on its own. These days, thankfully, most doctors are aware of the dangers of prescribing unopposed estrogen and no longer do so. However, what they do prescribe—progestogen—is not safe either. Very few are yet aware that estrogen's bone-protecting capacity is not all it is cracked up to be. Busy with their practices, they often do not have time to examine the scientific literature closely.

Again, it was Jerilynn Prior and her colleagues reporting in the *New England Journal of Medicine* who confirmed that estrogen's role in osteoporosis prevention is only a minor one. In their studies of female athletes, they found that osteoporosis occurs to the degree that they become *progesterone* deficient even though their estrogen levels remain normal. Prior also made an extensive review of published scientific evidence in this area. It confirmed that it is not estrogen but *progesterone* that is the *bone trophic* hormone—that is, the bone builder. Prior and her team were even able to identify progesterone receptor sites on osteoblast cells. Nobody has even found osteoblast receptors for estrogen. The only mechanism of action that estrogen has on bone is that it helps inhibit osteoclast resorption, but it can do nothing to build new bone. The bottom line is that it is in women with *progesterone deficiency* where bone loss occurs.

Awakenings

It was pressure from hundreds of women with osteoporosis whose bone density tests only showed that they were getting worse that triggered Dr. John Lee's experiments with progesterone. Many had already had one or two fractures, and many were already on estrogen replacement. Other patients he knew couldn't take estrogen because of a past history of breast cancer. Some were already on a good diet and were trying to get enough exercise, yet still they all had progressive osteoporosis. Even in the core of women without a history of breast cancer, Lee, like so many conscientious doctors, had been deeply concerned about the possible long-term side effects of giving estrogen replacement. Since estrogen is still produced by postmenopausal women, he asked himself, "Could progesterone alone be enough to prevent and/or reverse osteoporosis?"

Tender Mercies

Lee began to test his hypothesis on women with postmenopausal osteoporosis using transdermal progesterone cream together with a program of dietary changes, vitamin and mineral supplements, and modest exercise. Some of his patients were also given very small doses of estrogen, particularly if they suffered from vaginal dryness. Lee carefully monitored his results, keeping records for more than ten years. When at last they were finally published, his findings turned out to be nothing short of revolutionary. He had been able to accomplish the impossible. The natural progesterone cream had been able to halt bone loss whether or not the women taking it had been given estrogen as well. More remarkable still, his patients showed an improvement of approximately 15 percent in bone mineral density over a three-year period.

This had never been done—not with estrogen, not with other drugs like calcitonin or the diphosphates, nor with anything else. Patient after patient got better. Even more surprising, the women with the worst bones improved fastest. Some of them showed much greater than average improvement—a 30 to 40 percent increase in bone over the three-year period was not uncommon. Those women whose bone density was fairly good when the experiment began improved more slowly until finally each woman (no matter what condition her bones had been in at the start of the study) had reached her optimum bone density and then kept it.

Witnessing the effect of progesterone on bone was one of the most dramatic things that Lee had ever seen in his long family practice. It has a similar impact on other doctors who gradually became aware of what Lee had been doing, including a number of orthopedic surgeons who had been used to receiving referrals from Lee for his patients with broken bones. His patients stopped having fractures if they fell. Gradually, by word of mouth, the news spread. Before long, Lee had treated hundreds of women successfully with a progesterone cream and simple lifestyle changes. Out of a group of 100 of his treated patients, selected at random, only three had experienced fractures. One fell down a flight of stairs carrying a television set and broke her humerus. She refused to have it set in plaster, put it in a sling instead, and to the amazement of her orthopedist, found that it healed beautifully in under five weeks.

Another was a woman in her 70s who had been involved in a serious car crash. Driving a little Volkswagen, she had been crushed between two trucks. The accident demolished her Volkswagen and fractured both her knees. The orthopedic surgeon who had screwed the broken pieces together and then watched them heal swiftly commented that it was the best bone that he had ever seen in a 76-year-old. The third fracture, the result of a minor accident, was equally simple to heal. The other women treated with progesterone and a lifestyle change program simply didn't have fractures anymore.

An End to Osteoporosis

So there was Lee, a simple country doctor, with hundreds of patients who had been going through his office for some ten years, for whom he had records showing that their bones were greatly improved. He had women patients who had increased their bone mineral density even up to 50 percent.

Some of his patients were 45 years old, and others were 75 years old when they started treatment. Age did not matter; their bones were hungry for progesterone. The benefits his patients reported from progesterone and lifestyle change didn't end with osteoporosis prevention and the reversal of bone loss either. Women also reported a decrease in fibroids where they had been present, an increase in energy, a decline in aches and pains, and the disappearance of many other negative symptoms associated with PMS or menopause.

Hungry for Change

Although the successes of doctors like Lee who use topically applied natural progesterone constitute great news, it might be tempting to think that all you need to do to prevent osteoporosis is to rub on progesterone cream every day and then sit back munching on junk food, certain that all will be well. The trouble is it just doesn't work that way. How you eat and live are equally important and need to be addressed if you are to have a future free of bone loss and avoidable fractures. A good treatment and prevention program for osteoporosis needs to include carefully chosen vitamins and minerals that play an important part in osteoblast activity—vitamin D, vitamin C, beta-carotene, zinc, and magnesium—as well as weight-bearing exercise for at least 15 minutes, preferably half an hour or more, at least three times a week. Without adequate exercise, calcium cannot be incorporated into the bones, since it is only when bones are put under physical stress that calcium is demanded. A good program also emphasizes a way of eating that includes lots of calcium-rich leafy green vegetables and limits red meat to no more than a couple of times a week. It cuts down on alcohol and cuts out all "sodas" and manufactured soft drinks, for each of these in its own way affects the way calcium is used in the body. Many forms of purified protein, such as casein, lactalbumin, and egg whites—regularly used in slimmers' meal-replacement drinks—cause calcium loss, too. In fact, crash dieting of any kind is a common contributor to bone thinning in women.

Calcium Connections

In every case of osteoporosis, calcium loss from the bones lies at the core of the problem. Calcium is the most abundant mineral in your body.

It is vital for strong bones. So is phosphorus. After calcium, phosphorus is the next most prominent element in bone. The ratio of calcium to phosphorus is around $2^1/_2:1$. About 99 percent of the calcium in your body is deposited in your bones and teeth, although the remaining one percent has some very important jobs to do. It helps regulate nerve and muscle contraction, for instance. It is related to the parathyroid function and involved with blood-clotting and the metabolism of vitamin D. Calcium also enables your body to use iron properly and activate a number of important enzymes that help to regulate the passage of nutrients into and out of the cells. Finally, calcium is frequently called on—and called *forth* from bones—to balance the pH of your blood, rendering it more alkaline when it has become too acid from long-term stress, eating a lot of meat, or drinking a lot of coffee.

If this makes you think you need to rush out and buy a bottle of calcium pills, think again. Despite all the vitamin manufacturers currently pushing calcium supplements, research shows that taking calcium supplements is of little help in preventing osteoporosis. It may even make the problem worse. Taking higher doses of calcium supplements can contribute to kidney stones and interfere with the metabolism of zinc and magnesium, both of which play central roles in building strong bones. The best way to get your calcium is to eat the right kind of foods, particularly green leafy foods and sea plants, which are loaded with it in a form that is easy for the body to assimilate. The whole calcium issue is enormously complicated, yet it is very important to understand.

Metabolic Keys

For calcium to function properly in relation to bone building, it has to be accompanied by phosphorus—but not too much phosphorus—as well as magnesium, vitamins A, B6, C, D, E, and K. Zinc is also important, since zinc is a co-factor in the intracellular conversion of beta-carotene to vitamin A, which in turn helps manufacture the collagen matrix of bone. Zinc has to be present in sufficient quantities for the body's enzymes to make the conversion. Even the trace elements boron and silicon, needed only in the most minute quantities, play important roles in bone strength.

Forget the Milk

We have been led to believe that all you need for strong bones is to get lots of calcium—either by popping pills or drinking huge amounts of milk. Millions have been spent to propagate this fantasy. Yet, after three generations of milk promotion, osteoporosis has now reached epidemic proportions in the West, while in countries where milk is not drunk it hardly exists. So negative an effect can milk and milk products, such as cheeses, exert on a woman's health that if you would care to experiment by leaving all milk products out of your diet for three weeks, you are likely to find your looks and energy levels transformed for the better. This is not all that easy to do, since milk in one form or another finds its way into most convenience foods. It is in breads and biscuits and sauces. It is even in many nutritional supplements.

Milk is a food designed by nature for a very specific purpose—to feed young mammals until they can feed themselves. Cow's milk is made for cows, and human milk for humans. As we grow up, our bodies gradually lose the ability to produce *lactase*, the enzyme that digests the sugar in milk. This creates what is known as a lactose intolerance. Studies show that three out of every four adults in the United States have some degree of lactose intolerance. They are unable to digest milk properly. If they choose to include dairy foods in their diet, they find that their energy levels are lowered, their bodies can produce more mucus in an immune reaction, and that they experience food sensitivity reactions with symptoms that may include mood swings or depression, as well as aches and pains, often with no sense of what may be causing it all.

Milk is the most common food allergen in the Western world (wheat follows close behind it). Yet you find milk in one form or another just about everywhere—in cheese, cream, cream sauces, yogurt, ice cream, breads, and other commercially prepared food products. There is also mounting evidence that milk, the pure white food that we are continually told will give us good bones, strong hair, and plenty of energy, may actually be toxic to adults. At Harvard Medical School, Dr. Daniel Cramer discovered that using milk products increases the risk of ovarian cancer in lactose-intolerant women. After extensive analysis of lactose-intolerant women in 36 countries, as well as meticulous examination of human and animal studies, researchers concluded that *galactose*, one of the sugars in lactose, is toxic to the ovaries and interferes with fertility. Some believe it may even trigger birth defects. Far from turning to milk as a source of calcium, most women who value well-being would be better off clearing out milk and milk products from their diet altogether. If you are going to cut milk out of your diet, you need to get rid of anything that might contain milk products, such as milk solids, sodium caseinate, sodium lactate, milk fats, whey, or lactose. So read labels carefully.

As for taking pills, a number of scientific reports have shown that calcium supplements do little to stop the loss of cortical bone tissue and have virtually no effect at all on trabecular bone in the spine and the hip where most osteoporotic fractures occur. Yet most people still believe that the best source of calcium is milk or milk products. The question that they rarely ask is where does the calcium in milk come from in the first place? Cows get calcium from eating green foods—grass, silage, herbs, and plants. These are not the only plants that can take the calcium from the soil and turn it into a form available for absorption by animals. Beetroot tops, Chinese leaves, rocket, lettuce, seaweeds, herbs, and broad-leafed green vegetables are all excellent sources of calcium. A cup of any of these vegetables supplies as much calcium as a cup of milk. And this kind of calcium is easily assimilated, along with a collection of other important minerals and trace elements from such foods—all without having to deal with possible negative side effects of using milk products. Include plenty of organic leafy green vegetables in your meals, and you need never give calcium another thought. Incidentally, the reason why taking calcium supplements or drinking masses of milk has very little effect in halting—and none at all in reversing—osteoporosis is because it is usually not an *absence* of calcium in the body that is the problem so much as a *disorder in calcium metabolism.*

A Delicate Process

Calcium metabolism is a very complex process. The absorption of calcium from water or mineral salts in general tends to be highly inefficient. Only somewhere between 20 and 30 percent of the calcium you take in through processed foods will actually be absorbed. Most of that then gets filtered through your kidneys and then excreted in urine and sweat or eliminated through the feces. Many factors influence just how much calcium you will absorb at any time. When you are growing rapidly or when you place stress on your bones by doing weight-bearing exercise, your absorption of calcium is increased. When your body is in great need of calcium, it is also absorbed more effectively. In fact, the smaller the supply of calcium available from your foods and the greater the need your body has for this mineral, the more efficient calcium absorption becomes. The opposite is also true. When large quantities of calcium are available—say if someone has been drinking a lot of milk or has taken masses of calcium supplements—then the absorption of calcium is markedly decreased. It is worth remembering that in the United States, where the consumption of calcium supplements and milk products is the highest in the world, so is the incidence of osteoporosis.

Acid Test

For proper assimilation, calcium needs an acid medium in the digestive tract. As people get older, the hydrochloric acid content of the stomach tends to decrease. With this decrease comes a further decrease in your body's ability to assimilate calcium. Calcium absorption requires adequate vitamin D, too, which, together with parathyroid hormone, regulates the level of calcium in your blood. An adequate supply of the right kind of fat in the gut also facilitates the absorption of calcium. The mineral phosphorus is also essential to build bone. But if either calcium or phosphorus is taken in excess—as happens in the case of phosphorus in a typical Western diet that includes processed meats, colas, and diet drinks—then neither element can be used efficiently, and bone loss increases.

Your body deals with any excess calcium that you take in by dumping it wherever it can in an attempt to restore a healthy balance between calcium and other minerals present. Chemical calcium supplements taken over a long period of time can bring about an increase in calcium plaque in the arteries, as well as result in the calcification of soft tissues, but they won't make for stronger bones. Researchers at the University of Kentucky have found that calcium salt megadoses can actually decrease bone strength, as well as induce internal bleeding. Studies show that animals fed calcium as salts at a dietary level of 2.7 percent will die from profuse internal bleeding. Others report that pigs fed excess calcium have diminished bone mineral mass and lower bone-breaking strength. Taking drugs such as laxatives, diuretics, antacids, and tetracyclines also impedes calcium absorption. So does coffee drinking. Like taking in too much protein, it causes calcium to be leached from your bone and carried out of your body.

Once you begin to sense the enormous complexity and synergy involved with calcium absorption and use, you begin to understand why it is probably best to get the calcium you need from a good diet. If you still feel you *must* take calcium supplements, make sure they are low dose and in a form more readily absorbed than the usual calcium lactate or calcium carbonate, which are cheap to make and form the basis of most calcium supplements. As far as oyster shell calcium or dolomite is concerned, avoid them like the plague. They can be filled with dangerous heavy metals.

The Magnesium Connection

What surprises most women—doctors, too, for that matter—is that it is taking extra magnesium that can make the greatest difference to good calcium metabolism. Magnesium is another element essential for the proper metabolism of calcium. Magnesium probably acts as a catalyst for more enzymes in the body than any other metal. Magnesium is plentiful in properly grown whole grains—brown rice, buckwheat, millet, whole wheat, whole rye, and in legumes such as beans, lentils, and peas, but low in highly processed foods. Adequate magnesium helps the body absorb calcium. Where there is a magnesium deficiency, not only can osteoporosis develop easily, but so can joint and soft tissue calcification. Low intracellular magnesium undermines immune functions, too, causing susceptibility to infection, and conditions where women with low intra-cellular magnesium have been found to have unnaturally shaped bone mineral crystals.

Magnesium deficiency is common in women with or without osteoporosis. Milk is a relatively poor source of magnesium—another reason why it is a poor food for protection against osteoporosis. Magnesium deficiencies are particularly widespread in women over the age of 35 who have long been living on a Western diet. PMS expert Dr. Guy Abraham showed that giving women 600 mg of magnesium a day could bring about a significant increase in bone mass in nine months, although the women he treated were also given other vitamins and minerals as well as HRT, so it is impossible to determine just how much of the improvement was due to the magnesium. In a recent Israeli study, however, where 31 postmenopausal women were given 250 to 750 mg of magnesium a day for two years, bone density increased one to 8 percent in 75 percent of the cases and remained unchanged in the remaining 25 percent, while women who refused magnesium supplements altogether experienced losses in bone density of one to 3 percent.

According to many recent studies, vegetarians have stronger bones and less osteoporosis than do meat eaters. A good, unrefined vegetarian diet that includes whole-grain breads, cereals, legumes, and fresh vegetables is also moderate in protein and rich in magnesium, zinc, silicon, and other bone-strengthening minerals. By contrast, meat is high in protein. When you eat an *excess* of protein, calcium is drawn from your bones to help neutralize the acidic protein waste products. This creates a negative calcium balance. When forced to metabolize excess protein, the body carries calcium away from bones and excretes it. Eskimos whose traditional diet was very high in protein (250 to 400 grams a day) with a high calcium intake of 1,500 to 2,500 mg a day were found to have the highest rate of osteoporosis of any group of people. By contrast, the Bantu in Africa, who consume only 47 g of protein a day and get less than 400 mg of calcium—mostly from plant foods—remain free from osteoporosis. Of course, they also get plenty of exercise. Without adequate exercise, calcium cannot be incorporated into the bones.

Kids' Teeth, Yes—Women's Bones, No!

For strong bones into your 90s, steer clear of a diet that is excessively high in protein, avoid diuretics (and if you are on them, ask your doctor to take you off them), steer clear of fluoride, and don't drink fluorinated water. Fluoride is still wrongly recommended by some doctors as a substance that can help build bones; although fluoride encourages the development of bone mass, at the same time it decreases bone strength. A large body of research links even low levels of fluoride in water with an increased incidence of fractures. In people undergoing fluoride therapy, nonvertebral fractures have been shown to increase by 300 to 600 percent.

You should also avoid an excess of alcohol or sugar, which creates metabolic acidosis and leaches calcium from the skeleton.

Osteoporosis prevention is best started early, preferably in the teens, 20s, and 30s, while the density of bone is still increasing. It is easy to build good, strong bones and establish lifestyle habits that can carry you through the second half of your life with no trouble. If osteoporosis has already begun, you will probably want to make use of topically applied progesterone to restore normal bone density and keep you permanently osteoporosis-free. Finally, just in case all this sounds like a tall order, take heart.

The benefits that an osteoporosis-protective lifestyle can bring to overall health are immense. Such a lifestyle also helps to keep your immune system functioning well, helping to protect you from illness, countering early aging, and enhancing your energy all around.

CHAPTER NINE

PHOENIX IN THE FIRE

Hot Flashes, Deep Cleansing,
and Spiritual Transformation

ne day, an ordinary day like any other, almost imperceptibly you sense something strange is happening in your body. A tiny flutter of heat begins to rise and sweep up your torso, neck, and head. Then the strange feeling passes away again almost as quickly as it has come, and you find that you are now feeling just a bit chilled. Or maybe one night at 3 A.M. you awaken to find yourself drenched in sweat for no reason. "Am I ill?" you ask, making a quick check through your body, only to find that no, you do not feel ill. Then what on Earth is happening?

The most common herald of menopause is the appearance of hot flashes. They are virtually synonymous with it in the experience of many women. An adjunct to hot flashes are night sweats, where women awaken drenched in sweat, so much so that they not only need to change their night clothes, but also the sheets on their beds. Both night sweats and hot flashes can be disconcerting, particularly if a woman is fearful of them. Although a lot can be said about hot flashes, only two things are absolutely essential to know. First, they are *completely harmless*. Second, hot flashes are virtually the *only* symptoms among long lists of things usually attributed to menopause that genuinely belong to it. This was established by research carried out at Oxford and reported in the *British Medical Journal*. It compared midlife women with midlife men in an attempt to find out which of women's complaints were genuinely menopausal. Scientists reported that among those symptoms generally lumped together under the menstrual label—including aches in joints, migraine, depression, and the rest—only hot flashes show a direct relationship to menopause itself. Another interesting study carried out in Canada by Pat Kaufert found that despite all the discussion over hot flashes, most women still look upon them as normal and believe that having them doesn't detract from seeing themselves as generally in good or excellent health.

Cross Currents

Menopausal women are not the only people who get hot flashes. They can also be common during pregnancy, as well as just after giving birth. Men, too, will experience them after any kind of rapid withdrawal of sex hormones. Women of all ages get them especially strongly when their ovaries are removed surgically, and men when the testicles are taken out. So do people who for any reason have been given drugs antagonistic to gonadotrophin-releasing hormones. Such drugs cause testosterone levels in men and estrogen levels in women to fall rapidly. At the time of menopause, thinner women tend to experience more drastic alterations in their estrogen levels and are therefore more likely than their bigger sisters to experience stronger hot flashes.

The standard medical treatment for hot flashes is estrogen. And it is quite true that extra estrogen will relieve the symptoms just like all the little leaflets tell you. What they don't tell you is that if you decide to go on estrogen for a few years "to get you through the rough patch," when you come off it your hot flashes are very likely to return in force—whether getting off HRT turns out to be 3 or 4 years, or as many as 15 or 20 years later. Extra estrogen does not "cure" hot flashes. It only masks them for a while. In any case, there is nothing to "cure," for hot flashes are not a symptom of disease. They are a *normal bodily change* associated with the transition between the menstrual years and menopause.

Many physicians who work with natural methods of healing believe that, far from being a negative event, hot flashes can actually help cleanse the body. They can also be an indication of considerable vitality in the woman who has them. Most hot flashes happen without anybody ever knowing except the woman herself. Women always think they are more evident to the outside world than they are. And even if they are, so what? Why should a woman agree, even tacitly, to buy into the general consensus that menopause—like the swollen belly of pregnancy or the flow of menstrual blood—is something ugly to be hidden. To me, all three seem to be proud badges of womanhood. If, as many women fear, men are troubled by the evidence of them, that is their problem. They are probably the kind of men who find it difficult to contact their own deep sexuality and who therefore feel uncomfortable with the birth-death-regenerative nature of life. Bless them, and send a little prayer that one day they grow up.

No Great Matter

Back in the 19th century, hot flashes were known as "hot blooms." Even then they were recognized as the most common symptom associated with menopause. The physiology of the hot flash is not yet fully understood. Medical dictionaries define flashes as "vasomotor symptoms of the climacterium—sudden vasodilation with a sensation of heat, usually involving the face and neck, and upper part of the chest; sweats, often profuse, frequently following the flash." During a hot flash, blood rushes into the capillaries, the pulse rate rises, and skin temperature goes up. Hot flashes do not appear to affect blood pressure, but they are often followed by a chilling phenomenon. Both estrogen and progesterone play a role in internal temperature regulation. Hot flashes are triggered by the hypothalamus, which among its many responsibilities holds overall control for body temperature, as well as for directing the release of pituitary hormones. They can occur when a sudden lowering of the central hypothalamic thermostat takes place. The body trying to adjust its core temperature to this new setting produces heat loss by activating vasodilation (as blood flows through all the capillaries at the surface of the skin) and sweating.

At or near menopause, the ovaries are programmed to decommission themselves. They no longer respond to the secretion of FSH from the pituitary as they used to by secreting estrogen. The result is that the hypothalamus raises its production of GnRH—and its voltage. Finally, the electric excitation spills over to affect an adjacent limbic nucleus involved in temperature control, causing a reaction that produces rapid temperature changes in the body. The capillaries are affected by consequent chemical or hormonal changes that take place in the tissues, causing them to dilate and the nerves to be highly reactive.

Because hot flashes arise from neuroendocrine activity, heightened stress tends to make them worse. Similarly, placebos can often make them better through the complex interactive mechanisms of the immune, endocrine, and central nervous system by which mind and body are linked. In most women, hot flashes are at their most intense during the last year or so before menstruation ceases and during the first year or so afterwards. What do they feel like? This can differ just about as much as individual women do. Generally, there is a flash of heat that sweeps your torso, neck, and head. You feel the need to take off your sweater or jacket for a few minutes, then you'll probably want to put it back on again since the body's reaction to vasodilation can leave you feeling a little chilled afterwards. Sometimes hot flashes can make your skin go red and even blotchy. Sometimes they are followed by perspiration, which can either be no more than a little glow or as much as a torrent of water. Usually a hot flash lasts from a few seconds to a couple of minutes. Very rarely they can last as long as 15 minutes or more.

How often they come is another highly individual thing. A very few women seem to experience hot flashes—at least for a short period of their life—every hour or two. Others get them only at certain times of the day or night. Some women report up to 30 hot flashes a day, while most experience only one or two. A few women don't get them at all. Most of the studies done on menopausal women are carried out in Western countries where it is said that on average, 75 percent of women experience hot flashes. However, their prevalence in the whole world—bearing in mind the bias toward studies done in the West and the fact that in some primitive cultures, women don't get them at all—appears to be that between the ages of 40 and 60, the number of women who get hot flashes ranges from 24 percent upwards, depending upon the country of origin, diet, and lifestyle of the women. Very few researchers have investigated at what age hot flashes begin, but one study reports that in 60 percent of the women who experience them, they arrive on the scene sometime between the ages of 40 and 50, while in 10 percent of naturally menopausal women (that is, those who have not undergone a hysterectomy), they began before the age of 41. The prevalence of hot flashes is virtually 100 percent among women who have gone through an artificially induced menopause as a result of surgery. After surgery, symptoms are much more intense, and the flashes come much more frequently than they did before.

Factors that predispose women to hot flashes have also been little studied. What is known is that there is no correlation between hot flashes and socioeconomic groups, employment status, or medical status. The incidence of hot flashes is also not at all to be related to the age at which a woman began to menstruate or to her age at menopause nor to the number of children that she has had. The one factor that does appear to correlate with hot flashes is that women who get them tend to have a lower body weight than women who do not.

Some of the most interesting work looking at the incidence of hot flashes has come from examining the effect of diet and cultural attitudes. In Indonesia and Japan, women experience very few hot flashes, particularly compared to women in Western societies. Mayan Indians in Mexico report no symptoms whatever at the approach of menopause other than the menstrual cycle becoming irregular. It would appear that there are significant dietary differences operating here. Japanese women eat lots of soya products, which contain a high level of plant sterols. Urinalysis of Japanese women shows that elevated levels of estriol—the good-guy estrogen (compared to Western women with a diet high in natural phytosterols)— has the capacity to alleviate the symptoms of menopause. This could also explain the very low incidence of hot flashes amongst Mayan, Indonesian, and Chinese women.

The Real Thing

Certain plants are high in estrogenlike hormones—beetroots, potato root, parsley root, and yeast, for instance, all of which contain around 70 to 80 picograms of these natural phytohormones per 100 grams. Natural unheated honey contains significant amounts, while dry sage boasts 6,000 IU per kilogram. Clover is also high in phytohormones, as is alfalfa, fennel, celery, anise, and licorice. A diet that includes these foods should supply a much higher level of protective natural hormones to a woman's body and can help a great deal to alleviate hot flashes.

Research has also shown that estrogen levels tend to be lower in premenopausal women with hot flashes than those without hot flashes. However, it is quite clear that low estrogen levels, although they continually get the blame for hot flashes, are by no means all that is involved in their production. It is the sudden drop in estrogen that is the issue. And once the hypothalamus and pituitary accustom themselves to lower levels of estrogen, most hot flashes gradually diminish. Sometimes low estrogen is not involved in hot flashes at all. A small number of women go into menopause in their teens and 20s as a result of genetic abnormalities. These women seldom experience hot flashes. Hot flashes only happen to these women if they take supplementary estrogen in HRT for a time and then stop. There are many postmenopausal women with low estrogen levels who never have hot flashes, while others continue to have them.

Prior to puberty, when estrogen levels are very low, girls do not have hot flashes. On the other hand, hot flashes are reported by some women during pregnancy or immediately after giving birth when estrogen levels are high. At John Bastyr College and the National College of Naturopathic Medicine in the United States, a recent study of menopausal women showed that a formula of botanical substances rich in phytohormones was able to relieve the severity of menopausal symptoms, including hot flashes, in 100 percent of the women studied, reducing the total number of symptoms by 71 percent. Hot flashes were the most favorably affected of all symptoms despite the fact that estrogen levels *decreased* in the treatment subjects during the period of the study.

Allergy Connections

There are certain things known to contribute to the incidence of hot flashes. If you are troubled by their intensity, you might like to stay away from cigarette smoking; caffeine; and hot, spicy food. An overactive thyroid can cause hot flashes, too, as can untreated diabetes. Least recognized but in many cases also important, according to Dr. Ellen Grant, author of the courageous book *Sexual Chemistry*, hot flashes may be the result of allergic reactions, particularly to foods or chemicals in the environment. The high levels of steroid hormones used in HRT tend to suppress certain vascular responses such as those connected with allergies and with the body's attempt to detoxify itself. When estrogen decreases rapidly in a menopausal woman or in someone who has been taking extra hormones, then, according to Grant, the underlying allergy/toxicity or vascular reaction that was being masked by the hormones is exposed. Hot flashes can result. At the Charing Cross Hospital Migraine Clinic, Grant requested that her patients explore for themselves which foods gave them reactions such as migraine, headaches, and rises in blood pressure, as well as hot flashes. She found, as have many clinical ecologists and doctors well versed in the treatment of food sensitivities, that when an offending food such as milk, wheat, cheese, chocolate or oranges is removed from the diet, hot flashes will either cease or diminish significantly.

The Power Rises

From an energetic viewpoint, according to Eastern religions and traditional medicine, the experience of a hot flash is looked upon as a rapid release of *kundalini energy*—the cosmic creative energy that is said to rise up the spine, refining the nervous system and activating the chakras or energy centers, each of which is associated with a different organ or system in the body, as well as with different psychic or spiritual developments. The first chakra at the base of the spine is associated with survival energy, for instance, while the second chakra in the pelvis is connected with biological creativity. The fourth chakra in the center of the chest is linked with the heart and with feelings of compassion, the sixth between the eyebrows governs clairvoyance and far-sightedness, while the seventh chakra is known as the thousand-petaled lotus. When activated, it is believed to give the highest spiritual illumination. It is the seventh chakra that is responsible for the halo depicted around the heads of the saints, Jesus, and the Buddha.

When the kundalini fire rises in the body, it refines the nervous system so a woman becomes capable of carrying powerful healing energies, energies of wisdom, and of peacekeeping—all of which throughout history have been viewed as the responsibility of the postmenopausal woman or crone. It can be useful to view hot flashes from this point of view. It is often helpful to see them as life energy. I have worked with many groups of menopausal women by approaching hot flashes in this way. We have looked at them not as something to be feared or concealed, but rather as a sign that the creative fire of individual spirit, often long ignored, is demanding attention. Once you heed its call, not only can hot flashes cease to be a problem, but the most phenomenal energy is often made available for whatever purpose a woman wants to use it.

I Lie Burning

The long tradition of European natural medicine views hot flashes as a means the body uses to detoxify itself as well as to enhance immunity. Recent research shows that even a slight raise in temperature in the body can be instrumental in doing both. A few months before she died, I interviewed Dr. Dagmar Leichti von Brasch about menopause. A vital woman in her 80s and mother of five, Dr. Leichti was director of the world-famous Bircher Benner clinic for 40 years and niece to Max Bircher Benner himself. When I asked her from the point of view of natural medicine what hot flashes are all about, she told me that, like night sweats, they have always been considered the means by which a woman's body deep-cleanses itself and refines itself for new physical and spiritual tasks. I also questioned Dr. Leichti at some length about her own experience of menopause and about the experiences of the thousands of midlife women patients she had cared for during the more than half a century she spent practicing medicine. She told me that she believed from a spiritual point of view that hot flashes and awakening in the night in sweat can be important events in a woman's life. "They stop us from carrying on 'as normal,' which women are so apt to do—fulfilling their social roles. They demand that we pay attention to our bodies and to our lives," said Dr. Leichti. "This is exactly what menopausal women are supposed to do."

A vibrant and healthy woman, Dr. Leichti ran the clinic in Zurich while fulfilling her role as wife and mother. She had the same experience during her menopause that so many perimenopausal and menopausal women have of awakening night after night in the wee hours of the morning for no apparent reason. When this happens, it often occurs between 2 A.M. and 3 A.M. She told me she would find herself flooded by tears in the deepest sorrow. She would try to go back to sleep without success, so she lay in bed night after night with tears streaming down the sides of her face. For a very long while, Dr. Leichti could not work out why she felt so sad—especially since every morning she would rise and go about her duties at the clinic feeling perfectly normal. Finally, after several months of this, she decided that instead of remaining in bed, she would get up and go to her study to write down what she felt. "Before long," she told me, "I realized that I had begun to tap into new ideas which were exciting, to sense new possibilities, and to see the world in new ways. It was during those early morning hours that I dreamed new dreams about my future." Afterwards, when Dr. Leichti spoke to other women who'd had similar experiences—waking in fear or grief, anger, or frustration—she discovered that if they were able simply to allow themselves to feel whatever feelings arose from within, they discovered that hidden beneath these feelings lay wells of untapped creativity and bridges to the soul.

It is almost as though, from a spiritual point of view, hot flashes are like the Promethean fire of creation rising up within a woman, demanding that she pay attention to who she is and find outlets for this fire.

I believe that Dr. Leichti is right, for I have observed that over and over again when a woman experiencing hot flashes overcomes her fear of them and begins to listen to the dictates of her soul, both the intensity and the frequency of hot flashes diminish. As one woman who had originally had severe flashes said to me when I asked her about them a few months after she had taken up dancing and drumming, "Hot flashes? Oh, those. Yes, I guess I still have them. Most of the time I am so busy doing other things I love doing that I don't even notice."

Living in Time

I, too, have had the experience of waking up night after night. I would awaken like clockwork at 3 A.M. to lie in bed in a state that can only be described as a mixture of terror and frustration. I could never go back to sleep for another couple of hours—some nights not at all. I kept feeling that I wanted to get up and *do* something. I had a strange desire to leave my house and walk barefoot down the path through the woods to the sea. Then the fear would arise, a fear of doing something so unconventional—something different from what I was used to doing. Perhaps it was a fear of madness, I don't know. At that time I had no idea that what I was feeling had to do with my coming menopause. I was menstruating normally and had only begun to have the odd hot flash, which did not worry me or seem particularly strange since it felt very much like I feel during vigorous exercise. Later on, just at the point of my periods stopping, I began to venture out at night. I would go into my studio, turn on the lights, and work. At that time, I was finishing my first novel. Then after two or three hours, I would climb back into bed again and sleep for an hour before getting up to send my youngest son off to school. I relished that hour. Such a deep and blissful sleep came then—a sleep full of dreams and new visions. Later I was to discover, as Dr. Leichti had, that the work I did during my night vigils was the most creative work I had ever done.

Since then, having spoken to dozens of women who report similar experiences, I have come to believe that hot flashes, night sweats, night awakenings, and many of the other events associated with menopause often bring to the surface parts of ourselves that we are not living out fully. In Leichti's case, it was old sorrow; in my own, it was profound frustration about my work and a great deal of fear. In other women, it can be resentment, grief, sadness, or even wonder and a new kind of joy. Don't try to batten down the hatches and carry on "as normal." All of this is not to say that if you have severe hot flashes you should not do something to alleviate them, however.

It is worth consulting wise-woman lore. Recent research into the effects of a number of so-called old wives' treatments for hot flashes and other menopausal conditions strongly support their effectiveness. Still, much of how you experience something depends on your point of view.

The mythologist Joseph Campbell used to tell a story about a conversation he once had with Alan Watts, the writer on Zen Buddhism. He had told Watts about a problem he was having with his wife. She was always late. Campbell said that invariably he would make an appointment to meet her somewhere, then he would have to sit and wait for half an hour or more before she arrived. After a while, Campbell assumed that this was the normal thing for men to do because, after all, it takes women a long time to get out of the house. The problem was, he told Watts, that he always became irritated by having to wait. He would get so aggravated that when she finally did arrive, he had a tendency to be unpleasant. Watts told Campbell, "Well, your problem is that you want her to be there and you're wishing for a situation which is not the one you're in. Just realize that you are ruining the experience that you could be having while waiting by thinking it should be otherwise." After that, Campbell transformed waiting for his wife into a spiritual exercise. "The place where I was became so goddamn interesting I wasn't bored at all. Oftentimes it made me hope that Jean would make me wait a little longer," said Campbell. "That would have been impossible until Alan suggested shutting out any thoughts that my situation should have been otherwise."

Within each woman lies a similar ability to transmute that which seems frightening into a source of power. The phoenix is a mythological bird who, when consumed by fire, is born anew and rises from the flames to soar to greater heights than before. But the secret of the phoenix is always hidden, waiting for a woman bold enough and persistent enough to uncover it.

CHAPTER TEN

DOUBLE INDEMNITY
Plant Magic from Phytohormones

lants hold powerful medicine for women. Even to state such an obvious truth seems absurd since every culture in the world from the beginning of human history has turned to herbs and foods as medicine. Yet as women in the postindustrial world, we find ourselves in the absurd position of having to rediscover our medicinal and health-promoting heritage, not only by unearthing long-neglected local practices passed on verbally from woman to woman, but also by investigating herbal traditions from other parts of the world—Tibet, China, India, Japan, and Native America. The benefits of making medicinal plants a part of your day-to-day life become more obvious when you realize that the origins of most drugs lie in plants.

Quinine (the core antimalarial drug) is derived from cinchona, also called Peruvian Bark, for instance. It is the white willow that first sup-plied the analgesic acetyl salicylic acid, which has now been replaced by its chemical analog, aspirin. The lovely foxglove yields digitalis for ail-ing hearts. Morphine, ephedrine, codeine, and atropine all have plant ori-gins. And when it comes to preventing or treating women's symptoms—from PMS to hot flashes—little works better or is more long lasting than the gentle art of plant power. It is an art with two branches. First is the use of botanicals either singly or in a combination *medicinally* as treat-ment for specific problems. Second, less well known but equally important, is the health-promoting benefit of incorporating plants rich in minerals, enzymes, fiber, phytohormones (plant-derived), and other beneficial phytochemicals, as *foods* in your normal daily diet.

Secrets of the Yam

When it comes to using a plant to benefit women, the Trobriand Islanders from Papua New Guinea have a few secrets well worth knowing. The Trobriands are a little group of flat coral islands not far from Northern Australia. The author Paul Theroux visited them and then reported on his visit for *National Geographic* in 1992. In these islands, a form of wild yam grows in abundance. It is central to the island's social activities and forms the basis of the islanders' diet. Trobrianders, as it happens, have an almost perfect diet. It is low in fat, with no fried foods, and just about everything they eat is fresh. Their yams are grown in fields, then carried to the villages and stored in beautiful wooden houses built in the center of each village, which look a bit like small cathedrals. In most of these yam houses, a four-foot giant specimen is suspended in a frame of lashed poles. The yam represents not only food to the islanders, but also prosperity and the powers of life—in much the same way that corn was revered in Native American cultures. So sacred is the yam considered to be in this matrilineal society that men are not allowed to harvest the vegetable. If a man even accidentally comes upon a procession of women bringing yams from the fields, he is attacked and sexually ridiculed. His clothes are confiscated by the women, and he is sent back to the village stark naked—a laughingstock.

Masters of self-reliance, the Trobrianders have little interest in the outside world. They greatly value the preservation of their own culture, however. They also value sexuality, which is treated in a natural, matter-of-fact way and around which there is no guilt. They encourage teenage sex, and boys and girls aged 14 or 15 share *bukumatula* (bachelor houses) in which they are given complete privacy. Each year, at harvest time, a month-long yam festival is held during which all marriage is suspended and yams are eaten—prepared in a myriad of ways, from creamy porridge drenched in coconut milk, to boiled, steamed, and baked dishes. "For a reason that no one can explain," reports Theroux, "the birth rate is lower than might be expected." After the Theroux article appeared in *National Geographic,* the editor received a number of letters from readers. One was interesting. It came from a physician in Caracas, Venezuela, Mely Lechtich de Révai, M.D., who wrote: "Yam of

Dioscorea was long known by certain Mexican Indians to have a contraceptive effect. In 1939 Dr. Russell Marker, an American chemist, determined the molecular structure of diosgenin, a steroid substance with progesteronic effect derived from the yam root. Based on this information, Organon, a leading producer of contraceptive pills, uses the diosgenin from the Mexican yam roots as the raw material for some of its products."

Diosgenin, you will remember, is the stuff from which the natural progesterone used in progesterone cream is derived, as are any number of other patented hormones sold as drugs by pharmaceutical manufacturers. Not only is the progesterone derived from wild yam a cornerstone of the bloodless revolution, but, like the Trobriand Islanders' sacred vegetable, certain yams such as *Dioscorea villosa* and *Dioscorea Mexicana* are also useful as food supplements or natural medicines in the treatment of PMS and menopausal problems. Rich in phytohormones or their precursors, they can help protect against cancer and against the estrogen dominance that underlies female ailments. In the future, wild yam may turn out to be the best method of natural birth control available. It appears to work well for most women who have tried it, and, unlike contraceptive drugs, it has no negative side effects. Indeed, it boasts a long list of positive benefits.

Contraception au Naturel

Willa Shaffer is a remarkable woman, a Texas midwife who has dedicated her life to serving women's health and who trained in nutrition, midwifery, and reflexology. She has for decades used plants to enhance the health of women of all ages. Shaffer first experimented with wild yam some 15 years ago as a means of staving off threatened miscarriages and eliminating PMS and menopausal miseries, and found she got excellent results with it. Wild yam could be taken daily month after month, year after year, so long as it was needed to counter a woman's negative symptoms. Shaffer reports, as have others who use this plant regularly, that in addition to banishing the symptoms for which it is being taken, wild yam can improve a woman's energy levels, enhance digestion, eliminate aches and pains normally associated with aging or rheumatic conditions, and balance emotions. It also appears to be a perfect antidote to lost libido, helping to restore a woman's capacity for sexual pleasure when it has been lost. But most interesting of all, and potentially revolutionary if controlled studies are ever carried out on it, is Shaffer's rediscovery of the secrets of wild yam used for birth control.

Shaffer had been continually faced with recurrent symptoms and serious health problems caused by birth control pills in the women whom she looked after. Then in 1976 she came upon an article in a small American magazine called *The Herbalist*. The article talked about the healing properties traditionally associated with the wild yam and about its use as a contraceptive. Excited by the possibility of a benign alternative to the Pill, Shaffer passed the article around among her patients. They were eager to try the plant. After some initial difficulty, she was able to locate a source of dried wild yam in capsule form. She began to test it on scores of women. Then in 1986 she wrote a little booklet about her experience with the yam: *Wild Yam, Birth Control Without Fear*. It makes fascinating reading.

The ages of the women whom Shaffer tested ranged from 17 to 47. They came from many different backgrounds—some were black, some Caucasians, others were Latin Americans or had Native American blood. During her four-year test period, no negative side effects to the plant were reported by any of the women. There was no evidence, for instance, of weight gain, cramps, hormonal changes, swelling, or any of the other unpleasant symptoms associated with prescription birth control. Out of the first 75 women who tried it, 56 were still using it as their sole source of contraception four years later. Of the 19 who did not continue, three decided to get pregnant so they stopped taking the yam and had babies, six forgot to take it or did not take it as directed (that is, they took too little or did not continue steadily), and ten dropped out of the experiment or were lost track of. Only one woman became pregnant despite the fact that she *religiously* took the wild yam—possibly, Shaffer believes, because her own specific requirement for the plant for use as a contraceptive was much higher than average so she should have been taking more. She was a woman who had always said of herself, "Every time my husband just hangs his pants on the bedpost, I get pregnant!"

Dosage Decisions

In the beginning, Shaffer had no idea how much wild yam to use for birth control. Working together with a doctor who was familiar with the plant, she settled on three capsules in the morning and three at night, which would supply a total of 3,000 mg or 3 g a day of the powdered dried root. Shaffer discovered that it is important to take the wild yam for eight weeks before relying on it as a sole source of contraception. Should a woman forget to take the herb for one day or more, she needs to use an alternative method of birth control, such as a condom or diaphragm, along with the yam for a couple of weeks before relying entirely on the wild yam again. In the course of experiments with the yam, Shaffer also found out that all sorts of menstrual and menopausal problems are resolved by its use, including painful menstruation, irregular menstruation, mood swings, depression, and hot flashes, together with scores of other supposedly hard-to-treat conditions. Almost by chance, Shaffer had rediscovered what the Trobriand Islanders, the Central and South American Indians, and many other primitive cultures have known since ancient times—in several species of the wild yam is to be found an inexpensive, totally beneficial plant capable of giving a high degree of protection against unwanted pregnancy while enhancing women's health. It is quite a discovery—one that needs serious scientific investigation—yet the average doctor remains totally ignorant about the wild yam.

The women I know who use wild yam for birth control take 3 to 3.5 g of powdered root a day—either *Dioscorea villosa* or *Dioscorea Mexicana*—in other words, 1.5 to 1.75 grams in the morning and in the evening. Just how many capsules this amounts to if you choose to take it in capsule form depends upon the weight of the capsules. They report, so far without exception, that the wild yam they are using for birth control has also eliminated PMS, made heavy periods lighter, enhanced their energy, and helped to balance their emotions. Whether proper scientifically controlled studies will ever be carried out to validate Shaffer's anecdotal evidence depends more than anything else upon ordinary women becoming vocal enough to demand them. And if trials did validate wild yam as a reliable method of birth control, it could not only literally save millions that might be used in other ways (for contraceptive drugs are pricey and plants very cheap and widely available); it could also protect hundreds of thousands of women from the potential side effects of pharmaceutical contraceptives.

For two generations, feminists have quite rightly insisted that women's bodies belong to women themselves and that each woman must have the right to choose whether or not she becomes pregnant. As we women have decided to exert control over our own lives, we have, perhaps, been too ready to back drug-based contraception complete with all of its negative side effects because there seemed to be no alternative. Our doing so has too often wreaked havoc in our lives. Drug-based contraception still continues to disrupt the biology, long-term health, and emotions of millions of women in the world. Now seems an appropriate time to reevaluate our position. As

Shaffer herself says, "Can you imagine the change it would cause if wild yam would be used on a large scale? So many severe problems caused by the controversial birth control pills would be extinct. Let's all pray that people become more aware of the safe herbal remedies and preventatives that are available."

She then goes on to muse, "John Heineman states in his book that recent clinical evidence has shown that when the extract of mallow flower was administered to dogs (which have male reproductive organs that are anatomically similar to men), it causes substantial infertility by inhibiting the production of sperm in the testicles."

Finally she adds, "Now if I could only get my hands on some mallow flower..."

Like wild yam, many of the plants and botanical products most useful to women are rich in phytosterols—compounds whose molecular structure is akin to the body's own hormones. Vegetables and herbs that fall into this category include celery, fennel, ginseng, alfalfa, licorice, and red clover. Hops (*Humulus lupulus*) are so rich in plant sterols that exposure to them can affect the onset of menarche in girls. "It was girls and women picking hops who first drew attention to the fact that hops have an effect on the genital organs," says Rudolf Fritz Weiss, author of *Herbal Medicine*. "Before machines were introduced, hop pickers used to spend several weeks at this work, and it had always been known that menstrual periods would come early in young girls while they were there." The fresh hop plant contains significant quantities of plant hormones similar to a woman's own estrogen. They not only affect the menstrual cycles of women, but can also suppress libido in men. This is the cause of *brewer's droop,* familiar to beer-drinking men, and what has given beer its reputation for raising expectations while inhibiting performance. It is also why the *British Herbal Pharmacopoeia* suggests hops as a treatment for persistent erection.

Mission Impossible

All sorts of supposedly impossible healing tasks can be accomplished when phytosterol-rich herbs are used medicinally. But, sadly, few women know much about how to use them since so many of the old herbal protocols have been all but forgotten in the last 50 years. When I began to research the use of herbs for menstrual and menopausal problems, I was surprised to find that when you examine the scientific literature on phytosterol-rich plants, surprisingly few of the known benefits are listed. Most of the information we as women need in order to take control of our health and future life still has to come from other women by word of mouth. Occasionally, however, I come upon a book that is genuinely useful. Susun Weed's *Menopausal Years* is a real gem. Weed spent three years talking to more than 10,000 women about their menopause and then produced a handbook replete with practical advice and simple wisdom. She has, in effect, gathered many wise-woman practices and made them readily available to women. So has Willa Shaffer, whose knowledge not only of wild yam but many other useful plants comes from half a century of working with women and finding ways of helping them through every kind of health challenge.

Author of *Midwifery and Herbs*; *Wild Yam, Birth Control Without Fear*; and also the soon-to-be-published *Diary of a Country Midwife*; Shaffer learned her skills in childhood when plant treatments were the order of the day in dealing with almost any kind of illness. As a child, she had suffered from bronchial disorders and pneumonia, and she was usually given lobelia along with other plants. But then in her teens, in the early 1930s, she found she could no longer locate supplies of common plants for medicinal purposes, because pharmacies were by then busy converting their stocks of natural products into drugs. (It was then, by the way, that in North America, pharmacies began to be known as "drug stores.") From then on, Shaffer spent some 30 years in poor health, until in desperation she turned back to plants to help, and was at last able to heal herself. This prompted her to learn everything she could about medicinal plants, nutrition, and reflexology and to use what she had learned in her practice as a midwife. Shaffer now has women from as far afield as Central America and Europe consulting her for help. Like every wise woman worth her salt, she gives of her knowledge freely to any woman who needs it. Both Shaffer and Weed draw heavily on plants rich in phytosterols for the herbal treatments they recommend.

Green Afternoons

"Usually," says Susun Weed, "phytosterols are most concentrated in perennial roots (such as dandelion and ginseng), leaf buds (such as briar rose and blackcurrant), and hard berries (such as vitix and saw palmetto)." Unlike highly concentrated chemical hormones and drugs, plants such as these work gently and holistically in their effect on the body—many of the nonsteroid components of a particular herb support the actions of the active phytosterols. "Your body's access to phytosterols," Weed insists, "is increased when glycosides, saponins, minerals, and flavonoids are also present in a plant. Renowned hormone-balancing herbs such as Dong Quai/Dang Gui, black cohosh, and sarsaparilla contain a dozen or more of these constituents, each of which offers slightly different hormonal building blocks."

Among the most widely used phytosterol-rich foods and herbs are sage, red clover, sarsaparilla, and sassafras, licorice root, alfalfa, hops, wild yam, and yarrow. Phytosterol-rich rhubarb root and hops have been used for generations by doctors and herbalists in the treatment of menopausal symptoms, including hot flashes, vaginitis, and secondary amenorrhea. Now, in Britain and Europe, these two botanicals are sometimes given in the form of a product called Phytoestrol. Made by Pharmazeutische Fabrik Goeppingen Carl Mueller in Germany, this botanical consists of 90 mg of extract of hops and 4 mg of rhubarb-root extract. Doctors who use the product insist that, unlike drug treatments, it carries no negative side effects. One enthusiastic advocate of Phytoestrol is British naturopath and homeopath Dr. Harald Gaier, who uses the product regularly with women patients. Says Gaier, "It is not as fast acting as conventional hormones, but Phytoestrol brings lasting improvement to many women, and they have no drug interaction dangers or incompatibilities or side effects that accompany them."

A three-month double-blind placebo-controlled pilot study was carried out in the United States and reported in the *Newsletter of the Office of Alternative Medicine of the National Institute of Health* in 1993. It looked at the hormonal and symptom-relieving properties of a combination of traditional botanical medicines on perimenopausal women, including *Glycyrrhiza glabra* root (licorice), *Arctium lappa* root (burdock), *Dioscorea villosa* root (wild yam), *Angelica sinensis* root (angelica), and *Leonurus cardiaca* (motherwort). These botanicals were given in capsule form in equal parts. After three months, all participants in the test groups showed a reduction in the severity of menopausal symptoms, compared with only 6 percent of women in the placebo group. Seventy-one percent of the test group reported fewer symptoms—of which hot flashes, vaginal dryness, insomnia, and mood changes were the most common—as opposed to 17 percent in the placebo group.

Plant sterols are also known to act either indirectly or directly on the cells of connective tissue including bone cells. This may be one of the reasons why postmenopausal women living on processed foods—which are very low in sterol hormones—have a significantly higher level of arthritis and osteoporosis than other women. Dr. Joseph E. Pizzorno, Jr., and Dr. Michael T. Murray of John Bastyr College in Seattle are enthusiastic about the use of plant-based sterols as opposed to conventional drug estrogen in the treatment of female ailments, including osteoporosis. "Menopausal women commonly receive estrogen to help allay the hot flashes, nausea, bone loss, and other symptoms of this decrease in the body's own natural hormone level," they write. "While generally effective, both synthetic and natural estrogen may pose significant health risks, including the risk of cancer, gallbladder disease, and thromboembolic disease. Phyto-estrogens have not been associated with these side effects."

The general consensus among doctors aware of plant power and familiar with the use of botanical substances and foods rich in phytohormones is that the right plant foods and treatments can help balance estrogen dominance and maintain health, while at the same time preventing premature aging, degenerative diseases, and the hormonal disruptions that manifest as women's ailments.

Hormones—Good and Bad

Phytohormones act upon the body in very different ways from synthetic drugs and the xenoestrogens that pollute our environment as well as our bodies. Hormone drugs and estrogen mimics in our environment are very strong. Typically, when they bind with the body's receptor sites, they interfere with metabolic processes, since unlike natural hormones and their precursors, they are incapable of being changed by the body's own enzymes into other useful compounds. Nor can they be easily eliminated to restore hormonal balance where necessary. On the other hand, phytosterols or plant hormones are weak in their actions. They usually come to us through our foods in the form of precursors, which the body can then make use of to synthesize whatever hormones it needs. As John Lee says:

> Phytohormones are very different from the xenoestrogens which have an excessive estrogenic effect on a woman's follicles and are responsible for the widespread estrogen dominance now developing in women. They are gentle compounds which can be substituted for the body's estrogen. They occupy the same receptor sites but with less and less effect. As such, they tend to protect a woman from the xenoestrogens doing damage. These phytosterols "fit in" to a woman's metabolism. Her body recognizes

them and knows how to use them. I consider them a very benign and help-ful source of hormones.

At the Dunn Nutrition Unit at Cambridge, the work of Adene Cassidy and her team confirms Lee's assertions. Phytoestrogen does indeed compete with human estrogen, blocking the stronger estrogen from stimulating cells. This is why a diet high in soybean products such as tofu plays such an important part in protecting Japanese women from hormone-mediated diseases.

When weak estrogens from plants bind with receptor sites, they also help *protect* the body from both negative hormones and hormone-like influ-ences by encouraging the elimination of these "bad" sterols and allowing the body to readjust its own hormonal balance naturally. The vitamins, min-erals, and phytosterols in fresh foods eaten as close as possible to the state in which they come out of the ground—or carefully and naturally ferment-ed as the Japanese do—can bring to a woman's diet a supply of phytohor-mones sufficient to mitigate most of the female symptoms that plague us in industrialized countries. Kay-Tee Khaw, professor of Clinical Gerontology at the University of Cambridge, is another expert who voices enthusiasm about natural phytohormones from plants and stresses the importance of a wholesome diet of natural foods in preserving and enhancing a woman's health. Khaw believes such a diet may help lower the risk of osteoporosis, breast cancer, and heart disease. Quoted by Gail Vines in an article called "The Challenge to HRT" in *The New Scientist,* Khaw says:

> We have become so obsessed with looking for magic potions...that we are not asking the real questions about lifestyle that can have profound effects. Clinical medicine is the end of the line. Everyone asks, how could this have been prevented? We need to understand what causes some peo-ple to be healthy, and others not. If people today had the same fracture rate as existed in the 1950s in Britain, one in two hip fractures would not hap-pen. We need to understand what is going on.

The Wilder Shores

When it comes to eating, the best protection from menstrual and menopausal problems is a "primitive" diet of fresh foods; one that is low in fat and high in raw fruits, vegetables, and whole grains and legumes in their unprocessed form, plus a few fresh seeds and nuts. It is also important to include plenty of foods rich in phytosterols, such as soya products, sprouted seeds, and grains. Such dietary change is not some wishful action to carry out in the hope that it just might make a little difference to your life. In a study carried out in Britain where women were switched to a diet rich in phytohormones derived from soya flour, red clover sprouts, and flaxseed oil, researchers reported that the menopausal symptoms of 25 women were significantly reduced by such alterations alone.

In another study carried out in Scandinavia and reported in *The Lancet* three years ago, researchers discovered that Japanese women (who, you will recall, have a very low incidence of breast and uterine cancer and experience very few menopausal or menstrual problems) who eat large quantities of phytosterol-rich foods, including soya products, eliminate an astounding 1,000 times as much phytoestrogen in their urine as do Finnish women. In effect, their bodies have become saturated with phytohormones that both trigger the elimination of the bad sterols and also spill over themselves as waste. With this kind of phytoestrogen intake, researchers reported that the risk of breast cancer is only a fifth what it is among American women on a typical Western diet.

In the United States, studies of Seventh Day Adventist women on vegetarian diets show that they not only have a very low incidence of breast cancer, they are recognized as the healthiest people in the Western world. Studies also show that they have low levels of estrogen in the blood, and they excrete much higher levels of estrogen in their urine than do meat-eating women.

The Emulators

A high-raw way of eating, such as that outlined in *The New Raw Energy*, which my daughter Susannah and I researched and wrote, has long been used by doctors and health practitioners trained in natural methods of healing—both to protect from and to counteract menstrual and menopausal symptoms that have resulted from hormonal imbalances. In part, this is because such a diet—in which 50 to 75 percent of your foods are taken fresh and raw—supplies a very high level of essential nutrients and enzymes, which encourage optimal metabolism and help detoxify the body of whatever might be interfering with metabolic processes. But a raw energy way of eating is also high in phytohormones from raw seeds, nuts, vegetables, and fruits to help the endocrine system rebalance itself. And because these foods are mostly eaten fresh, the beneficial plant substances they contain are easily assimilated when you eat them.

But foods do need to be fresh. You can lose 50 percent of the vitamin C in a fresh cabbage within the first 24 hours after picking. After 48 to 72 hours, you can end up with a mere 5 percent of what was originally present. Just as vitamin levels decrease when foods lose their freshness, so too are the levels of phytosterols in natural foods diminished when a food we buy has been grown in a faraway country, harvested before it is ripe, and shipped thousands of miles before it ends up on our table. After picking, the synthesis of phytosterols within a plant ceases, while oxidation processes that destroy vitamins and hormones speed up.

Green Magic

Some of the best hormone-rich foods to add to your diet—both as a protection against trouble and for the sake of overall vitality—are the green foods: spirulina, chlorella, the seaweeds, sprouted alfalfa, and green barley. Eating some of the green foods every day can slowly, over a period of several months, help replenish what may have been lost for many years. It is something that is very difficult to do any other way, for in order for minerals to be well assimilated, they have to be highly bio-available—your body needs to easily make use of them. Most vitamin mineral supplements are not bio-available. Seaweeds, chlorella, spirulina, and green barley are also wonderful cleansing foods to help detoxify the body of excess estrogen and other pollutants such as lead, mercury, and aluminum, which may be interfering with metabolic processes. They are excellent energy enhancers. Try ten days on green foods coupled with other high-raw phytosterol foods such as those included in Miso Detox and Buildup (see chapter 26), and you may be delighted that so much benefit can come to you so quickly. The body is always attempting to strengthen and heal itself and is hungry for those elements from foods that can help it do so. Green foods have much to offer.

Age of Treason

Orthodox medicine's almost total disregard for the use of phytosterol-rich plants in the treatment of women's ailments is of recent origin. It is as though with the coming of patentable drugs, centuries of traditional methods were dismissed with the wave of a hand. "Uterine tonics" made from sterol-rich herbs and plants were used for centuries to treat all different kinds of female complaints. They still work. Once you get to know the actions of various herbs, you begin to develop a feel for the character of each botanical and a skill that enables you to call on the plant or plants you need just when you need them. But it is important to remember that plants are slower acting than drugs, so you need to be patient. It is often necessary to use an herb for a few weeks or even longer before you will experience its full benefits. Having said that, I have frequently found that an herb will bring almost immediate relief.

One big advantage of using botanicals is that many, when taken over a period of time, will do the job for which they were being taken so well that you no longer need to use them (see chapter 25). Another important thing to remember when using herbs is that they often work well in combination, and there are some good combinations on the market (see Resources for what is available).

It is essential that the supply of herbs you are using is clean—preferably organically grown. Some herbs on the market today have been grown in countries where pesticides and herbicides are sprayed heavily. Others are not fresh or have been irradiated or are contaminated with chemicals. Often, suppliers themselves are not even aware of how the dried plants have been handled. Once you have your herbs, it is a good idea to keep them in airtight jars in the refrigerator so they stay potent for as long as possible. Having worked and played with plants, herbs, and tinctures for many years, I have developed the deepest respect for their beauty and their power. Each plant has its own unique personality, which you can turn to for health or strength when you need it. I keep herbs in my garden, cut them fresh in summer, and use them dried in winter for everything from cooking a soup and making a salad to healing a cough, banishing a headache, or clearing a room of negative energies. I also keep a whole row of liter and half-liter bottles of plant tinctures just behind my desk in the room in which I work and call on them frequently when help is needed—for energy, to calm stress, or to ward off an impending infection. The support that plants can give a woman going through her passage to power is nothing short of miraculous.

ORDER OUT OF CHAOS
Eating for Radiance and Well-Being

ife feeds upon life. Modern practices destroy food's *wholesomeness.* Wholesomeness is a property very hard to measure except in terms of the degenerative effects that eating foods without it has on our bodies. Destroy a food's wholesomeness, and you destroy its integrity as well as its ability to support health at the highest levels. And once the health-giving integrity of any food has gone, it has gone for good. It can never be compensated for by vitamin and mineral supplements or by eating cereals to which extra fiber and vitamins have been added. You can analyze every bit of information available about an apple, break it down into its chemical constituents, and quantify the level of each one. You can then gather all its constituents together again, but you still won't be able to make an apple. Only *life* can do that.

The secret to eating for high-level health is making use of wholesome foods radiant with life energy that increase mental and physical energy and protect from premature aging, while restoring hormonal order. The theory is simple; the practice gets more complicated. The first step is forsaking, once and for all, convenience foods with all their fragmentation and hidden fat and sugar for a life-generating way of eating based on simple wholesome foods grown on healthy soils, and eaten as close as possible to the state in which they come out of the ground.

Next comes incorporating foods rich in phytosterols. They include raw foods, concentrated green foods, and naturally fermented high-chi foods

from the Orient, such as miso. You also need to be savvy about body energy—what enhances it and what depletes it—and about food allergies, and
how they can undermine health and vitality, and about how to avoid them.
It is important to become streetwise about fats, too, since nothing can foul
up a woman's hormonal system like processed fats in foods, and *junk fats*
are just about everywhere these days. Finally, you need to address the question of nutritional supplements. The decisions you make about how and
what you eat from the age of 35 onwards largely determines the kind of
menopause you will have and how protected you are from osteoporosis.
These same decisions are responsible for how slowly or rapidly your body
ages and how much energy you have to do whatever you want to do with
your life. Much of what follows I have investigated in previous books—
Lean Revolution, for example—but it is so central to understanding how our
bodies function that it is worth restating here. Let's tackle energy first.

Witness to the Fire

Carbohydrates are your body's main source of energy for all its functions. However, just any old carbohydrate won't do. Only *complex* carbohydrates—fruits and vegetables, unrefined grains, and sea plants and
legumes—provide steady, lasting energy throughout the day. They also protect you from blood-sugar problems, mood swings, and the chronic fatigue
that is prevalent in the lives of many women over the age of 35, which leads
them to binge on sugar or coffee or pep pills just to keep going. Sugar cravings are common with PMS, and indulging them can be dangerous to a
woman's long-term hormonal health. Women with PMS eat three times as
much refined sugar as those without. Eating sugar causes your body to
excrete magnesium and interferes with the liver's ability to deactivate
harmful estrogen. Adequate magnesium is essential in preventing PMS and
menopausal symptoms, as well as in keeping immunity high. It helps the
body to deactivate excess estrogen, clear painful menstruation, and reduce
lower abdominal and back pain. Many of the ill effects of dairy products
also appear to involve magnesium. Dairy products are nine times higher in
calcium than magnesium. Eating them regularly can upset the
calcium/magnesium balance, interfering with the metabolism of important
B-complex vitamins and making PMS symptoms worse.

One of the major energy problems caused by eating processed foods
full of *simple* carbohydrates such as white flour and sugar is that it brings

about a progressive decline in your body's ability to metabolize sugar. Unlike natural foods full of protective fiber, refined and processed foods are highly concentrated foods. Fiber is no longer present to dilute their concentration and to slow down the rate at which the simple starches and sugars they contain are absorbed into your bloodstream. Such foods are far more *calorie dense*. When you eat them year after year, they begin to overwhelm the body—especially the pancreas—causing blood-sugar problems and mood and energy swings that wreak havoc with your health.

Refined and highly concentrated convenience foods devoid of their natural fiber make your blood-sugar curve rise steeply, as a lot of sugar is pumped quickly into your system, then they force it to drop off quickly. After a couple of hours, you get an energy slump and feel hungry again. It is little wonder. Believe it or not, each teaspoon of sugar in the jam you ate was refined out of 6 to 12 feet of sugar cane, and in the processing all the protective fiber and other nutrients, such as chromium, which your body needs for its proper assimilation, were lost. So a couple of hours after breakfast, you have to reach for a bar of chocolate to keep going. If the snack you choose is, say, a couple of biscuits or a sweet roll, you take in another 4 spoons of sugar—the sweetness of 9.6 meters or 32 feet of sugar cane—which you get in one big bang with no protective fiber to slow down its release into your blood. This jolts the pancreas, forcing it to respond quickly by producing more and more insulin to keep your blood sugar from going too high.

The Dark Is Rising

Continue to eat concentrated foods full of simple carbohydrates year after year, and your blood glucose levels will tend to get higher and higher, as the pancreas is continually forced to release more and more insulin in an attempt to control it all. Even though insulin is still being produced in high concentrations, your body will have become insulin resistant— that is, your cells no longer respond normally to insulin, and the body's ability to control blood sugar is lost. When this happens, the calories from your foods are more and more easily converted into fats, or triglycerides, which are then laid down as fat stores on your belly, hips, thighs, and bottom. You'll also increase your likelihood of getting heart disease and other degenerative conditions.

Simple carbohydrates such as white sugar, white flour, cornflakes, and white bread are *high* on what is known as the *glycemic index*. This means that they cause the blood-sugar level to rise quickly, contribute to insulin resistance, sometimes disturb appetite, and make energy maintenance difficult. Foods high on the glycemic index are foods to avoid. They include glucose, most packaged breakfast cereals such as cornflakes, instant mashed potatoes, maltose, white rice, white pasta, white bread, sweet biscuits, potato chips and most processed packaged foods. For lasting energy and good health, it is important to choose natural foods that are lower on the glycemic index—fresh vegetables, apples and nontropical fruit, oats, brown rice, sea plants, whole wheat spaghetti, soybeans, lentils, sweet potatoes, lima beans, and kidney beans; as well as fruit sugar from apples and oranges. These are foods that you can feel comfortable eating a lot of. Don't get misled by the nonsense that is written on the packaging of foods you buy, either. Read the ingredients carefully, and watch for hidden sugars that could interfere with the fat-burning process in your own body—glucose, sorbitol, invert sugar, corn syrup, maltodextrin, dextrose, barley syrup, and malt sugar. Even many products that claim to be sugar-free contain one or more of these, all of which are just another name for sugar.

Caffeine Freedom

What place do coffee, tea, and soft drinks have in a healthy way of eating for women with menstrual problems or passing through menopause? Very little. Certainly they should not be drunk every day. Quite apart from the negative effects of caffeine—an ingredient in coffee, tea, and many soft drinks—drinking coffee messes up blood sugar. Caffeine, technically known as trimethyl xanthine, is a habit-forming drug. It has been shown to be responsible for headaches, insomnia, nervousness, anxiety, and that familiar wired mental state that keeps you buzzing for a time intellectually but tends to disconnect you from your instincts, and, in some women, even from having a good grip on reality. Caffeine gives you a quick lift and the illusion of energy, only to let you crash down a couple of hours later when you are inclined to reach for more.

Caffeine has a mutagenic effect, too—that is, it is capable of crossing the placenta to cause permanent damage to an unborn child, as well as breaking apart the chromosomes in your own cells and interfering with the repair of DNA. Drinking coffee stimulates the secretion of acid in your stomach, disturbing natural appetite-control mechanisms and making you far more likely to end up with an ulcer than your noncoffee-drinking cousin. Actually, caffeine acts as a stimulant to the central nervous system in a rather curious way. It makes you *feel* more mentally alert. But tests show that in reality, it creates more confusion and nervousness. In animal experiments, very high doses of caffeine have been shown to create psychotic behavior. Coffee also tends to raise blood pressure and to increase the risk of coronary thrombosis. Drink five cups each day, and your heart attack risk goes up by 60 percent. Coffee also makes the blood more acid, which, in turn, draws calcium from your bones to try to reestablish a healthy acid/alkaline balance. Drinking more than two cups of coffee a day is one of the things you should not do if you want to prevent osteoporosis.

And tea? It too contains caffeine—100 mg to coffee's 120 mg in a regular-sized cup. Tea also contains tannic acid, which is an irritant to the digestive system. There is also evidence that drinking tea in quantity interferes with iron absorption from foods. Even if you have always been a committed six-to-eight-cups-a-day tea or coffee drinker, after a couple of weeks on good water, you will find you don't miss it. Then when you have an occasional cup, it becomes a simple pleasure rather than an addiction.

Cut the Soft Drinks

The average intake of soft drinks in the West has risen to 8 to 12 cans a week in some countries—between 400 and 600 a year. Women and children are the biggest users. Many colas and soft drinks also contain caffeine. And they are far too high in sugar. They bring nutritionally empty calories into your body that you can ill afford. A 12 oz. (330 ml.) can of cola contains 7 teaspoons of sugar—about 40 grams. Colas are full of chemicals to pollute your body and preoccupy your liver's elimination processes. As for the "diet" varieties, quite apart from the proven fact that drinking them will do absolutely nothing to help you lose weight, they are an even more chemically unpleasant cocktail, full of excess phosphorus and additives that only pollute your body and further contribute to calcium loss from bones. Stay away from them. They are also full of phosphoric acid (the chemical used to etch glass), which, when your body tries to eliminate it via the kidneys, combines with calcium—leaching this vital mineral from bones, teeth, nails, and hair. Fizzy colas are major contributors to osteoporosis in women.

All Fats Are Not Equal

Now let's look at the issue of fats, for the kind of fats you eat greatly determines the hormonal health of your body. Each of us in the West consumes about 175 grams of fat a day. That makes 63 kilograms a year. Between 40 and 50 percent of our food calories come from fat. The cookies you buy in your local supermarket are well over 40 percent fat, and the munchy-crunchy snacks that masquerade as health bars seldom contain less than 50 percent. For long-term good health, you need to reduce your fat intake down to between 15 and 25 percent of the calories you eat. You also need to take great care to make sure that these fat calories are the right kind. This is not always easy to do.

All fats and oils in our foods are made out of fatty acids. A fatty acid is a molecule that contains an acid part and a fat part. Chemically, it consists of a chain of carbon and hydrogen atoms to which one oxygen atom is attached. A molecule of fat differs from a molecule of carbohydrate (which is also made out of carbon, hydrogen, and oxygen) by the fact that the fat contains a lot less oxygen. This makes it highly concentrated and is why there are nine calories to each gram of fat, while only four calories in each gram of carbohydrate or protein.

Fats can be roughly divided into two groups—saturated and unsaturated. A saturated fat is a fatty acid with a molecule where each carbon atom is connected to a hydrogen atom so that there are no empty *spaces* to allow one or more of the carbons to reach up and join together with molecules of other substances in your body. Because of this, saturated fats (found in meat; dairy products such as cheese, ice cream, and milk; and tropical oils such as palm kernel oil and coconut) are stable, inactive, and virtually inert in your body. Their major *raison d'être* is to provide calories in a concentrated form that can later be burned as energy. Eat too many foods full of saturated fats, and they do their best to lay themselves down as fat stores. You will get as much saturated fat as you need from your food without ever giving it a second thought.

Unsaturated fats are different. They are made up of fatty-acid chains that *do* have empty spaces—carbon atoms with open arms that are not connected directly to hydrogen atoms. Unsaturates come in two forms: *mono*-unsaturates, such as olive oil; and *poly*-unsaturates, found in corn, sunflower seeds, peanuts, and many other foods from which they are extracted. Thanks to their free spaces, mono-unsaturates and poly-unsaturates are much more biologically active, more able to easily take part in important biochemical changes in your body that produce energy, create hormones, and help burn stored body fats. The right unsaturated fats are essential to a woman's hormonal health all through her reproductive life and beyond. That is, the right *kind* of unsaturated fat. But there is a lot of hokum spread about unsaturated fats by sellers of margarine and producers of processed junk foods. Just because a label says "unsaturated," it doesn't mean the food in the packet is good for you. Ninety-eight percent of them are not. You have to be shrewd about what you buy and really know the ropes. This means going a bit deeper into the whole fat issue. Bear with me. An understanding of good and bad fats can revolutionize your health.

Bare Essentials

Your body can make all the fat it needs for daily metabolic processes except for two essential fatty acids: linoleic and linolenic. These are found naturally in fresh foods, in seeds and nuts, in vegetables and fish, and even in wild meat such as game. For optimum health, you need no more than two to four tablespoons of these essential fatty acids a day, yet despite our high-fat intake in the West, they can be as hard to find in modern convenience foods as the proverbial hen's teeth. These two unsaturates help you burn body fat and build energy; they also help your body manufacture important hormones. Linoleic and linolenic are called essential fatty acids because that is exactly what they are—essential to human life and health.

The moment you remove an unsaturated fat from the food in which it comes, you produce what is known as a *free-fat*. A free-fat is any fat that has been separated out from the food in which it occurs in nature—corn oil, for instance; peanut or groundnut oil; sunflower oil; safflower oil; as well as any margarines or biscuits or other foods containing them. Free-fats are something women should avoid like the plague. Through complex operations involving the use of heat and unpleasant chemical solvents, food manufacturers turn our natural fatty acids contained in wholesome fresh foods into highly artificial fat products that damage health. It takes an amazing 12 to 15 ears of corn to produce a mere teaspoon full of the golden oil. All the protective "packaging" of fiber, vitamins, and minerals gets thrown out in the process or fed to pigs. Advertisers are continually promoting products full of "polyunsaturates" as though they were healthy. It is a lot of rubbish. Most polyunsaturated fats are not at all healthy.

Let me give you an example of what I mean. In addition to the common process "hydrogenation" that turns an unsaturated fat into a saturated one—making an oil into a solid fat like margarine by adding extra hydrogen atoms to spaces on the fatty-acid chain—there are other processes commonly used in food processing that degrade or completely destroy the health-giving properties of whatever essential fatty acids a polyunsaturated fat may contain.

The Good Guys and the Bad Guys

Natural, unadulterated, unsaturated fats for health come in a chemical configuration known as a *cis* form. This is the *only* form a woman's body can use for anything except pumping up her fat stores. Cis fatty acids are destroyed by modern processing procedures such as bleaching, hydrogenation, heating, and deodorizing, which turn out the golden oils that shimmer from the shelves of our supermarkets and with which the mass-produced foods we eat today are riddled. These procedures alter our healthy cis fatty acids into unhealthy *trans*-fatty acids by rotating the hydrogen atoms on the fat molecules so that they change sides. Cis fatty acids—the good guys—are rather like "gloves." Like natural hormones, which key into hormone receptor sites, they fit perfectly onto the "hands" of the molecular fat receptors in your body. Trans-fatty acids are bad guys. Like the drug-based hormones and xenoestrogens, they don't properly fit into your body's metabolic machinery. Their presence can even block fat receptor sites, interfering in your body's ability to produce important hormones involved in reproduction, causing PMS and menopausal miseries.

Since trans-fatty acids don't occur in nature, like many hormone drugs, your body has never developed any mechanisms for making use of them. It treats them as foreign invaders rather like toxic wastes and does its best to try to protect you from any detrimental effects they can have on your body (such as furring up your arteries) by laying them down in fat tissues. A first principle of trouble-free menstruation and menopause is to *eliminate free oils, hydrogenated fats, and processed foods from your diet*. Every processed fat contains unhealthy trans-fatty acids. Not one mass-produced margarine on the market is genuinely health-promoting despite all the advertising designed to convince us to the contrary—nor are all those golden oils, salad dressings, and biscuits, breads, or ready-made meals containing them healthy. So don't be misled by the words *contains polyunsatu-*

rates. Margarines and cooking oils are *junk fats.* Your body cannot use them for health, and, because their presence actually blocks the uptake of cis fatty acids, eating them can lead to fatty-acid deficiencies and hormone chaos. The ordinary saturated fat that you find in steak or chicken is healthier than such artificially produced, hydrogenated, unnatural fatty acids. It is important to read every label, and anything that says it contains hydrogenated vegetable oil or partially hydrogenated vegetable oil, leave on the shelf.

Don't assume you can believe everything you read on food labels either. Look on any packet that lists the protein, carbohydrate, fat content, and calories per serving, and make some quick calculations to tell you what percentage of the calories in the food are fat calories. Here's how to work it out quickly.

Say that a particular package of cookies contains 145 calories per 100-gram serving, made up of 4 grams of protein, 19 grams of carbohydrate, and 7 grams of fat. Multiply the amount of fat by ten (rounded up from fat being nine calories per gram); that is, add a zero to the number of grams of fat per serving, to give you how many of the calories per serving are in the form of fat. Then compare this figure with the total calories. In this case it would be 7 x 10 = 70 calories of fat in each 145 calories. Now divide 70 by 145 and you get 0.48—the fraction of those calories per serving that comes from fat. This tells you that the cookie calories are about 48 percent fat calories. As this is way above the limit of 25 percent for optimal health, reject the packet.

As far as the golden vegetable oils that you find on supermarket shelves are concerned, don't use them. On your salads, instead of using salad oils, use *cold pressed extra virgin* olive oil. This oil is not a polyunsaturate with many free spaces on its molecules, but a *mono*unsaturate, with only one free space that makes it highly stable. It is the best overall oil for salads. You can also use it in tiny quantities for wok-frying vegetables.

So just where do you get the important unadulterated essential fatty acids you need, and how do they work? The answer to the first question is simple.

Essential fatty acids are found in abundance in nuts, beans, grains and seeds, and soya products, as well as in olives and other plant foods. Soybeans are an excellent source; so are grains such as wheat and barley and oats and maize. What happens in your body when you eat these foods is that the linoleic and alphalinolenic acid they contain are converted into other fatty acids that are needed for various purposes, provided, of course, that your diet is not full of junk fats that prevent these conversions from taking place. It is important to buy your foods really fresh. Reject any grain or seed or nut that does not taste and smell absolutely clean, and keep your nuts and seeds in the fridge. With the exception of avocados, nuts, and olives, most of these whole plant foods have a low fat content. Animal foods, however, have a much higher fat content. Even the leanest steak boasts 50 percent of its calories from fat, while the more delicious fat-marbled variety can be as high as 80 percent. Butter and cream go even higher, offering 100 percent of calories from saturated fats, none of which you need for health.

Clever Conversions

In your body, the essential fatty acid, linoleic acid, is converted by an enzyme called the delta-6-desaturase enzyme into gamma linolenic acid, or GLA. These days it has become well known as a way of improving the skin and as a treatment for female problems including PMS. GLA is, in turn, changed into prostaglandins, and different fatty acids such as arachidonic via other metabolic steps. Linolenic, the other essential fatty acid, is present in pumpkin seeds, flaxseeds, soybeans, and walnuts, as well as in oily fish such as wild salmon, mackerel, sardines, and wild trout. Because of the way they are fed these days, farmed fish such as trout and salmon contain more and more saturated fat and less and less linolenic acid. Linolenic is similarly converted through the action of an enzyme called delta-5-desaturase into eicosapentanoic (EPA) and then on to docosahexanoic acid (DHA).

A major reason why GLA from evening primrose oil, borage oil, or starflower oil has such a positive effect on the body is that, because our Western diet is high in junk fats or trans-fatty acids, we often have difficulty making the conversion from linoleic to gamma-linolenic. Similarly, in recent years, fish oils containing EPA and DHA have been prescribed—particularly for athletes and people at risk from heart disease—because as we get older, there appears to be a decline in the enzymes that are necessary to make these conversions. One of the best ways of getting extra quantities of essential fatty acids is to buy vacuum-packed flaxseeds, pulverize them, and sprinkle a teaspoonful or two on your cereals or salads every day.

Cry Wild

More than 50 years ago, Hans Eppinger, chief doctor at the First Medical Clinic of the University of Vienna, discovered that a high-raw way of eating leads to increased cellular respiration. This it does in a number of ways by creating a kind of positive feedback loop where one thing in turn stimulates another until cell metabolism is heightened. It eliminates accumulated wastes and toxins from cells and tissues. It supplies the level of nutrients essential for optimal cell function. And, perhaps most important of all, it heightens the microelectrical tensions associated with cell vitality so that even cells in a particularly sluggish and neglected system are revitalized. They become better able to burn calories in the presence of oxygen and to produce energy efficiently both for overall vitality and for carrying out the housekeeping on which the health of your body depends.

Capillaries are minute blood vessels that form the vast network of microcirculation throughout your body. It is their responsibility to deliver oxygen-rich blood for it to be used by the cells. So important are these fine vessels that nature has supplied you with incredible lengths of them. If you were to attach all the capillaries in your body end to end, they would measure some 60,000 miles in length—more than twice around the world. The state of your body as a whole depends to a great extent on the condition of your capillaries, for they are the arbitrators of cell nutrition, respiration, and elimination. It is through these capillaries that nutrients and oxygen are carried. Each of them has tiny "pores" that allow plasma but not red blood cells to seep through and pass into the body fluid. This is how nutrients are delivered and wastes eliminated from tissues. Without good microcirculation, metabolism cannot take place efficiently. That is why the capillaries play a vital part in the successful elimination of excess fat deposits with all their stored toxins.

Unfortunately, over the years, the capillaries of women living on the average Western diet become twisted, distended, and highly porous. When they do, proteins seep through and deposit themselves between the tissues and the capillary walls, where they interfere with proper oxygen exchange and impede nutrient delivery and waste elimination. This can gradually starve cells, tissues, and organs of all they need to function properly and can also lower cellular metabolic activity. Such changes in microcirculation lower overall vitality, since none of your body's parts are receiving the oxygen and nutrients they need for healthy metabolic functions. They also predispose you to degenerative illness and rapid aging. A high-raw way of eating helps restore normal microcirculation and thereby not only heightens metabolism, which is necessary for rebalancing hormones, maintaining good energy, and maintaining normal weight, but in a very real way it also rejuvenates your body.

Life-Generating Diet: **Low-Fat, Low or No Dairy,** **High-Fiber Natural Foods**	**Western Diet:** **High-Fat, High-Protein,** **Convenience Foods**
Normalizes weight	Promotes overweight
Stabilizes emotions	Promotes emotional instability
Alleviates breast tenderness	Exacerbates breast tenderness
Reduces breast cysts	Increases breast cysts
Relieves PMS	Exacerbates PMS
Lowers risk of osteoporosis	Increases risk of osteoporosis
Lowers risk of cancer in breast, ovaries, and womb	Increases risk of cancer in breast, ovaries, and womb
Protects from diverticulosis	Encourages diverticulosis
Reduces risk of heart disease	Increases risk of heart disease
Alleviates heavy periods	Exacerbates heavy periods
Relieves endometriosis	Exacerbates endometriosis
Protects skin and body from premature aging	Encourages premature aging of skin and body
Reduces risk of varicose veins	Increases risk of varicose veins
Lowers risk of gallstones	Increases risk of gallstones
Eliminates constipation	Encourages constipation
Relieves chronic fatigue	Exacerbates chronic fatigue
Reduces risk of bowel cancer	Increases risk of bowel cancer

Sacred Hunger

Ideally, the foods you eat on a high-raw diet should be chosen from fresh, organically grown vegetables and fruits, for these foods offer the highest complement of substances of nutritional value to an organism. But for me, as for most people, this is just not possible. I grow my own herbs and a few fruits and vegetables in my garden in the country, but half of the time I live in an apartment in the city, where I have little access to anything that has been organically composted. Making at least one meal a day a big raw salad made out of sprouted seeds and grains and all sorts of raw vegetables—from raw beetroot to raw herbs, carrots, cauliflower, or whathave-you—solves, at least in part, the dilemma about organically grown foods. Since you've grown the sprouts yourself, you *know* that they haven't been subjected to any chemical treatments, and because you have used (or should have used) spring water for them, you know that they do not contain any undesirable minerals or other chemicals. Your salad is also an excellent source of top-quality protein, essential fatty acids, and natural sugars. When seeds are sprouted, the starch in them begins to be broken down and turned into natural sugars that are easy to assimilate and provide energy to heighten your mood.

Finally, and probably most important of all, remember that homegrown sprouts are brimming with life energy. This life energy is as yet little understood; it is only beginning to be measured by sensitive instruments. There are no better raw foods than sprouted seeds and grains. Clive McCay, professor of nutrition at Cornell University, once researched the sprouted soybean and declared that he had discovered an almost perfect food: "a vegetable which will grow in any climate, will rival meat in nutritive value, will mature in three to five days, may be planted any day of the year, will require neither soil nor sunshine, will rival tomatoes in vitamin C, will be free of waste in preparation and can be cooked with little fuel..."

Red Dragon

The Japanese are without question the healthiest of any industrialized nation. Sadly, this is now changing thanks to the invasion of Western convenience foods and eating habits into their culture. However, there is still much we can learn from them. Unlike 20th-century Western medicine and nutrition, which are both limited by their linear chemical thinking, the

Asian approach to health and nutrition takes into account the importance of manipulating life energy, or chi, in order to create the balance and harmony in the body on which good health depends. Their whole approach to food selection is traditionally energetic in character. It is a balancing of yin and yang energy in food selection and of the various tastes—sweet, bitter, sour, burnt, and so forth—which are said to influence the energy flows that regulate the secretion of hormones and the function of the various organs and systems. Whole grains, legumes, and vegetable foods are good foods for *centering* energy (the body's chi), while sugar and meat and dairy products are very far from the perfect balance of yin and yang and so tend to render their energy off-center and unbalanced. Meat and dairy products are very *yang* (dense and contracted in nature), while sugar and sweet things are *yin* (very expansive and cooling to the body). When you eat sweets, the body, needing balance, begins to crave meat and vice versa. For optimal health, choose *centering* foods—the same wholesome grains, vegetables, local fruits, and legumes that contemporary researchers and clinicians from Pritikin to Ornish have discovered help heal the body even of long-standing chronic conditions.

According to traditional Japanese nutrition, the major cause of women's health problems in the West is our consumption of dairy foods, excessive sugar and meat. The Japanese and Chinese have never included milk products in their diet. They have always insisted that the human body was not designed to consume cow's milk and that eating milk products year after year causes the body to degenerate. Increasingly, Western nutritionists are beginning to side with the Asian view. The two most common foods to which people tend to be sensitive are milk and wheat. This is not surprising, since convenience foods are replete with these two foods. There is much we can learn from the Asian approach to food and health.

In Japan, there is as yet little awareness of a high-raw way of eating for healing and enhancing health, but this is compensated for by the tradition of slow, natural food processing and preservation they use to create their staple foods—miso, kuzu, umeboshi, and brown rice vinegar. Unlike our high-tech food technology, the Japanese traditional methods of handling foods for preservation and the creation of dishes such as miso actually improve a food's health-giving quality by enhancing its chi. Traditional miso is made by combining *kogi* (cultured grains or soybeans that have been fermented) with soybeans, salt, and water and then letting it ferment naturally from between three months to two years. Many naturally processed foods such as these play an important part in the modern system of macrobiotics, which, like the high-raw approach to health, has been credited with an almost infinite ability to support the body's healing of itself.

Nutritional Supplements

One of the most common questions women ask is: Provided my diet is good, do I need to take nutritional supplements? Ideally no. The best sources of vitamins and minerals are organically grown foods. No supplements can or ever will compete with them in health-promoting properties. Certainly no amount of nutritional supplements, no matter how wisely chosen, will ever replace a good diet. Many large-scale studies show that women in the Western world are deficient in nutrients such as zinc, some of the B vitamins, magnesium, and others. For women who have been exposed to high levels of xenoestrogens and who for years have eaten the standard supermarket fare while living stressful lives, specifically chosen vitamins, minerals, trace elements, and certain essential fatty acids can greatly enhance health.

The best nutritional supplements are the superfoods such as spirulina, seaweeds, chlorella, green barley, and wheat grass. They contain complexes of important vitamins, minerals, and trace elements in a form that is balanced and easily assimilated by the body. Antioxidant nutrients and metabolites such as vitamin C, vitamin E, beta-carotene, coenzyme Q10, and selenium can be helpful, too. They improve the immune system's function and are helpful in warding off illness and degeneration. Magnesium is vital for good immune function and hard to come by in processed foods, while zinc strengthens the immune response. Women who are athletes or who do a lot of physical activity need greater quantities of magnesium than others and almost certainly more zinc as well, and these can only be supplied by nutritional supplements. So do older women.

Every woman is a complete biochemical individual, so only the roughest guidelines about nutritional supplements can be given. Specific nutritional programs are best devised with the help of a skilled nutritional advisor, since most doctors receive virtually no nutritional guidance in relation to their medical training (see chapter 28 for guidelines and suggestions).

Finally, although to my knowledge nobody has done any hard research into the subject, from the experience of women themselves, it seems obvious that many women's dietary needs and desires change after menopause. Most women find they feel better on a mostly or completely vegetarian diet that eliminates dairy products, caffeine, and meat. There are exceptions, however, so it is important to experiment. A few women actually need meat and do far better if they eat it during and after menopause. Certainly if you decide to eat meat, it needs to be from healthy animals (see chapter 27) and low in fat.

———⊷≍⊶———

CHAPTER TWELVE

BODY HEAT

Exercise As the Key to Personal Freedom

or a few women, exercise is such a normal part of their lives that they do it regularly without thinking. It makes them feel good, so they run or swim, play tennis, do yoga, row, or attend dance classes. For most of us, however, heavier exercise is something that can seem rather daunting—especially if you haven't done any for 30 years. From our earliest introduction to physical activity in schools, our perception of exercise gets colored by the confusion that exists between sports skills and fitness. Being skillful at a particular sport does not necessarily have much to do with being fit. Many women who discovered in school that they were not natural athletes are still put off by the idea of taking up some form of regular activity, because they feel they lack physical prowess or that they will simply be "no good at it."

Being good at something is completely irrelevant. What matters is simply that you use your body by setting it in motion and letting it experience the kind of movement for which it was made. It can be useful to look at whatever your own unconscious assumptions may be regarding exercise so you can clear away any cobwebs, for exploring the possibilities of what exercise can do to change you for the better is a life-expanding experience. It can be one of the most exciting journeys a woman can take at any time, but especially in the middle of her life. And this is particularly true if, like me, your natural tendency is to curl up into a ball and flop onto the sofa.

Dr. Walter Bortz of the Department of Medicine at the Palo Alto Medical Clinic in California published a fascinating paper in which he reviewed more than 100 studies showing that the sedentary lifestyle that has developed in the past 50 years in the West causes bodily damage. Disuse through inactivity increases levels of cholesterol and triglycerides, for instance. It also reduces *vital capacity*—that is, your ability to take up and use oxygen. Bortz found that the average sedentary 45-year-old has lost half of the ability to take up and use oxygen. With that loss comes all sorts of degenerative changes to the body that even most doctors still think are a part of normal aging. What is so wonderful is that when a sedentary person gets into regular exercise for a year, he or she can restore the ability to take up and use oxygen to that of a 25-year-old. The benefits of restoring vital capacity are superior to any drug or medical treatment in existence. This is particularly true for women in midlife and beyond. As one of the world's foremost authorities on exercise, nutrition, and good health, Dr. Michael Colgan says, "There is no longer any doubt: Exercise can save your life, while couch potatoism creates an existence that is nasty, sick and short...*exercise directly prevents disease*." (The italics are mine.)

Numerous studies show that most bodily changes associated with age have little to do with years passing. They are, instead, the result of negative shifts in what is known as our Lean Body Mass (LBM)-to-fat ratio—that is, decreased muscle mass in relation to fat—which occurs as a result of simple disuse. There is a widespread belief that as women get older, their body metabolism naturally slows down and therefore it is normal that we grow steadily fatter. Yet here, too, inactivity is the culprit.

Your Lean Body Mass is always shifting. Being inactive makes it shrink. So does going off and on slimming diets. Crash dieting causes you to shed muscle tissue. Yet when lost weight is regained, it is regained in fat, forever decreasing the weight of your LBM. This is why the more you diet, the flabbier your body becomes. And because crash dieting shrinks LBM, it also shrinks your metabolism so it becomes harder and harder to stay thin until finally you need to starve yourself (and often ruin your health) to keep the scales right. It is little wonder that when your muscle tissue is good, as it is in a wild animal or a healthy child, your own brand of radiance shines through.

What I didn't know until recently, however, is that the more you strengthen your LBM, the easier it is to get rid of psychological hang-ups, fears and all those other niggling things that hold you back. When it comes to using exercise as a bridge to freedom for women in midlife, it is muscle you need to work with. To do so brings about a fascinating metamorphosis and a highly individual one. It will not change you in any intrinsic way, nor will it turn you into someone else's idea of who you should be or what you should look like. It will only help make you more what you are. As you work week after week with the right kind of exercise, even a body that may have been distorted over the years through stress, poor eating, and lack of movement metamorphoses into the true form that is hidden within it. That is where resistance exercise comes in, and the best form of resistance exercise is weight training.

Catalog of Rewards

Working with weights does not mean that you will end up with a killer body. Quite the contrary. Exercising in order to build muscle, using light weights and many repetitions, is the most effective way of enhancing LBM. It chisels and defines arms, legs, torso, hips, and bottom, even if they have been neglected for many years and have lost their natural tone and shape. So good is this kind of body-building at improving LBM that until recently no one considered that it might be an excellent form of protecting against degenerative illnesses such as coronary heart disease as well.

There was a time when aerobic exercise was considered king for health, fitness, and longevity. Now, thanks to new research into the effects of weight training at prestigious centers such as McMasters University in Ontario, we know that aerobic exercise combined with weight training is the very best you can get for health, fitness, and longevity; as well as good looks, stamina, and energy. As a result, the much-respected American College of Sports Medicine has recently revised their long-standing assertion that aerobic exercise holds the ultimate key. Their new program advises a minimum of two sessions of weight training a week using ten different exercises to enhance the large muscles of the chest, back, and legs, as well as three sessions of aerobic exercise. Ideally, I think three sessions a week are needed, each between 30 minutes to one hour in which you combine resistance movement with some aerobic activity to warm up and cool down (see chapter 29). Then you get the best of both worlds. Be sure, also, to walk as much as you can in the open air.

The right exercise also helps prevent degenerative diseases such as cancer and heart disease. An eight-year study that followed more than 10,000 men and 3,000 women and was reported in the *Journal of the American Medical Association* looked at the long-term effects of physical fitness. It found that sedentary women have a 460 percent higher mortality rate than those that exercised more regularly. Men in the low fitness category had a 340 percent higher rate.

Exercise Brings Benefits	Disuse Brings Trouble
Builds strong bones	Renders bones porous and fragile
Increases life expectancy—on average by seven years	Precipitates deterioration of arteries
Clears anxiety and depression	Lowers noradrenaline levels
Enhances mental clarity	Induces fuzzy-mindedness
Enhances immune functions— increasing the levels of lymphocytes, interleukin 2, neutrophils, and other disease-fighting components of the immune system; also lowers cancer rates in women	Encourages aches and pains to develop as the cells accumulate lactic acid after even the mildest exertion and suppresses immune function
Encourages more restful sleep and greater relaxation	Fosters emotional instability
Improves both mental and physical flexibility	Makes ligaments and tendons lose strength and flexibility so you are more easily injured
Increases mental and physical energy	Causes muscle and brain cells to lose the enzyme capacity for maintaining energy
Increases insulin sensitivity, helps to maintain energy levels and protect against diabetes	Undermines energy and encourages blood sugar disturbances and disorders in glucose metabolism
Improves the elimination of wastes	Contributes to the development of constipation, hemorrhoids, and varicose veins, and can lead to disturbances in bowel function

Alleviates symptoms of PMS	Exacerbates symptoms of PMS
Lowers cholesterol—especially the "bad" low-density lipoprotein (LDL), one of the best predictors of cardiovascular disease	Increases levels of cholesterol, LDL, and triglycerides
Encourages good Lean Body Mass-to-fat ratio	Encourages flabbiness and the laying down of fat stores in the body
Normalizes blood pressure	Fosters rising blood pressure as the years pass
Keeps sex hormones at optimum levels	Causes sex hormones to decline, which affects skin, psyche, and libido

Caterpillars into Butterflies

I have always been fascinated by the idea of transformation—you know, frogs into princes, Cinderella becomes the belle of the ball. Most people believe that in *real* life, transformation is not possible. They have obviously never worked with muscle. Quite apart from all the mind-boggling new research into how the *right kind* of exercise can rejuvenate your body, in the past year I have discovered for myself that exercise is a great deal more than something you do to counteract aging or protect yourself from heart disease. It can foster personal metamorphosis of the deepest order—physical, emotional, and spiritual. Not only is such transformation possible, it is virtually guaranteed—provided you are patient and are willing to put real *muscle* behind it.

A year ago, I made a decision to explore just what kind of transformation was possible for me by working intensively with muscle. I had just finished writing a book, *Lean Revolution*, which examines in depth a way of regulating normal weight in the body. In the course of my research, I had come to understand the enormous importance of enhancing Lean Body Mass (LBM). I knew that *skillful* weight training (not the slap-about kind you see carried out in most gyms) is the fastest and most efficient way to do this. So I searched out someone who could work intensively with me as a trainer to shift the LBM-to-fat ratio in my own body. I found a Welsh champion weight lifter, Rhodri Thomas, who said he would take me on. When we began to work together, I was scared to death that after the first two hours I would collapse in a heap. After all, I am no athlete. However, I was eager to find out for myself just how change happens through muscle, so we trained for six days a week. Every day we would work with weights backed up by aerobic exercise such as running, swimming, and cycling, interspersed with other activities like squash and tennis—just for relaxation. I found to my amazement that I did not collapse. Instead, I watched as all sorts of deep changes began to take place. Muscles I didn't know existed slowly and quietly began to surface through my flesh.

I discovered that the psycho-physiologists are right—feelings, thoughts, and past experience are indeed held within our own flesh. All sorts of old memories, feelings, and fears seemed to be encoded in some mysterious way in my muscles. As you work muscle intensively, sometimes these rise to the surface to be lifted off, much as the body is detoxified of physical toxins on a fast. Frequently, I found myself pushed to my absolute limits. Then the gym floor would be covered equally with my sweat and my tears. Still, thanks to Rhod's presence and a will that came out of somewhere deep inside me, I kept working.

Now, a year later, I am glad that I have. I have discovered that working with muscle in this way transforms the body in an outer way by changing LBM-to-fat ratio and reshaping your body, which has all sorts of wonderful rewards. It also, in many ways that are even more wonderful, helps develop from within a slow but steadily growing sense of self-confidence, clarity, and independence. For many, myself included, this is a deep change that would have been virtually impossible to come by any other way. It now seems to me that working with muscle slowly and steadily day after day builds a powerful bridge between one's inner and outer world. So now when I think back to all those fairy tales about transformation, about frogs and princes, for the first time in my life I feel I am beginning to understand them and to understand what real transformation through the body is about. It is not all glitzy like they say in the movies. It is slow and inexorable. Yet it brings in its wake gifts far beyond our wildest dreams.

CHAPTER THIRTEEN

THE ALCHEMY OF ENERGY
21st-Century Energy-Based Medicine Is Here Now

*M*any years ago, the brilliant Nobel laureate Albert Szent-Györgyi, who isolated vitamin C, was prone to asking a peculiar question at dinner parties: "What is the difference between a living rat and a dead one?" According to the laws of classical chemistry and Newtonian physics, there should be no fundamental difference. Szent-Györgyi's reply to his own question was simple yet revolutionary: "Some kind of electricity." Living systems are first and foremost energy systems. And the "electricity" of which Szent-Györgyi speaks is the mysterious life energy, which distinguishes us from inanimate things in the universe. The alchemy of energy deals with the means of enhancing it.

The biochemical approach to natural menopause that we have been looking at so far involves things like the manipulation of hormones, changes in diet, and the use of selected botanicals that aim to bring about changes in the body's functioning through *physical* or *chemical* means. And they are terribly important. There is no substitute for supplementing a natural hormone like progesterone where it is needed, or for using botanical products to shift hot flashes, restore emotional balance, and banish insomnia, just as there is no effective way of improving bone strength and density unless, in addition to any hormonal support needed, you exercise and follow a wholesome diet, ensuring that the vitamins, minerals, and trace elements your body needs are optimally supplied. But there is another equally essential dimension to health, emotional well-being, and spiritual development that such approaches only address obliquely, if at all. In the linear, drug-based thinking of the late 20th century, this dimension of health and healing is too often neglected: the *energy* dimension.

The Order of Energy

Your body is not just a collection of physical and chemical events. Like all living systems, it is a unified collection of energy fields. Take action to alter the quality of these fields, and you can change the way your body functions for ill or good. You can even change how you think and feel. In a living organism, it is energy, not chemistry or physical form, that is *primary*. Shift it and the organism will in turn alter itself chemically and physically. This is how acupuncture works and why practicing certain martial arts can so affect health and personal power. And this is what lies at the core of energy medicine.

A great deal of the most advanced diagnostic equipment used today in orthodox medicine—from ECGs (electrocardiograms) for looking at heart function and EEGs (electroencephalograms) for examining brain function, as well as MRI (magnetic resonance imaging) and EMGs (electromyelograms)—already make use of the principles of energy medicine. Rather like Dr. McCoy's approach to healing on *Star Trek*, the new energy medicine goes way beyond mere diagnostic techniques such as these. It looks set to become the medicine of the 21st century.

Sometimes an energy approach to health and healing employs mindshifting techniques such as meditation and body movement (like Tai Chi) to improve the way the body feels and functions. At other times, it makes use of external energy carriers such as homeopathic remedies or space-age equipment that subject the body to external fields of some sort (magnetic, sonic, acoustic, electrical, light waves). Whatever its source, the aim of all forms of energy treatments—from the use of something as simple as the Bach Flower Remedies to actions of the advanced light beam generators—is to enhance life energy by restoring energetic *order*. Energetic order is the key to high-level well-being. It lifts vitality and intensifies mental clarity, enhances spiritual awareness, and triggers self-healing, while at the same time improving the specific function of the body's various organs and systems. After an energy treatment, the liver works better and can metabolize hormones well, and the adrenals are strengthened so a woman is better able to handle stress. Reestablishing energetic order improves the function of the pituitary and hypothalamus, which are responsible for the control of hormones, and makes the assimilation of nutrients and micronutrients from the foods we eat more available to us. But to understand a little of how the energy dimension works, we need to leave behind for the moment the biochemical world we have been exploring and move into the realm of high-level physics—the interface between consciousness and physical reality.

Negative Entropy

Two of the most important laws of physics are the laws of thermodynamics. Simply put, they are attempts to understand events in the universe by studying the kind of energy changes that accompany them. The First Law of Thermodynamics states that the quantity of energy in the world remains constant. Energy is neither created nor destroyed; it is simply transmuted from one form to another. The Second Law of Thermodynamics is central to an understanding of why energetic order lies at the core of physical and spiritual well-being and how energy medicine can be used to enhance health. It is best formulated in terms of *entropy*. Entropy is a measure of *disorder*.

This Second Law is known as the *law of entropy*. It describes the way that, left to their own devices, all things in the world become disordered—iron rusts, buildings crumble, dead flowers decay, and so forth. In short, everything tends toward *maximum* entropy, a state of maximum disorder in which all useful energy has been decreased. But what is remarkable about living organisms, including our own bodies, and what still puzzles the world's finest scientific minds, is that, despite the law of entropy, so long as we are alive, our bodies maintain themselves in a state of fantastic improbability. In the words of Albert Szent-Györgyi, who spent most of his life trying to penetrate this mystery:

> Life is a paradox...the most basic rule of inanimate nature is that it tends toward equilibrium which is at the maximum of entropy and the minimum of free energy. The main characteristic of life is that it tends to decrease its entropy. It also tends to increase its free energy. Maximum entropy means complete randomness, disorder. Life is made possible by order, structure, a pattern, which is the opposite of entropy. This pattern is our chief possession; it was developed over billions of years. The main

aim of our existence is its conservation and transmission. Life is a revolt against the statistical rules of physics. Death means that the revolt subsided and statistical laws resumed their sway.

Of the Highest Order

In a way that no one has ever been able to explain, living organisms, unlike things in the inorganic world, are superbly equipped to maintain energetic order. This, in turn, supports physical and biochemical well-being. It is something that makes virtually no sense within the paradigms of chemistry and Newtonian physics. Where, by rights, there should be little difference in the chemical and physical processes taking place within a living body and those that occur in a corpse, in reality there is every difference in the world. Living systems create for themselves a high degree of *negative entropy*— despite the fact that events in the universe as a whole are running wild to destroy it. For, in spite of the innumerable destructive processes continually going on in and around us, we have the power to resist entropy and to maintain energetic order. Indeed, there is every indication that so long as we live, we are continually involved in the process of creating even more order. This we do both individually in the repair functions of our cells and enzymatic systems and also from an evolutionary point of view, since living organisms appear to continue to differentiate into ever more complex and highly structured organisms as time passes. And the better the quality of order in our bodies, the healthier and more vital we remain, regardless of age.

Negative Entropy Means Menopausal Freedom

From an energetic point of view, aging is the process that transports a woman's body from a highly ordered internal state toward maximum entropy—that is, death. There are two ways in which this can happen. Either energetic order or the biochemical harmony that depends on it is steadily eroded so that the body and mind slowly but surely degenerate (as they do in most people these days), or we can take informed action to support energetic order and maintain negative entropy to the highest degree.

By taking the second route, we are able, in effect, to *die young late in life*. But such a goal can never be accomplished entirely by manipulating chemistry alone. One of the first scientists to recognize this was another

Nobel laureate, the physicist Erwin Schrodinger. He took a close look at the scientific contradictions implicit in the living state and concluded that so long as the human body is alive, it resists entropy and avoids decaying into an inert state of equilibrium through metabolism—by eating, drinking, and assimilating various kinds of information from the environment.

As far back as 1944, Schrodinger wrote:

> Every process, event, happening—call it what you will; in a word, everything that is going on in Nature means an increase of the entropy of the part of the world where it is going on. Thus, a living organism continually increases its entropy—or as you may say, produces positive entropy....What an organism feeds upon is negative entropy...which is in itself a measure of order. Thus the device by which an organism maintains itself stationary at a fairly high level of orderliness really consists in continually sucking orderliness from its environment.

From an energetic point of view, a woman's body is an *open living system.* As such, it is constantly processing energetic and chemical *information* that comes to us not only through the kinds and combinations of foods we eat and the way we prepare and process them, but also from the air we breathe, the ideas on which we allow our minds to play, and the electromagnetic environment in which we live. In effect, as Schrodinger believed, and as a long tradition of natural medicine both in Europe and the Orient has taught, to ensure a high degree of vitality and to protect ourselves from degeneration, we need to "suck order" from our environment. To maintain the kind of energetic order that best fosters health and spiritual development during menopause and afterwards, we need a constant supply of the right information from the outside world.

Biophotons and Quantum Magic

Long ago, quantum physicists established that wave particles such as electrons, atoms, and molecules in living systems behave as biophoton energies. These energies appear to help regulate and control enzyme activities, cell reproduction, and other activities in living systems. Experiments such as those reported in the March 1995 issue of *Scientific American* by Brumer and Shapiro has well established the existence of these particle/wave reactions in organisms. Like lightbulbs, atoms give out radiant bio-energies that can either act constructively or destructively on the body's own molecules. Scientists are beginning to define how the interference wave forms generated both by internally manufactured toxins and by environmental pollutants—another name for life energies—on which health and protection from premature aging depend work constructively to support health and vitality. Within the next decade, we are going to hear a lot more about these biophoton energies and their effects on our health. For now, we can still make practical use of the knowledge already available on how to influence them for healing and regeneration.

Energy Consciousness

From the point of view of quantum physics, as human beings we are not only immersed in an energy field, but our bodies, our minds, and our selves *are* energy fields. These fields are constantly expanding, contracting, and changing as our thoughts, diet, and lifestyle change. The aim of any form of natural treatment—from dietary change and detoxification to hydrotherapy, exercise, and meditation—is first to enhance positive bio-energies in an organism, and second to help to balance them and create order.

Many researchers now work with bio-energies and the kind of transformations they can bring about. Medical intuitives such as Caroline Myss, international lecturer on human consciousness, are capable of clairvoyantly examining subtle energy states in a person and of pinpointing where his or her bio-energies are being dissipated. In doing so, Myss helps people learn to work with their own bio-energies to bring about self-healing.

Sheer Radiance

Meanwhile, in University Parapsychology Research Laboratories such as the one at UCLA, scientists such as Dr. Thelma Moss have experimented with techniques such as Kirlian photography to examine, record, and analyze the unique energetic patterns that living things emanate. Kirlian photography is one of the methods whereby ordinary nonvisible force fields around and through living and nonliving things can be recorded visually and studied. Kirlian photographs are extraordinarily beautiful. Researchers find they get consistent results when working with the Kirlian method to photograph plants and foods when comparing cooked foods with their raw counterparts, for instance, or the leaf of a healthy plant to the leaf of a damaged one. The luminescent energy corona recorded on film from a living thing such as a healthy plant, or one of the superfoods such as organically grown herbs, wild crafted algae, organic green juices, or plant enzymes, is significantly stronger, more radiant, and wider than in that of a processed food. The corona produced by well-harvested spirulina or an organic raw carrot or cauliflower is dramatically reduced when these foods are cooked or processed. Uncooked vegetables and fruits radiate brilliant spikes of light, harmoniously surrounded by geometric shapes. Cooked and processed foods show only the dimmest evidence of corona discharge. Foods, plants, and herbs with a wide corona carry a lot of the life energy useful for rejuvenation.

Etheric Forces

Chromatography is another tool useful for studying energy. It is widely used in chemistry, biology, medicine, and industry as a way of analyzing complex substances such as the amino acids in a protein or for detecting impurities in a compound. The use of chromatography to measure energy differences between living things and between natural and synthetically made substances was originally developed by European chemist Ehrenfreid Pfeiffer.

Early on in his career, Pfeiffer was asked by the German mystic Rudolph Steiner to find a chemical reagent that could be useful in charting the quality of life energy—what Steiner called the *formative etheric forces*—in living matter. After experimenting with many different substances, Pfeiffer discovered that when he added extracts of living plants to a solution of copper chloride then let it evaporate slowly, it would produce a beautiful pattern of crystallization typical of the species of the plant used. Radiant form and shape consistently indicated the life strength of the plant. Pfeiffer established that strong crystallization patterns indicated health, while weak ones indicated ill health.

Nowadays, scientists working with techniques such as chromatography, Kirlian photography, photomicography, and polarized light field photography—as well as clairvoyant healers who can actually "see" changes in energy patterns around plants, people, and animals—confirm that certain foods, herbs, and plant products carry high levels of harmonious bio-energy. They can be used to enhance the beauty of a living organism's energy patterns.

So can techniques of breathing, meditation, and deep relaxation, as well as the laying on of hands or spiritual healing, hydrotherapy, bodywork, and autogenics. That is why all of these things can be so helpful in the rejuvenation process.

Healing the Impossible

One of the most interesting researchers to look into the area of life force–energy treatments for healing and regeneration is the American healer Mitchell May. At the age of 22, May was in a car accident that rendered him profoundly damaged. He lost several inches of bone from his legs, and the tissue and nerve damage was extensive. He lay in insufferable pain. His physicians told him he would never walk again and that it was necessary to have his right leg amputated. They also informed him that his immune system would be permanently compromised and that his health would be severely restricted for the rest of his life. May was lucky enough to have been hospitalized at one of the most important medical research centers in the world, the University of California Medical Center at Los Angeles. There, he became part of a special study involving ongoing experiments into life-force healing and extrasensory perceptions, using skilled spiritual healers working under strict scientific controls. He met and worked with a very gifted healer named Jack Gray. Gray had a great gift in his ability to activate powerful and natural healing life-force energies within a person. Within a week of Gray's having begun a simple laying-on-of-hands treatment, May discovered that he was able to turn off and on his experience of excruciating pain using the techniques Gray taught him.

Energy Healing

May became fascinated with the whole area of life-force healing and became an apprentice to Gray. He developed an interest in states of consciousness, subtle energy, and in discovering ways to enhance life force through the use of spiritual healing, plant foods, and biological compounds—those which have a particularly high quality of energetic radiation. May's own story is one of the most well-documented tales of impossible recovery in medical annals. Not only did his body heal, he was able to learn to walk again and now, almost 25 years later, he has full use of his body. In the process, he has also become one of the most respected and acclaimed healers in the world.

During the period of his recovery, May worked intimately with Gray, and with Thelma Moss in her Parapsychology Research Laboratory at UCLA, photographing energy patterns around foods and other nutritional substances. He also carried out wide searches of scientific literature and conferred with physicists, health professionals, doctors, and practitioners of natural medicine, trained in both Western science and Eastern health traditions. He set out to discover, test, and record information about specific foods and plant compounds that can enhance human health—not only chemically by supplying an abundance of vitamins, minerals, phyto-antioxidants and immune enhancers, but also by providing an abundance of life force. May wanted to find ways of making it possible to help people live at their fullest energy, vitality, and wholeness, in maximum health and well-being.

Entranced by Beauty

Before long, May became totally fascinated by the beauty of energy patterns certain foods and plants emitted. He also became convinced—as had many researchers before and after him—that the fundamental processes of healing and rejuvenation depend on intensifying the life force within an individual and then helping to bring about a harmonization and balance of its movements within the living system. He saw that there was so much potential to help people by working in an energetic way. He also discovered (as have practitioners of natural medicine) that it is not just food and plants that are able to enhance the life force. He experimented with many forms of meditation and breathing, shifts in attitudes of mind, and various healing modalities, energy-shifting exercise such as Tai-Chi, yoga and the martial arts, which enable us to awaken the life force within.

Most of all, he loved working with plants. Slowly, painstakingly, he identified plants, algae, mushrooms, sprouted seeds, and grains, all of which carry an abundance of this life energy. He also found they could be used to intensify a person's own life energy and help create coherent and harmonious patterns of energy within. As early researchers into the healing effects of living foods such as Dr. Max Bircher-Benner and Dr. Max Gerson had insisted, plants are holders and emitters of *quantum sunlight*— life force that we can use to our advantage, either taken fresh and live or when grown, harvested and dried properly, since these plants are able to transfer their life force to us.

Perfect Balance

May's highly practical experiments were carried out over 20 years, during which he conferred with the very finest medical practitioners in Western medicine, as well as experts in Chinese and Ayurvedic medicine, and spiritual healers. Slowly, painstakingly, he was able to identify foods and plants—organically grown—with a particular abundance of life force and to develop ways of further heightening their powers for healing by combining them in a carefully formulated synergistic way, so that the energies of each balanced and enhanced the energies of the others. Out of this, he developed what I believe to be the most remarkable and potent nutritional supplement that I have ever come across. It is called Pure Synergy. Its combination of 62 of nature's most potent and nourishing components include organically grown freeze-dried herbs, organically grown immune supporting mushrooms, plant enzymes, freeze-dried royal jelly, wild crafted algae, organic green juices, and many other natural ingredients, and is the finest superfood made so far (see Resources).

Bodymind

By no means does all energy medicine come in the form of foods and plant products. Practitioners of Ayurvedic medicine, qi gong, yoga, and meditation have throughout the ages insisted that consciousness plays the central role in governing physical and psychological health. For generations, the power of the subtle energies of consciousness or the mind to influence the body have been preached. Only recently, however, have researchers begun to draw scientific maps of how this occurs. Much of their new knowledge comes out of a fascinating medical and biochemical discipline with an absurdly long name—*psychoneuroimmunology*—or PNI, for short. Far from being two separate entities, mind and body are more like opposite ends of a *bodymind* continuum—two aspects of a living being— and PNI is the scientific study of the bodymind. Western scientists working with mind/body medicine such as Dr. Joan Borysenko and Dr. Candice Pert, former Chief of Brain Biochemistry at the Clinical Neuroscience Branch of the National Institute on Mental Health in the United States, have been charting in measurable physical terms some of the pathways by which mind influences energetic order for better or worse. They have also been exploring ways and means of empowering people by discovering mental and physical techniques that can enhance that order.

PNI first rose to prominence in the late 1970s, then broadened its base to include high-level physics and psychology, out of which a new science of consciousness is being forged—another way of looking at life and health from the point of view of energetic order that creates the underlying patterns of the universe. It sees human beings as part of a universal energy field, interconnected with all of life, and recognizes that the action of hormones in your body plays a central role in bodymind functions and the way in which thought, in turn, affects hormonal balance.

Leading researchers in the field of PNI have discovered that the human mind, which includes our conscious thoughts and unconscious impulses, as well as what could be called our superconscious or transcendent mind and our emotions, are all elaborately interwoven with every function of the body via nerve pathways and chemical messengers, such as the endorphins, neuropeptides, and hormones. A powerful hormonal/nerve relationship exists between your sex steroids, such as estrogens and progesterone via the pituitary, the adrenals, and the hypothalamus. Known as the *hypothalamic pituitary adrenal axis*, it links thoughts and emotions with physical responses. New evidence even suggests that a few of the body's chemical messengers may be made of a single molecule whose configuration can actually be altered by a person's mental, emotional, and spiritual state to create new forms.

Bodymind Maps

With each passing month, more scientific maps of bodymind are being drawn. They show how what you think and feel powerfully influences the level of vitality you have, as well as how slowly or rapidly you age and the shifts of hormones in your body. It is because of these connections that so many hormonal disturbances in a woman's body have psychological or emotional components—from endometriosis (where the lining of the womb proliferates out of control) to PMS, dysmenorrhoea (painful periods), and amenorrhoea (the absence of a menstrual period). A woman's hormonal symphony, which is an important element of her bodymind, is such an important piece of music that it ideally should not be tampered with. The introduction of an artificial hormone or drug to a woman's body can be like trying to add an African rhythm to a baroque fugue. When the various receptors of hypothalamic and pituitary hormones are faced with having to cope with synthetically altered hormones, this can distort the balance in the endocrine system and disturb energetic order in the body as whole. Via the hypothalamic-pituitary-adrenal axis, it may also lead to a disturbance in a woman's thinking functions and to her emotional balance—so, by the way, can the mental and spiritual stress of her feeling trapped in a job or a relationship that she hates or that offers her soul no nourishment.

By contrast, the regular use of a meditation technique; of an energy-based exercise practice such as the Chinese Tai Chi; of biofeedback, through which one learns to exert conscious control over bodily processes; or of regular prayer; is a way of bringing energetic order back to the body— not only through the mechanisms of PNI, but in other ways so far only partly understood by doctors and scientists working in the fields of PNI. This, too, is an important branch of energy medicine.

Homeopathic Energetics

Energetic products can also be used to help restore harmony and order in the body. Take homeopathic medicines. The latest research into the ways in which homeopathic remedies work shows that their actions belong not to the realm of chemistry, but to the domain of quantum physics and the field of energy medicine that is taking shape out of it. In using ordinary chemical medicines and drugs, generally speaking, the higher the dose, the greater will be the effect. Just the opposite is the case with homeopathy, where the more a medicine is diluted, the higher its energetic potency becomes. Homeopathics are made by a process that entails diluting a substance or compound again and again in alcohol or water and then *succussing* it— shaking it vigorously. Lower doses of homeopathic remedies still contain traces of the substance from which they have been made even though their primary actions lie in the way the particular remedy's energy resonates with the energetic order of the person or animal being treated.

But, once any homeopathic is diluted one in 124 times or more, no trace remains of the compound or substance from which it was made. Examining such remedies, using nuclear magnetic resonance (NMR) imaging, researchers are able to do readings of their subatomic activity.

One researcher who has looked closely at the mechanisms by which they act is German biophysicist Dr. Wolfgang Ludwig. Ludwig has demonstrated in other ways that homeopathic remedies emit measurable electromagnetic signals and that the nature of dominant frequencies in these signals are specific to certain remedies. So are the Bach Flower remedies. These inexpensive and effective products for restoring harmony, and mental or emotional balance, can be very useful to women in their menstrual and menopausal years.

The homeopathic remedies most commonly used in menopause and hormonal complaints tend to be *Lachisis, Sepia, Pulsatilla, Apis, Aconite, Calcarea Carbonica, Cimicifuga racemosa, Sulphur,* and *Phosphorus.* But in the hands of a good homeopath, a remedy prescribed is always determined by a total picture of a woman's constitution and symptoms. This is one of the reasons that research validating the actions of homeopathic remedies can be hard to carry out. Unlike drugs, which are constantly given to any patient with a particular complaint, in homeopathy the same condition may call for completely different remedies according to the constitution of the person being treated. That being said, there was an interesting open study published in 1992 that investigated a German homeopathic combination remedy for menopause and PMS known as Mulimen. Made from *Agnus castus,* black cohosh, sepia, and St. John's wort, it was given to women over a three-month period. Out of 82 women treated, around 49 experienced significant relief from their symptoms from this alone. Half of the women who had been experiencing hot flashes became completely free of them.

Energetic Soul Alignment

If I could choose only one health-enhancing product for use year in and year out, it would be Vita Fons II. Vita Fons II is a second-generation version of something known as *Vita Florum,* developed by Elizabeth Bellhouse as a vehicle to carry what might be described as the energy of perfect balance and order. According to Bellhouse, each human being consists of seven different and interdependent levels of being: *body, soul, brain, emotions, and mind*—all of which are meant to communicate freely with the *divine core* via the *spirit.* When, for any number of reasons, the human spirit does not resonate in harmony with its divine core, a person's energetic order becomes distorted, energetic order is undermined, and optimal well-being becomes degraded. This can manifest in many ways—physical illness, emotional disturbances, or spiritual pain. When used on the body, Vita Fons II products are designed to help restore resonance with the divine core of an individual—the only element within each of us which is said to be totally perfect. This, in turn, strengthens a person's psychic and spiritual bodies and heightens an organism's natural abilities to maintain order, which in turn helps create physical health or restores it where it has been lost. It also encourages each individual spirit to create conditions that allow the perfection of his or her divine core to influence all aspects of a person's life.

Since the power of Vita Fons II is entirely nonchemical, its energy can be carried to the body in a number of different mediums—in water, in a tablet, in an ointment, lotion, massage oil, salve, or talcum powder. It is used over any areas of the body where there is discomfort, as well as over energy centers at the navel, heart region, solar plexus, and forehead. Because it is the energy in Vita Fons II and not the material substance from which it is made that does the work, it is not the amount of any Vita Fons II product that you use that is important, but rather the frequency with which you use it. When well, a woman of, say, 50 years old might use the water six times a day to maintain order. If she were ill, she would increase the frequency of use depending upon the severity of the illness.

The company that produces Vita Fons II is controlled by a nonprofit charitable trust whose purpose is to make available this high order of energy product to all who want it. The products are available throughout the world either by mail order or through appointed importers. Reports of the positive transformation and physical healing from users are by now legion. Bellhouse has written an interesting book, *Life's Flowering*, that delves into the subtle nature of Vita Fons II, how it works, and what the value of this very special energy is in the modern world.

Energetic Rejuvenation

Mitchell May, and others like him, such as Dr. David Peat and two-time Nobel nominee Robert O. Becker, have delved deeply into the field of subtle energies. Their work is helping to build bridges between orthodox, chemically based allopathic medicine (which until recently paid little attention to the energetic aspects of healing) and the ancient traditions of medicine that have always viewed healing as primarily an energy art. Breathing, movement, thoughts, and dreams, as well as the metabolism of the foods that we eat, all contribute to active energy "information" or life "intelligence" capable of bringing about a continuous circulation of harmonious energy to transform and heal the body. Energetically speaking, illness and degeneration are viewed as some sort of misalignment or blockage that interferes with the natural flow of energy, perverting its natural balance or siphoning energy off from its natural vital function of supporting the body.

DISTANT THUNDER
Personal Health, Autonomy, and All That Challenges It

Since the Industrial Revolution, we have been steeped in para-digms or models about health and medicine that are frequently in opposition to the basic principles of natural law—principles that have been affirmed throughout history by all the great religions of the world and recently validated by scientific discoveries in high-level physics. They include an awareness of *wholeness* that implies the interrelatedness of all things, an acknowledgment of the *energetic nature of life*, and an appre-ciation that health and illness are not two separate states (the former to be preserved at all costs and the latter to be wiped out as quickly as possible), but rather opposite ends of the life continuum. What each of us experiences at any moment in relation to health and illness is nothing more than a par-ticular degree within a multiplicity of degrees at some point along that con-tinuum, an expression of the birth-death-regeneration cyclical nature of life.

Our Western health/medical paradigm or model looks upon the phenom-enon of the universe, at life itself, as an accidental occurrence, nothing more than a complex but ultimately explainable series of chemical and physical reactions to be studied, classified, and manipulated to our advantage. Such a paradigm or model, unconscious though it is in most of us, has led to our con-sidering both doctor and ailing patient as separate from the health/disease process. It has also led us to ignore any relationship between mind or spirit and an organism's state of health. Finally, it has created a tendency toward treating disease as a measurable, quantifiable, pathological state affecting specific tissues, organs, or systems that has little relationship to the thoughts, feelings and lifestyle of the sick person—that illness arises entirely as a result of outside events such as trauma, infection, or simply bad luck.

Science of Fragmentation

Such a model has had value. It has provided us with an elaborate science of diagnosis enabling us to identify innumerable disease conditions. It has also made possible the study of specific effects of a myriad of chemicals and drugs, which may be used to "fix things"—to kill the microbe or wipe out the symptoms. Unfortunately, it has also resulted in our losing sight of the woods by confronting only the trees. By listening only to the tumor or the infective agent present in a disease state without reference to the overall condition of the person who is sick, we have become deaf to whatever possible "messages" may be being spoken from the unconscious or superconscious mind. We have eliminated the possibility, through listening to these messages, of learning more of the "language" of illness and health, and of how to work with the body's own processes to help transform the former into the latter. Instead, our modern way of operating with illness has become to eradicate a symptom, to replace a defective part, or to suppress a pathological process. It is an approach described by theologian Paul Tillich as "unhealthy health."

Such is the thinking behind most conventional treatment offered women for menstrual and menopausal problems. In an attempt to alleviate symptoms, regardless of long-term costs to the physical and spiritual health of the woman being treated, there has as yet been little attempt to identify the reasons why female complaints have taken on epidemic proportions in the 20th century. Nor, too, are questions much asked about the relationship between the health of the individual and the health of the planet. Until, as women, we demand that they be asked; until we come to the point where, instead of looking at disease from a linear, masculine point of view as an entity to be suppressed or destroyed at all cost, we begin to see it in a female way as an expression of the cyclical nature of life fully connected with a human being's feelings, dreams, disappointments, and the environment in which we live—we will have to content ourselves with makeshift half-solutions to complex female problems.

Growing Market

During the first half of the 20th century, menopause was viewed as a natural physiological occurrence that rarely required medical intervention. Only after synthetic hormones (the estrogens and progestogens) were developed, did it come to be described as a hormone-deficiency disease. The medical profession has gradually extended its scope of action way beyond that of the diagnosis and treatment of disease that used to be its purpose—to encompass the "control" and "management" of what was considered a perfectly normal event in a woman's life. One doesn't even need to fall into the paranoid trap of suspecting conspiracy to wonder about the coincidence between the demographic emergence of the post-war baby-boomer market—more than 100 million women in the United States and Europe alone coming of menopausal age—at the same time that menopause has been labeled a deficiency disease. The potential market for hormone drugs is the largest in history. Pharmaceutical manufacturers have only begun to tap in to it.

Once you define menopause as a disease, then you need to find a "cure" for it. In making use of the cure (HRT drugs), you are putting the body at risk of cancer and numerous other side effects, no matter how infrequently they occur. If, instead, you choose to define menopause as a natural change in a woman's life, a passage from one stage of her life to another physically, emotionally, and spiritually, then you are faced with an altogether different challenge. You are not trying to *cure* anything. You are instead in the business of affirming this change as natural, and looking out for information and techniques that can not only make it as easy as possible (as we already have with natural childbirth), but also of helping each woman use her symptoms whether they be emotional or physical as roads to further empowerment. There is no money in such an approach, and most of the men and women who are the trailblazers in the natural menopause revolution are neither wealthy nor selling anything other than the truth.

A Complex Web

The practice of medicine and the training that any doctor receives has to be constantly updated because things change so rapidly. Every doctor is faced with choices about whether to go for further education after leaving medical school. In organized medicine, both in Europe and the United States, most information and continuing medical education offered to doctors comes from pharmaceutical corporations. Doctors' lives are very busy. They are filled with the demands of their patients. It is not all that easy for them to keep up with the constantly evolving scientific research that can enable them to make shifts and alterations in the treatment methods employed.

Most of the post-graduate education that our doctors receive after they leave medical school (even our specialists, such as endocrinologists and gynecologists) comes not from the experience of other doctors nor even from reading scientific journals, but straight from the medical-industrial complex. This is a close-knit association of pharmaceutical manufacturers, organized medicine, and medical regulatory agencies at government level. But the medical-industrial complex has its limitations. It does not have to be corrupt to be vulnerable to the same weaknesses and human prejudices that the rest of us suffer from. The manufacture and distribution of drugs to the public is a multinational business on which medical research itself is dependent for some of the billion-dollar grants offered to doctors, biochemists, university scientists, and other organizations throughout the industrialized world to enable them to carry out their research. This creates a complex web in which the medical establishment, pharmaceutical manufacturers, and government regulatory bodies are closely connected to one another, so much so that many people at the top of their profession in one group will shift, often more than once during their career, to another group.

The goal of a pharmaceutical company, just like the goal of any business, is to make a profit. In this case, profit comes from the sale of drugs that carry a patent—that is, drugs that are chemically unique. When a patent belongs to a particular company, the company is protected against any of its competitors selling the same product. Such a company is quite naturally not interested in carrying out research on nonpatentable medicines, such as widely available herbs or natural progesterone, regardless of how great their health benefits may be. Neither are they going to inform doctors about the potential such natural compounds might have for improving human health. To do so would undermine their own sales. Instead, the flow of research money out of pharmaceutical manufacturers tends to be directed toward establishing the efficacy of patented drugs. As a result, scientists working in research, as well as doctors whose largest source of information after leaving medical school comes from the medical-industrial complex, tend only to have experience with the use of patented drugs. They remain largely unaware of natural products or techniques that can be used but are nonpatentable. This is the main reason why it is not surprising when a government official, industry-supported consultant, or academic expert speaks out against some natural form of treatment. Be it hydrotherapy, acupuncture, or the use of a compound such as natural progesterone, he or she is likely to dismiss its value. Such people often have very little, if any, personal knowledge of the subject.

In many ways, it is little wonder that doctors are so ill informed about differences between the actions of natural progesterone and those of the progestogens with which it is so often confused, especially when even the medical references to studies inaccurately refer to various synthetic progestogens as "progesterone" in discussing their actions and side effects. What does seem particularly sad is that occasionally even some of the most conscientious researchers—professionals who have spent much of their career informing the public about the long-term dangers of using hormone drugs—can fall prey to the same error.

What are the arguments against the use of natural progesterone, and who has come out strongly against it? Surprisingly, very few doctors, even very few gynecologists who prescribe HRT regularly to their patients, have even voiced an opinion—probably because they are still not aware of it as an alternative and because, like much of the medical literature on the subject, they wrestle to clarify the confusion between a synthetic progestogen and progesterone itself—the same molecule that is found in a woman's body.

So far, Britain's most vocal opponent of natural progesterone use has been the writer Dr. Ellen Grant—a researcher and expert in the use of a nutritional approach to female problems, from PMS to menopausal troubles. I have always had enormous respect for Dr. Grant's work. Almost singlehandedly, she has gathered material together and made public the long-term dangers of the use of contraceptive pills. Over the years, I have learned much from her. However, when it comes to the progesterone issue, Dr. Grant is vehemently opposed to it. In fact, she strongly opposes the use of *any* steroid hormones—natural or artificial.

A few months ago, in response to an interview with John Lee about natural progesterone, which appeared in the newsletter *What Doctors Don't Tell You*, Grant wrote an article called "Hormonal Mayhem," in which she expressed her opinion that natural progesterone supplementation, like the use of synthetic progestogens, is riddled with dangers. She claimed that John Lee had made three fundamental mistakes—asserting that progesterone supplementation is safe, regarding natural progesterone as any different from the synthetic progestogens, and claiming that osteoporosis is in some way related to progesterone. Grant writes that "even small amounts of extra progesterone, estrogen, or testosterone at key times during pregnancy can interfere profoundly with physical and mental development and sexual orientation," citing animal studies by Dr. Gina Schoental to support her statement.

Out of respect for Ellen Grant's opinion, and because it was important to me before incorporating the information on the use of natural progesterone into this book, I carefully examined the references on which she was relying to back up her assertions, including Gina Schoental's work. I was surprised to learn that, when contacted, Dr. Schoental confirmed that her work had never involved progesterone.

In the same article, Dr. Grant also warns of the dangers of progesterone use, claiming that progesterone suppresses immunity, that together with viruses and chemicals it acts as a co-carcinogen (cancer causer) and has a number of other negative actions. When a doctor colleague and I later examined in depth the papers cited by Dr. Grant to support her assertions, we were forced to disagree with many of the conclusions that she drew from them.

There are three ways in which the natural progesterone molecule that is chemically identical to the progesterone produced in a woman's body is a unique hormone. First, it is the main precursor of other important steroids such as the corticosteroids. Unlike the progestogens, it is not an end-product molecule. Second, it provides many important intrinsic functions in the body. Third, it is remarkably free of side effects such as those listed so extensively for the synthetic progestins. So far the lack of distinction between natural progesterone and their synthetic analogues appears largely a semantic problem wrought by the use of the word *progesterone* as a generic term for progestogens as a whole. It is little wonder that the average GP or gynecologist is likely to be ill informed on the subject of natural progesterone and its use.

However, it is my belief that in time—given the mounting numbers of women whose well-being is restored in part at least through the use of natural progesterone—even those who know little or nothing about it will come to see how much it has to offer. The people who are going to be most instrumental in bringing this about are the key players in the bloodless revolution—women themselves who report to each other, to the press, and to their doctors their experience of its use. After all, it was only through public awareness of the existence of food allergies and the profound effects they can exert on health that the medical profession slowly came round to looking at the issue and finally to taking it into account. So, I suspect, will it be with natural progesterone.

At the moment, many doctors—ignorant of xenoestrogens and unaware of the estrogen dominance to which they contribute—still insist that women need to take estrogen either together with a progestogen or on its own as menopause approaches. They tell you that the risk of cancer is minute in comparison with all of the protection that HRT provides and that it will automatically relieve the anguish of hot flashes and numerous other troublesome symptoms that are supposed to result from menopause. What they don't tell you is that there are other, safer, easier, and less expensive ways— both in terms of money and in terms of potential strain on the body and psyche. These include natural herbs, natural progesterone products, dietary change, homeopathy, and lifestyle change. And the reason they don't tell you is because, by and large, they do not know. In the face of the elaborate network that disseminates information about drugs, there is so far no economic or political pressure group that could even begin to compete in public-relations terms to give the other side of the story.

Beware of Watchdogs

In the Western world, it is the United States Food and Drug Administration (the FDA) which takes the lead in the approval of a food or drug for distribution. What the FDA decides today becomes a blueprint for action in other countries tomorrow. When, a few years ago, a poisonous batch of the amino acid tryptophan was discovered in America, the FDA took this amino acid entirely off the market. Country after country followed suit, and it has never returned. In 1962, the FDA was given broad powers to regulate "articles intended for use in the diagnosis, cure, mitigation, treatment, or prevention of disease in man or other animals" as well as "articles (other than food) intended to affect the structure of any function of the body of man or other animals."

There is a popular misconception that the FDA is an effective and efficient watchdog constantly looking out for the interests of people by testing the safety and efficacy of various drugs, nutritional products, and remedies. This is simply not the case. It is the pharmaceutical manufacturers—not the FDA—who test the products they have developed. They then submit their results to the FDA for its approval. The average cost of testing a single new drug today is phenomenal—over $200 million. Even if a product or drug receives FDA approval, this does not mean that it is safe. There are instances where pharmaceutical manufacturers have withheld information about side effects, and many more when serious side effects have been discovered only after years of a drug's use by hundreds and thousands of patients. Manufacturers of simple natural remedies are unable to afford the huge expense of applying for FDA approval. The safety and effectiveness of various botanical products and natural progesterone creams is well supported by clinical experience over decades. But these remedies are not publicized widely, and few doctors therefore know about them. There is also virtually no money available to carry out the tests necessary to receive FDA approval on a generic product that cannot be patented. So natural remedies and approaches to health often remain well-kept secrets—publicized, if at all, only by practitioners who have used them and know they work, and women whose lives have been changed by them.

Drug or Cosmetic

Remedies such as natural progesterone creams, pellets, and oils are effective and safe. However, companies that manufacture them—not only in the United States but in other countries—are in the absurd position of being unable to say anything publicly about their efficacy. With the exception of natural remedies already widely in use in the United States, when the major amendments to the Food, Drug, and Cosmetic Act were made in 1962 that demanded lengthy and expensive testing to prove a drug's efficacy, natural generic remedies could not be sold as such. In fact, manufacturers of natural treatment products and nutritional supplements are not even allowed to give their products names that suggest how they are to be used. This means that natural products need to keep a low profile.

You will find that natural progesterone creams will not even say "progesterone" on the label; they must speak in veiled language about "wild yam extract" instead. And they will be referred to as "cosmetics" simply because if they were correctly labeled, they would have to be categorized as drugs and could not be sold without a license. One of the unfortunate things about the position in which the FDA has placed manufacturers of these products is that there is no way of establishing the quality of one product as compared to another by being able to inform customers about a product's manufacture and what standards it maintains. So, together with the two or three best natural progesterone products, you can find some copycat second-cousin versions manufactured by companies without the best technology and without the real knowledge to produce a high-quality product. Meanwhile, the women who may have heard about natural progesterone cream, and want to try it, find it very difficult to know which is the best product to buy.

In 1994, a British company called Higher Nature began importing a good range of natural progesterone products into Britain. They were responsible and intelligent in the way this was done. The company provided seminars for doctors and other health practitioners, as well as talks for the general public and the press, inviting doctors of the caliber of John Lee to present their clinical findings, background information on progesterone, and protocols for use. Higher Nature set up a panel of trained nutritionists whom professionals and nonprofessionals alike could contact by telephone for further information and advice. They also made available research papers, as well as independently produced reports and books to anyone wishing to buy them. The reception for the new products turned out to be excellent, particularly since a growing number of far-sighted British doctors soon became highly enthusiastic about the results their patients were getting from their use.

Within a few months, the company was forced to stop selling the products except by prescription. This is how things have remained since. As it stands now, any woman in Britain wanting to make use of a good natural progesterone product has two options. Either she goes to a doctor who she knows works with them and hopes that, after examining her, he or she will prescribe them, or she can order the products—quite legally—from abroad for her personal use only. Yet the protocols for the use of these valuable products remain hard to come by for a woman who needs them. Meanwhile, the biggest irony is this: What few doctors are aware of is that the routinely prescribed combinations of estrogen/progesterone now used as HRT have in fact *never* been approved by the FDA for use as hormone replacement therapy for postmenopausal women. As Gail Sheehy says:

> I also found that Provera has never been approved for treatment of menopause by the U.S. Food and Drug Administration. Notwithstanding, the FDA's Advisory Committee on Fertility and Maternal Health Drugs stated in 1991 that this combination of hormones [i.e., estrogen progestogen combinations] may be used indefinitely by a woman with a uterus. Asked what proportion of the female population over age fifty would be suitable candidates for long-term consumption of estrogen alone or combined with synthetic progesterone [sic], the committee replied, "Virtually all. A blank check."

As Ellen Hodgson Brown who wrote the introduction to *Breezing Through the Change* says:

> The FDA has never approved the estrogen/progestin combination as hormone replacement therapy for postmenopausal women, so its long-term risks are unknown. What research does show is that progestins may reverse the cardiovascular benefits of estrogen; and they do *not* reverse its increased risk of breast cancer and may increase it. Synthetic progestins also come with a long list of side effects many women are unable or unwilling to endure.

In recent decades, women have taken greater and greater control over their own lives. We have exercised choice about whether and when to have children, about the kind of relationships we have with our men or with other women. Yet, what I see happening is that our assertion of choice and independence is being used and fed into the HRT mania that interferes with the very freedom of body, mind, and spirit that natural menopause can offer a healthy woman, for the process that Noam Chomsky has named "manufacturing consent" is most certainly taking place in the continued insistence that women at menopause are fundamentally in need of medical management. Meanwhile, the revolution in natural menopause continues to expand, its primary thrust coming from women themselves. After all, it is we who fought for our right to choose to bear children or to remain childless. It is we who demanded that our men be allowed into the delivery room and that we have the choice of a drug-free childbirth at home. And it is my belief that women will ultimately decide how to handle menopause or indeed just how much handling of it is needed.

As it once was with natural childbirth, the knowledge about how to use many of the best natural products and treatments for women can only come from individual scientists and, ultimately far more important, by word of mouth from women themselves—women who, having struggled to find their own way through menopause and out the other side with what information they could glean, pass on their knowledge to other women who need guidance and help. One day I hope there will be a self-supporting organization rather like La Leche League to give practical advice to women who need it. That kind of information is the best you can find anywhere, because it is information based not on theoretical ideas, but on practical experience and bonds of respect—not only for the female body and psyche, but for the magnificence of life itself. It also has nothing to sell except the truth.

PART II

THE SCIENCE OF MYTH

CHAPTER FIFTEEN

MOONSTRUCK

The Passion and Power of Female Rituals

*I*t is not easy to be female at the dawn of the new millennium. In the past half century, a woman's place as defined by society has undergone drastic shifts and revisions, many of which have offered us greater freedom of choice. Women have demanded, and to some degree achieved, equal opportunities at work with men. We have refused to spend all of our lives in supportive roles. We have sought out new ways of relating to our families, our work colleagues, and friends—as well as to ourselves. We have also gone a long way toward eroding long-standing negative assumptions about the female, the idea that as women we are too emotional, too unfocused, and too fickle to accomplish anything significant. We have proven that women have good minds and are capable of high achievement academically, in business, and in the arts. Yet being a woman in today's world demands that we be willing to live the life of a juggler. Each of us has become involved in a never-ending task of trying to keep the balls of our life's roles in the air—professional woman, mother, worker, lover, wife, achiever—while we get through each day, week, and year.

Daughters of the Father

Many women have chosen to walk away from the limited, self-sacrificing lives they watched their mothers lead—lives that too often produced

grief and bitterness as the menopause years approached. Instead of following in the footsteps of the traditional female whose primary role was concerned with nurturing, they have looked toward the male world for their
mentors and role models as a means of giving credence to their need for a
sense of purpose, for their ambition, intellect, direction, and definition of
success. They have opted for achievement in the world by becoming *daughters of the father*—women who identify with the traditionally male focus on
power, independence, prestige, money, and glamour, and for whom anything
less than carrying out "important work in the world" is simply not enough.

Other women have simultaneously tried to live out the male ambition
inherited from the world of their fathers and also to redefine their fostering
female energies in the hope that they will be successful in the world yet still
be able to raise their children and fulfill their sexual and emotional needs.
They try to make lives for themselves that they hope will not end in sorrow,
as the lives of countless generations of previous Western women have.

Still others have decided to reaffirm traditional values as *daughters of the
mother*. They have chosen to create lives for themselves dedicated primarily
to nurturing the ambitions of lovers or husbands, and devoting themselves to
the development of their children so long as they remain within the family.

These are only a few of the possible choices now open to women in a
world where shifting economic, social, and personal values have undermined the established social order and made choice possible. Whatever path
we choose, something deep within each of us searches for meaning and
longs for freedom—whenever we have time to think about it between caring for children, paying the bills, and trying to look like we have just
walked off the cover of *Vogue*. Such are the warp and woof from which our
lives are woven during our 30s and early 40s—lives that often include a
career as well as further education, motherhood, loverhood, and a myriad of
other things. Such is the ordinary world of today's woman.

So great are the demands on women now—many of them self-
imposed—that we are often in danger of losing track of our own souls and
of burning ourselves out. There is no place for the old female rituals in our
lives. In other cultures, among the Native Americans, for instance, women
would leave the tribe for a few days each month to enter the soul realms and
experience the Moon Lodge during menstruation. There, in the presence of
other women, they gave themselves permission to enter altered states of
consciousness, to restore their energies, and to express the wildness of their
own creativity—a creativity that at the dark moon time of menstruation has
nothing to do with nurturing or relating to men or children.

We have no such opportunity. Instead, many women, unaware of the value of venturing into the soul realms, choose to "control" their moods and cycles by taking hormones—not only to avoid unwanted pregnancies, but even to regulate events so that a business meeting doesn't come up in the middle of a menstrual period when they might not be as rational or as socially acceptable as at other times. Then, sooner or later, every woman gets moonstruck. When it happens, the ordinary world in which she has been living is rent asunder. She is being initiated into the mysteries of the dark blood. Menopause has arrived.

"Isn't it wonderful," the editor of the woman's page of a national newspaper said to me one day, "that science has finally conquered women's biology."

"What are you talking about?" I asked.

"Oh, you know," she went on, "it's great. We don't have to menstruate anymore, and we don't have to have babies, thanks to the Pill. We don't even have to go through menopause or get old now that we have HRT. At last, women are set free from their biology. I'd like you to write a piece on it."

It took me a few seconds to recover from the shock of hearing an intelligent woman voice an opinion so far from my own sense of what being female is about. I knew there was no point in even discussing the issue. I said that the idea didn't grab me and walked out of the office, literally stunned by how carelessly this poor frazzled daughter of the father could dismiss a million years of inherited woman power, wisdom, and blood. She had done it with the wave of a hand and the swallow of a pill. Then, almost as an obituary, she had proposed a 750-word article on modern women's newfound "freedom." At the door, I turned to look at her. There sat a haggard 35-year-old who looked 50, hunched over her computer, smoking cigarettes. Three years later, someone told me she had just had her womb removed.

Wasteland Echoes

The editor's sense of freedom, like much of the so-called freedom we hear about, is certainly of a very limited kind. Since all freedom is won at a price, I cannot help wondering how high a price we are paying and if it is real freedom at all. I know too many dynamic, successful women who appear to have everything. Yet, when you sit down with them alone, away from the glitter of their busy lives, they describe feeling out of sync with themselves. A sense of sterility and stagnation permeates their lives, and they carry a feeling of emptiness and even of betrayal, yet from what and by whom they rarely know. Many have aimed for the top and arrived. So now what? Where is the next challenge, the next battle to be won, the next social occasion? They tend to pack their days with duties and appointments, always wary that if they stop for a moment, they might let somebody down or their lives might fall apart.

Just as our mothers and their mothers before them embraced the expectations of their culture—that fulfillment would come through being a good wife, a good mother, or a good servant—women have now taken on another cultural stereotype. We have learned to do things logically. We have largely bought into a male stereotype based on the attainment of academic, financial, or artistic success. We have thrown ourselves headlong into the male world, and many of us have "made it" within that world's terms. However, in the wake of our success, we often find ourselves pursued by a confusing sense of barrenness and despair that further achievement in the world, new love affairs, or the prospect of a face lift can do nothing to cure. It is at this point that many women, myself included, first hear the call to adventure. It comes as a powerful challenge to leave the ordinary world in which we have lived decades of our lives and set out in search of answers. Why did this happen? What was wrong? What secrets have we forgotten, and what connections have we lost in our obsession with *doing* things and our tendency to opt for chemical control of our body's cycles? And what are we missing out on?

When I began the research for this book, these were some of the questions I set out to find answers to. The search led me down two paths that at first seemed so separate that I did not see how they could possibly meet—science and myth. First, I explored the biochemistry and physiology of a woman's body, entering the fascinating world of shifting hormones and trying to make sense of it. When I discovered the phenomenon of estrogen dominance and realized that most of the physical and emotional agonies of menstruating and menopausal women in the West have resulted from the same male-oriented, blinkered, linear view of reality that has poisoned our planet, it overwhelmed me.

How could we as women continue to buy into values and ways of living that not only did not serve to bring to fruition our own talents and our capacities for joy, but were inexorably destroying the earth? Where had all our real freedom and power gone—not power in the male sense of *power over*, but in the female sense of *power to*? I also delved deep into the past in search of archeological findings and archetypal connections that might give clues to just what as women we had lost and how any of these lost treasures might be rediscovered. This led me into the realm of myth and ritual. I discovered that the two worlds—the world of science, with all its shifting biochemistry and rising and falling hormones—and the world of myth, peopled with archetypes, symbols, goddesses, and rituals—not only meet, they are blended within a woman's body and psyche. And where they meet is a cauldron of blood.

Blood Mysteries

According to written records, since the beginning of human history, the power of creation was believed to reside in the blood that pours forth from a woman's body. It ebbs and flows with the waxing and waning of the moon. Blood has always been credited with magical power and with containing the essence of a person's soul—one's "life blood." Medieval physicians believed that a young woman's menstrual blood could cure leprosy and act as an aphrodisiac. For centuries, rituals for taking in spiritual powers involved ingesting menstrual blood; it was mixed with red wine and taken as an alchemical drink. Ancient Egyptians, Celts, Persians, and Taoists in China all held similar beliefs about menstrual blood and carried out similar rituals. In ancient Greece during planting festivals, women mixed their menstrual blood with corn seeds, then spread them upon the earth for fertility. In the 17th century, when William Harvey wrote his famous scientific treatise on the circulation, he referred to the flow of blood through the body as the *coursing of spiritual power.* Even our word *blessing* is derived from the Old English *bloedsed,* which means bleeding.

Menstrual blood and the blood of childbirth are the only blood given freely—that is, shed without wounding. Not only metaphorically, but speaking strictly from a scientific point of view, human life cannot be created without the blood in a woman's womb. So profoundly did an awareness of the power of a woman's blood touch the lives of primitive people that native words for menstruation carry connotations of spirit, divinity, and magic—of the supernatural and of the sacred. Ancient Hindus taught that all life is created out of the congealing of Great Mother's menstrual substance, which had been worked and thickened to form curds or clots from which the crust of solid matter emerges. Their goddess of creation, Kali-Ma, "invited the gods to bathe in the bloody flow of her womb and to drink of it; and the gods, in holy communion, drank of the fountain of life and bathed in it, and rose blessed to the heavens."

Moon Goddess

A woman's average menstrual cycle is 29½ days—exactly the length of the moon's passage from new to full and back to new again. In primitive cultures, where women live in close physical proximity to each other and their natural menstrual cycles are not disrupted by such things as exposure to unnatural light, electromagnetic fields, drugs, and hormones, they tend to menstruate at the same time. However, ovulation tends to occur when light is brightest, at the full moon; and menstruation begins during the moon's dark phase—at new moon. There is by no means anything pathological in any woman in the modern world not cycling in this particular natural rhythm, but it has been demonstrated that the menstrual cycle can be regulated according to the exposure to varying degrees of light that mimic the waxing and waning of the moon's phases. Under such circumstances, the three phases of the moon—waxing, full, and waning—correlate exactly with the monthly cycle of ebb and flow of female hormones—the estrogen-dominated proliferative phase, ovulation, the secretory luteal phase, and menstruation itself.

In the realm of myth and symbols, these three phases are superbly mirrored in the three phases of every woman's life: childhood, before the sex hormones begin to flow; the childbearing years, which begin at the menarche; and the postmenopausal years of the goddess in her crone guise. In ancient cultures, the moon was considered the source of fertility and birth. She ruled destiny and time, the secrets of the unseen world, transformation, death, and regeneration. It was the moon's power that quickened all of life. Sowing and harvesting were done in harmony with her ebbs and flows. It was the moon growing bright then darkening and disappearing altogether each month that taught people that nothing in life is constant. The only thing on which you could rely is change. The moon became a symbol of the cycle of transformation that makes its home in a woman's body, while woman came to rule all things that involved change.

Archeologist Marija Gimbutas, the late professor emerita at UCLA, is the acknowledged world expert on neolithic goddess-centered cultures in prepatriarchal Europe. Author of more than 20 books, she paints a richly detailed picture of their social structure, agriculture, customs, rituals, religion, and art. Much has been learned in recent years about the nature of the goddess-centered cultures that existed for literally tens of thousands of years in Europe and Asia. The miniature sculptures that have been unearthed in the past 20 years give insight into the great variety of female manifestation of the divine, which appeared as long ago as 27,000 to 25,000 years B.C. Three thousand of these have been found in Siberia alone. In *The Civilization of the Goddess*, a monumental encyclopedic book that has already changed history, Gimbutas writes:

> According to myriad images that have survived from the great span of human prehistory on the Eurasian continents, it was the sovereign mystery and creative power of the female as the source of life that developed into the earliest religious experiences. The Great Mother Goddess who gives birth to all creation out of the holy darkness of her womb became a metaphor for Nature herself, the cosmic giver and taker of life, ever able to renew Herself within the eternal cycle of life, death, and rebirth.

We learn from ancient sources that, like woman herself, the Moon Goddess has many faces. At the new moon, she is the Virgin Goddess wrapped in enthusiasm for new beginnings as seeds sprout and first shoots appear. When her second phase begins, so does puberty. Buds turn into flowers and flowers to fruits as virgin becomes transformed into Divine Mother in charge of procreation and sexuality. She is the pregnant goddess, mistress of animals, bringer of life, the madonna. As the moon begins to wane, woman passes through her next initiation to a time of harvest and a time of death, during which all that is old becomes compost for new life.

It is the Dark Goddess who rules the darkness of the moon, death, and rebirth. Ancient statues of the Dark Goddess carved in bone, marble, alabaster, or clay are often white—for white is the color of death. Bones are turned white by the elements. The big breasts and hips you find on statues of the Divine Mother are replaced by stiff nudes. The Dark Goddess is often shown without breasts, her hands either on her chest or extended along her sides. She is shown with an enlarged pubic triangle, for the Dark Goddess of the waning moon is not only goddess of death but of regeneration. She rules the time in a woman's life when all that has run its course, all that is outmoded or no longer meaningful, must be destroyed to make way for a more authentic life. She rules menopause.

Dark Goddess

Menopause is the initiation of the Dark Goddess. It is the passage during which a woman is asked to confront the possibility of her own death and probe the mysteries of decay, dismemberment, and regeneration. As menopause approaches, often a woman wants to spend more time in nature and to feel her spirit fed by the earth. The fear of menopause and the fear of the crone, so widespread in our society, are nothing more than a reflection of a fear of death itself. For in our modern world we have forgotten the great cyclical flow of birth, flowering, death, and regeneration that is hidden within the circle of the moon, as it is within all life and reflected in the circle of our own souls. Our patriarchal culture denies cyclical time and views events as linear.

In linear time, the end is not connected with the beginning, and birth and death are not two events in a continuing cycle of life but opposites—the one to be celebrated, the other to be resisted at all costs until the bitter end. It is no wonder that our society wants to blank out menopause and to reject the older female. It is the only way in the fearful fragmented world we live in that human beings can deny for a time their own mortality. And so the Dark Goddess remains a focus of fear and loathing in stereotypical male-dominated linear thinking. Any woman who does not break through the limitations of such thinking and move beyond it risks becoming so paralyzed by fear that she will look upon the crone as an enemy to be resisted. In truth, she is the archetype and medium by which the internal split that took place thousands of years ago between woman and her feminine nature can be healed.

The Dark Goddess is death's priestess. It is she that wipes out old patterns and then, acting the role of the midwife, gives birth to new forms of living. She can seem a terrifying figure to women approaching menopause. She has so long been repressed within our psyches that when at last her energy rises and she makes her presence known, it can sometimes arrive on the scene like an earthquake or a volcano—some eruption of nature that occurs when pressures held too long within the earth are released. Yet she has always been present in our lives; she has appeared each month as the moon grows dark and menstrual blood flows. Now, at menopause, the Dark Goddess at last comes to rest within a woman's being, for instead of being released each month, the dark blood of creative power is retained within a woman's body and made available for her use.

Spokeswoman for the Dark Goddess is the crone. Her presence in a woman's life is usually easy to spot. She appears whenever we experience any drastic and dramatic changes—the death of a loved one, loss of a job, disfiguration. She is the teacher who guides us through the transformation that is demanded of us. She is there in our deepest despair and at times when we connect most powerfully with our own creative fire. She is the handmaiden that nurtures us through dark nights once we are willing to make the descent into our own psyche and connect with whatever forms are sleeping there so that we can begin to live our own power. When these connections are made, she is present, too. She teaches us by her presence alone to become deeply and spontaneously sexual, assertive, straight, incorruptible, prophetic, intuitive, and free. All of these qualities are asking to arise at menopause, and all are gifts of the crone. They are, it must be said, also the qualities that most terrify the patriarchal culture in which we live.

Inexorable Nature

The crone is the irrational power of nature that causes all things to decay and be changed. The experience of change is terrifying to both men and women who have lived their lives believing that material reality is all there is and that reason is the ultimate means by which all our problems will be solved. Whatever else she may be, the crone is most certainly not reasonable. No more reasonable than the forces that cause leaves to decay when they fall in autumn, transforming them into leaf mold that will eventually bring new life to the forest. No more reasonable than the hurricane which, irrespective of man's wishes or longings, blows its course through city and countryside. No more reasonable than the earth herself as she quakes and trembles with the shifts taking place in the continental plates of her body.

It is little wonder that male-centered religions have diabolized the crone, for she is the ultimate destroyer, the emasculator of male reason. Nature and the crone aspect of the Dark Goddess become in men's minds the castrator—so much so that during the Inquisition, witches were accused of collecting severed penises in boxes or birds' nests. Yet even the male penis itself represented—and still represents—an instinctive power to the male, which most Western men feel uncomfortable with, for the penis seems to have a life of its own, quite separate from the man to which it is attached. Like the Dark Goddess, it defies man's sterile reason. As Barbara Walker says in *The Crone: Woman of Age, Wisdom, and Power*: "The conviction peculiar to males that sex organs have an uncontrollable, independent life of their own, is expressed in the churchman's belief that the stolen penises moved about and ate food in their captivity like animals." The penis, too, is an instrument of the Dark Goddess.

The Dark Goddess lives at a woman's core. She guards the self. She is the friend of the soul, whose purpose in your life is to fiercely protect and further the whole process of your learning to live authentically from your core. She never trades in deceit, she never lies, nor does she veil her power. She refuses to uphold any relationship that doesn't work, and she tears away at anything within us that is greedy or grasping or infantile. She continually urges us to reclaim our own power—the power to set limits and to shout "no," and the power to say, "This is what I will do and this is what I won't do" when we are faced with any sort of abuse or anyone trying to steal our power or dominate us.

Madness of the Imprisoned

But the Dark Goddess is far more than this. She is the female power so long rejected and repressed by Western civilization that when it rises to the surface, it may break forth in fury to devastate a woman's ordinary world. Sometimes when she forces her presence to be felt at menopause, she can well up inside and make us hysterical. Her frenzies—which in the male-dominated world of linear thinking are looked upon as something for which a woman should be tranquilized and kept under control—were once treated with the deepest respect as visitations from the gods. It was in such a state that the Pythia or Sibyl at Delphi prophesied the future and told secrets capable of turning those who sought her help into conquerors of nations. When we forget the power of the Dark Goddess—when we separate ourselves from her essential nature—then we experience her as the destroyer who arrives like a great snake to break up the structure of our lives, devour our relationships, and make mincemeat of our most precious self-deceptions. She can quickly cut through the patriarchal feminine image of being "pleasing," "submissive," "gentle," and "nice."

If a woman has so much control of her own behavior that the Dark Goddess is unable to arise when it is time for her appearance to be made, if she remains deeply suppressed, then a woman can experience her energies in the form of a life-threatening disease, depression, hopelessness, or despair. Or, she may find herself living in a wasteland and feel her life to be meaningless and without direction. It is only by finding ways to reconnect with her energy within that the powers of transformation are set free to work their magic and lead each of us on our own individual path toward freedom. As Demetra George says in *Mysteries of the Dark Moon*:

Whether we see the Dark Goddess as dancing ecstatically in a swirl of red flames, or enveloped in mist gazing into the inner pools of her psychic awareness, or throbbing with her orgasmic, magical creative energy, or embracing us in our grief, or furiously raging, screaming, crying, or desperately withdrawing into a stupor of denial or numbness, her ultimate purpose in each one of these guises is the same. She destroys in order to renew. The Dark Goddess of the dark moon is the mistress of transformation, and she exists everywhere there is change.

At the time of her appearance at menopause, the Dark Goddess demands that each one of us clears out of our lives whatever is no longer essential to our inner being, whether this be possessions, relationships, or jobs—anything that does not help us grow and fulfill our deepest needs. If we ignore her demands, she can become like a wild and unruly creature when thwarted, ruthlessly tearing apart whatever in our own lives is restricting the full expression of our souls. Her rise can threaten everything that in ordinary life we try desperately to hold on to—our self-confidence, our self-image, our sense of accomplishment, and our material possessions. All of the things which for many years may have supported us now come under the scrutiny of her gaze and the ruthlessness of her sword.

What can be hard to realize, while all this is happening, is that everything she does is done with love. We see such things as the breakdown of a marriage, the loss of a job, and the physical illness that can come at times of enormous change as evil and negative. We spend most of our lives trying to avoid a crisis at all cost. Yet, crises are often the only means by which we can be thrust forward to a new life. Were the energies of the Dark Goddess not to rise, we would remain stagnant. We might continue living out an artificial existence, while all the time trying to fill up the emptiness within with whatever we can lay our hands on, from drugs and sex to success and power in the world—yet never succeed. It is the Dark Goddess that gives us the motivation to change and brings us the power to be able to carry it out.

Migration of Power

She also pulls us away from the external world, asking us to withdraw to a place of stillness in which we can begin to hear the echoes of our own souls—sounds that for years may have been ignored or forgotten. She stirs our being at the deepest level. She asks us to enter our own personal dark-ness, calling us to make a vision quest, presenting us with pain over any issues in our lives that we have been denying. She asks us to face our fears and taboos, whether they be addictions, dependencies, or inadequacies, so that we can bring them into the open where they can be looked at and healed. Like the crone who is her messenger, the Dark Goddess has no adornments. She is naked and raw in her confrontations. She arrives to lead us into the labyrinthine recesses of our own being, and, if we consent, she offers us the courage and the strength to face our own personal demons. Either we acknowledge her call, retreat from the outer world, and begin to make our descent voluntarily, or she grabs us by the throat and drags us under. And, just in case we might be tempted to think when menopause arrives that sexuality is dead, she makes us think again. It has not died, but been transformed.

The sexuality of the postmenopausal woman is the sexuality of the crone. It is the sexuality of sheer instinct—wildness set free. It is she that calls a woman into the secret places of the woods and provokes her to dance naked in wild abandon. Hers is a sexuality to be used in any way a woman chooses—in union with another, or alone to generate the alchemical meeting of male and female within her own body. The sexu-ality of the crone belongs to herself alone. She will be what she is; she will have what she wants. She is neither passive nor submissive, and her sexuality has nothing whatever to do with bringing physical children into being.

The crone's eroticism is sheer ecstasy, lived for its own sake, and sheer creativity. She creates in an uninhibited, animated, fiery way that emanates from the soul of a woman. Such sexuality is the fuel for all creative powers in the world. It carries with it the energy of regeneration and of healing, not only for a woman herself, but for the world. It is the kundalini power—the rejuvenating cosmic illumination, the power of the serpent, the sacred fire that heals. As the crone gains entrance into the body and psyche of the menopausal woman, she illuminates one dark corner of her psyche after another, lifting away all that is old and dead and without meaning, the way kundalini energy rises up within a woman's body to illuminate each of the chakras. Her power becomes the power of the menopausal woman. It lies in her dark blood—the blood of creation that now, forevermore, will be retained within a woman's body.

Today Is Almost Over

Before menopause, before the Dark Goddess makes her appearance in our lives, our energies are occupied with the challenge of adjusting to the world and caring for others. At menopause, these energies are set free to shine forth with their own brand of pure beauty. A woman becomes aware of herself at menopause—as a living being separate from the collective life of work, of the family, and the community. Until menopause, most women in the so-called civilized world have lived under the guidance of the ego. We have sought to gain power over our external world and over nature in order to fulfill our personal needs. And to a greater or lesser extent, we have succeeded. What happens at menopause is that suddenly the way we have been living and the skills we have learned—getting on with people, getting ahead in the world—no longer work, or if they do work and we continue to get what we think we want, we often find that it no longer nourishes us.

Then all of a sudden as the moon reaches its fullest peak, like the woman who is coming to the zenith of her power, a shadow appears. The ancient Chinese insist that when the moon is almost full and at its brightest, this is the moment at which the powers of darkness are strongest within, readying themselves to break forth. So it is with a menopausal woman. Suddenly, the strength, the power, and the sense of control seem doomed to slip away from you. The ordinary world in which you have lived and been comfortable with no longer works. The world of safety begins to dissolve. As it dissolves, this rising of the shadow reflects in a stark way any weaknesses, deficiencies, or parts of us that still remain ungrown or unlived.

I was the daughter of a jazz musician. As a child, I didn't go to school. I grew up on the road with my father, traveling hundreds of miles a day from one job to the next. Many of the places where his band played were amusement parks. Amusement parks are wonderful places, full of all sorts of bright lights, games to play, things to do, and prizes to be won. However, I remember noticing, at the age of six or seven, that amusement parks in the stark light of dawn revealed every hidden scrap of paper, every surface whose paint had worn. A carnival the morning after is quite a different place from the one it was only hours before.

Often a woman's experience of menopause is like this. An amusement park in the stark light of dawn can be terrifying to someone who wants to go on, entranced by the illusory games it offered a few hours before. But to others who have grown tired of the games, it offers new textures and colors—a far richer and starker experience of reality and aliveness than any number of neon lights and whirling wheels could ever hope to mimic. "The party's over," the song says, and "the candle flickers and dims...now you must wake up." This is the challenge of the menopausal woman. In this challenge lies a choice—try to run back into the world of the carnival, which seemed so appropriate the night before but is no longer, or step forward toward the clear light of dawn? Gaze with steely eyes at the reality around you and ask the question: Where do I go from here?

CALL TO ADVENTURE
Menopause: Gateway to a Richer Life

he joy of menopause is the world's best-kept secret. Like venturing through the gateway to enter an ancient temple, in order to claim that joy, a woman must be willing to pass beyond the monsters who guard its gate. As you stand at the brink of it, it can appear that only darkness, danger, and decay lie beyond. And in a way, this is true—although most certainly not in the way most women believe. For having passed through the doorway of menopause into the realms beyond, I have come to believe, as thousands of women from all cultures throughout history have whispered to each other, that it is the most exciting passage a woman ever makes.

Of course, nobody told me this beforehand. It was a secret I had to discover for myself. Like most modern women, my head had been filled with the horrors of hot flashes, fainting spells, and dry vaginas; with memories of my mother's tears shed over a wrinkle that appeared one day to mar her perfect face; with the prospect of enforced celibacy—after all, no man can feel lust for an old woman, or can he? It was partly by accident, I think, and partly because—despite good health and secure family circumstances—my own journey through menopause was not an easy one, that I discovered the secret that throughout history women living in patriarchal cultures have guarded close to their hearts. The doorway of menopause that each of us is invited to pass through is a call to adventure. It connects the ordinary world in which we have been living to a numinous zone of magnified power. Within that zone are hidden treasures to match our wildest dreams. But, like every prize worth having, these riches can only be claimed and brought back if a woman is bold enough and persistent enough to answer the call. What is calling? Nothing less than her own soul.

Hero's Journey

This call to adventure that a woman hears at menopause can arrive in as many different forms as there are women to hear it. But, whatever shape it takes, its purpose is the same. It is asking her—imploring her—to leave behind the comfortable world of her ordinary existence and for a time to venture into a challenging, unfamiliar place. It is asking her to set out on her own hero's journey—a journey that is completely unique to her. Sometimes this entails making an outer journey to a real place, moving to a new job, or leaving behind a marriage that has outlived its usefulness. For many, the journey only takes place in the mind, the heart, and the spirit. Either way it is primarily an inner journey that takes a woman out of her ordinary world with all its ordinary assumptions to transform the way she thinks and lives—from weakness to strength, from grief to purpose, from despair to hope—and then brings her home again.

The word *hero* comes from a Greek root that means "to protect and to serve." Like "poet" or "teacher," it is a word that refers equally to a woman or man. A hero is someone willing to move through and beyond narrow thinking and familiar landscapes in order to discover the larger world of meaning—someone willing to sacrifice or to transmute her own fears and hesitation, anger, and sorrows into creative power. From a psychological point of view, the hero archetype corresponds to what Freud called the ego—that part of a woman which, in separating from the infantile bond to the mother, establishes her ability to function as a unique member of the human race. The hero archetype also represents the ego's search for its true identity—the self—and for wholeness. The task a woman faces at menopause is to call forth the hero within, and, by journeying with her, to identify and resurrect whatever parts of her own being and whatever creative potential is still waiting to be lived out. It could be said that the hero's journey as a whole is the process by which the ego (the hero), believing herself separate from the other parts of herself, comes to incorporate them in order to become the self. Well traveled, such a journey enables a woman to turn her potential into power and her dreams into reality. And on every woman's hero's quest it is the Dark Goddess who is her handmaiden, her sister, her guide, her destroyer, and her midwife.

Language of Myth

The transformation involved in a woman's passage to power is profoundly mysterious. It is an experience which, although a few things can be said of it in terms of psychology, ultimately defies analysis. One cannot speak of it in the same language we use to discuss the biochemistry of hormonal changes or the relationship between essential fatty acids and brain chemicals. This is because the linear, denotative language of science fragments and separates and therefore only helps us to scrutinize the surface of reality. It won't enable us to take even the first step past the guardians of the threshold when menopause arrives, let alone empower our journey. To speak of the nature of the hero's journey at menopause, we must leave behind the words and concepts of science and find a new language—or perhaps resurrect a very old one. For this we need stories, tales, rituals, and dreams. We need to call on the language of myth, for only myths reveal the eternal patterns of our souls.

Thomas Mann speaks of what it is like to look at the world through mythic eyes, about the way that a human being becomes conscious "proudly and darkly yet joyously of its recurrence and typicality....Myth," Mann says, "is the legitimization of life. Only through and in it does life find self awareness, sanction and consecration."

Joseph Campbell puts it another way:

> Myth is the secret opening through which the inexhaustible energies of the cosmos pour. The wonder is that the characteristic efficacy to touch and inspire deep creative centers dwells in the smallest nursery fairy tale—as the flavor of the ocean is contained in a droplet or the whole mystery of life within the egg of a flea. For the symbols of mythology are not manufactured; they cannot be ordered, invented, or permanently suppressed. Myths are spontaneous productions of the psyche, and each bears within it undamaged the germ power of its source.

Myths live forever in our fantasies, dreams, and relationships.

Mythological archetypes, symbols, and rituals are the stuff on which we need to draw and to which we can relate when exploring the meaning implicit in the changes that each woman is impelled to make when menopause arrives. By coming in contact with appropriate myths—myths that address the challenges we are facing and help us to experience the flavor of the worlds we are preparing to enter—the seeds of new awakenings can be sown. Jungian analyst Clarissa Pinkola Estés says in *Women Who Run With the Wolves:*

> If a story is seed, then we are its soil. Just hearing the story allows us to experience it as though we ourselves were the heroine who either falters or wins out in the end. If we hear a story about a wolf, then afterward we rove about and know like a wolf for a time. If we hear a story about a dove finding her young at last, then for a time after something moves behind our own feathered breasts. If it be a story of wresting the sacred pearl from beneath the clay of the ninth dragon, we feel exhausted afterward and satisfied. In a very real way, we are imprinted with knowing just by listening to the tale.

The Frog Prince

Once upon a time there was a king who had three fine daughters. The youngest of these was so beautiful that when the sun shone upon her, it smiled. She liked to play with her favorite toy, a little golden ball the queen had given her. Now gold is an incorruptible metal, and she loved her golden ball more than anything in the world. A golden sphere. The perfect circle of her soul.

Every day she would steal away from the castle, take her little ball, and wander down a path through the woods to the edge of an old well—the entrance to the underworld. There she loved to sit beneath a feathery willow tossing the golden ball into the air and catching it as it fell. Tossing and catching. Tossing and catching. One day while playing her little game and tossing her "soul" around, a shimmery dragonfly buzzed by. For just an instant, she took her eye off the ball. But that was all it took. Whoosh. The golden sphere flew straight past the lovely hand held out to catch it.

Splash, it hit the water. Down, down it went until the dark water swallowed up her beloved ball completely and carried it who knows how far beneath the earth. Gold is a heavy metal.

Heartbroken, the princess wept. She wailed. She cried. She stamped her feet. Alas, nothing would bring back her beautiful golden ball. Her "soul" had sunk to the bottom of the well. Of course everybody knows that when something gets swallowed up in the underworld, one of its inhabitants is sent to the surface. Sometimes it is a dragon, sometimes a wolf, sometimes a monster or a bear. This time it was a little frog that came plopping up out of the water. "What's wrong, princess?" he asked. "Why are you crying?"

"I've lost my golden ball, funny frog," she said.

He replied, "I'll go and get it for you." The princess was delighted. "But what will you give me in return?" demands the frog.

Of course, why did she not think of that before: Every kindness must be paid for. "I'll give you anything you want," she said. "My clothes, my jewels, even the golden bracelet I wear."

"I don't care for your clothes, your jewels, and your golden bracelet," the frog said.

"Well, then what *do* you want?" she snapped.

"I want to be your playmate," he replied. "I want to sit at your table and eat from your golden plate. I want to hop on to your bed and sleep at the side of your pillow. Promise I can do this, and I'll swim right down and fetch your ball."

The girl doesn't even stop to think about the deal. After all, she supposed he was only a useless frog, and there was no way a frog could be the friend of a princess. So she says, "All right, you can do that." True to his word, the frog dove down.

Now he has become the hero on an adventure. And so the story goes...

Every hero's journey begins as we meet the hero in her ordinary world. The ordinary world is the place where you know who you are, are familiar with how you have been living, and with the various roles you have been playing—mother, friend, worker, lover. Yet, we know before a dozen words are spoken that this ordinary world is going to change, just as a woman in her late 30s and early 40s begins to sense something pretty fundamental is about to shift. The hero never knows what it is, but we who are listening to the story know that her ordinary world is bound to be a vivid contrast to the strange new world she is about to enter.

In *The Wizard of Oz,* we are introduced to Dorothy's boring day-to-day existence in Kansas. In *Romancing the Stone,* we meet Joan Wilder at her desk in her drab little apartment, finishing off yet another romantic novel with not the remotest hint of romance in her own life. For the princess, living her ordinary life means sitting beside a well playing with her toy. Then something happens to disrupt a woman's life. It can be an illness, a death, the loss of a job, a love affair, or unendable ennui. Maybe the Fisher King has been wounded and the land is dying, as in the Grail legends; maybe some wrong has been perpetrated that needs to be put right. Maybe, as happens to the princess, the hero's attention is stolen momentarily, and her beautiful golden soul is lost.

Maps of Unknown Territories

A prime function of mythology is to supply the symbols that can transport a woman onwards. Whether they echo through the tale of Persephone and Demeter, the story of the Loathly Lady from the Grail legends, or films like *An Officer and a Gentleman,* all myths are like maps that guide you off their edges into unknown territory. Each story, like each woman's life and journey, is unique, yet the archetypes that underlie it are universal. They cannot be ordered or invented. Neither can they be repressed forever. When the time is ripe, they spring forth spontaneously from the human psyche, each bringing with them intact transformative power. At that moment, a story such as *Beauty and the Beast,* or the tale of Greek earth goddess Demeter and her daughter Persephone, becomes soul food to nourish, inspire, and focus a woman's energies in a way that reconnects her with meaning.

Myths and rituals help us define our rites of passage. In primitive societies, they are the ceremonies connected with birth, the naming of a child, puberty, marriage, menopause, and death. Each transition in the tribe was associated with specific rites and myths that went with them and would function as a formal exercise for severance. By letting a myth echo through one's being, it becomes easier for the mind to be radically pulled away from whatever attachments, attitudes, and patterns of living at any particular stage need to be left behind.

The Dark Is Rising

One of the curious things about mythic stories and rituals is that, if they are not supplied from the outside in the form of stories that carry power for transformation or rituals that help us gather these transformative powers and direct them, then they will come from within in the form of dreams or images. At the brink of a significant shift in my own life, I dreamed I was on a desert island. There were priestesses dressed in white robes carrying a bier on which lay a mummy wrapped in white gauze. They moved slowly under the sun. Dazzled by the light upon the sea, I watched them carry their burden across the sands toward me. It was as though I was mesmerized. As they drew near, one of them raised her hand. They stopped and set down the dead body on its bier right before me and began to unwrap it. One of the priestesses glanced up at me. Her eyes were dark and piercing. Suddenly, I knew with absolute horror that they were unwrapping the cadaver because I was supposed to eat the dead body—something so absolutely repugnant to me that I would do almost anything to avoid it. I awakened, trembling and swimming in sweat.

The dream that so frightened me was a unique product of my own mind, yet within it lay the archetype of transmutation—the same experience you find within the holy eucharist or communion rituals of the Catholic church during which wine and bread are transmuted into the blood and body of Christ. The deeper layers of my being were sending me messages through the language of dream that something in my life that had died and been embalmed now needed transmuting. The idea of eating a dead body was anathema to me. Yet through my dream, my soul was calling out to me, telling me not to run away but to face the task before me and learn to look at things with new eyes. Once I got over the first shock, I realized it was teaching me that in "eating" a dead body—that is, in consciously welcoming into my awareness what was moribund in my life and devouring it (instead of trying to avoid it as I had been doing), the old and dead could be transmuted into new life just as the dead parings from vegetables become compost to nourish spring flowers.

Whether they appear in dreams or stories, such myths and rituals that are available to us contain the symbols we need to carry our own lives forward. Without them, it is far too easy for a woman to become crystallized, transfixed in the habits of her past that tie her down and hold her back. At puberty, we need to break away from the absolute dependence we have known as children. If we do not do so, we find ourselves trapped in neurotic patterns that make it impossible for us to enjoy our lives and find meaning in them.

Motherhood, too, has its myths. Like the youngest child in the fairy tale, we must set out to find our fortune. So does menopause. Mythic symbols—the snake who forever sheds its skin and is born again, the Beast who becomes transformed through the love of Beauty, the Medusa's head which when looked upon turns men to stone—do not refer to something that is in any logical sense knowable or known. They speak of spiritual powers that move through our lives and can only be known by the effects they bring about. The function of the archetypal journey of the hero—so important in a woman's life at menopause—lies in its ability to help a woman blinded by the emptiness of material existence become transformed into someone who knows that in choosing to live for cultural and spiritual ends, she becomes connected at the deepest level with her own values and nourished by her own soul.

❀ ❀ ❀

The Tale Continues

In a jiffy, the frog came back with the ball in his mouth. The princess, without so much as a by your leave, took it from him and skipped back up the path home. The frog, in his floppy-frog way, followed behind her, crying, "Hold on. Wait for me." Plop, plop, plop. But of course, being a frog, he was very slow. The princess and her family were eating supper when at last he arrived at the castle. Plop, plop, plop, the king heard something coming up the steps. The princess squirmed in her chair.

"What is that?" her father asked. "Oh, nothing," she replied, "just some silly frog I met." "Did you make him any promises?" the king wanted to know. [All at once, morality enters on the scene.] "Yes," the princess replied.

"Then he better be let in," her father answered.

The small spotted creature came galumphing through the door, then leapt up on the table, plopping his funny feet on the edge of the princess's lovely golden plate and completely spoiling her dinner. Finally, she got up after eating nothing and went off upstairs to bed. But guess who was following her—plop, plop up the stairs—right up to the heavy door to her bedroom which was shut tight.

So the frog hurled his little green body against the door, crying, "Hey, princess, I want to come in." She opened the door. "I want to sleep in your bed with you," he said. By now, the princess had had enough of this disgusting intruder even if he did rescue her beautiful golden soul for her. So she picked him up and dashed him against the stone wall with all her might. The frog's body split open. Out of it stepped a handsome prince with eyes as blue as the summer sky. It seemed that he had been cursed by a hag who had turned him into a frog.

[Like the princess, he, too, had been stuck at the brink of adulthood unwilling or unable to move onward. One of the reasons I so love this tale is that in it each of them in a funny way is able to rescue the other.]

The next day, after the princess and the frog prince were married, a mysterious coach arrived at the castle gate to fetch them and take them back to the prince's land. They got in it and set off when suddenly there was a loud ping.

The frog prince shouts to the coachman, "What is that? What has happened?"

"It is just the sound of an iron band breaking," he replied. "It has been around my heart ever since you have been gone."

The coachman, like the land the prince left behind when he was forced to descend into the underworld and become a frog, had been suffering. His heart has been bound up while the land itself, deprived of the generating and governing power of the prince, had lain barren. Now that he was on his way home, the band was broken and the land was beginning to be fertile again. And the prince brought an even greater boon gathered on his descent—a wife as a gift to the world that had been longing for his return.

A myth is a special tale that can be told ten thousand times in a thousand ways without losing its power. It is a tale that will be received differently by everyone who hears it, yet will carry the same archetypal hook for all of us. In every myth, in every tale of power, each character represents a different part of the psyche. The maiden is the unawakened, innocent, sleepy female beneath which is to be found a warrior's heart and the ability to bear the pain of loneliness, difficulty, hurt, and betrayal in order to triumph. The king is the moral principle. He has a full knowledge of the underworld into which the hero falls or is dragged, as well as skills that can advise her and spur her onwards in her journey. The frog represents the nursery version of the great serpent that inhabits the underworld. He is consort to the Dark Goddess, who carries the life-generating powers of death and resurrection up from the abyss. He also represents all that has been rejected by the proud princess in her callow youth—all that is unadmitted, unknown, and undeveloped in the depths of a woman's consciousness, the treasures hidden in submarine palaces, the glittering diamonds waiting for the hero if only he or she will descend and claim them. The prince is the formative power of the hero destined through perseverance and single-mindedness to reclaim his power and regenerate his land.

Listening to the Whispers

Until recently, when the power of stories and rituals has begun to be recognized (thanks to the work of people such as Joseph Campbell, storyteller Clarissa Pinkola Estés, and astrologer Demetra George), the myths needed to help guide us had been all but forgotten. Sadly, they still play no part in our linear left-brain education, yet they are essential to our growth. Myths help us to see who we are and what we can become. They connect us to the archetypal or universal dimension of human experience. In doing so, they help free us from our own sense of personal limitation and from habit patterns that imprison us, for somewhere in the depths of our humanness the echoes of mythic archetypes that can empower us still sound. Hearing such stories helps us learn to stop and listen. Without the right myths, women at menopause can easily become trapped in an obsession to restore youth and to continue our blood cycles, even if only artificially, by taking hormones. Then, instead of taking up the call to adventure and facing our fear, like a prince and princess at the brink of adulthood, we refuse to move forward.

Thousands of women today are being denied the experience of a natural menopause. They have been seduced into believing that what is happening to their body and psyche is a disease, something terrifying that can only be handled by medical intervention. They have become disempowered by elements that would steal a woman's power for their own commercial ends, and they have become frightened by information in the media, by advertisements, and by doctors, whose only knowledge about menopause comes from "facts" disseminated by the manufacturers of hormones designed to "treat" it. So much fear surrounds menopause—fear of losing one's attractiveness, of getting old, and of no longer having the right to be called female. Like the Gorgon's head or the Medusa, menopause looms large in our society as something that must not be looked upon directly, lest we are turned to stone, for when we lose touch with the myths of menopause's hero's journey, we lose touch with its meaning.

This journey both echoes and is an echo of the hormonal, physiological, and biochemical changes taking place in a woman's body. So it is imperative that we become aware of how to balance our hormones and nurture our bodies. Then, the years beyond menopause can be lived in optimal health, and we are more easily able to manifest in the world the treasures we return with.

I have come to believe that the hero's journey we are called upon to make at menopause is the most important journey a woman ever takes: First, because it is taken with the greatest awareness, given her age and maturity; and second, because at the end of the childbearing years a woman has become biologically free of the need to channel her creative energies into propagating the species. Now, at last, she is free to use her creativity in any way her soul dictates. The power of creation has always been centered in the feminine. That is why poets turn toward the muse for inspiration. Yet few women in the last few thousand years have succeeded in making full use of those creative energies except in a biological way. We have been far too busy giving birth, raising children, and nurturing the creativity of others to be able to explore our own at very deep levels. The hero's journey at menopause offers the possibility of changing these patterns in our lives once and for all—first, by reconnecting with the creative fire within each of us; and second, by honoring our right to use it to accomplish whatever we want.

CHAPTER SEVENTEEN

HERO'S JOURNEY

Making Your Own Passage to Power

he hero's journey each woman takes is unique. Yet every hero's journey told throughout history follows the same archetypal patterns. The story begins in the ordinary world. We meet the princess doing what she always does—sitting in her favorite place playing with her golden ball. Then comes the call to adventure. Something happens to turn the ordinary world on its head. The hero is faced with a problem, a challenge, or a difficulty to overcome. Sometimes the call can come by sheer chance—a blunder (or so it would appear to the linear male world)— the way the princess's golden ball falls into the well. Except, of course, there are no chances in the cyclical realm of the female where the interconnectedness of all things is recognized. There are many ways in which the adventure can begin.

Frequently the call comes in the form of a challenge. It can be physical. Suddenly you wake in the middle of the night with hot sweats. It can also be psychological. You find one morning that your life no longer means anything to you. You wonder where you've been and where you're going. Something is definitely not right. In whatever form it comes, the call heralds the beginning of adventure. From now on, things are never going to be the same. It puts us on notice that destiny has summoned us, and our spiritual center of gravity has suddenly shifted out of the familiar world of society toward realms unknown.

Refusing the Call

Invariably, following closely in the call's wake, fear raises its familiar head. We want to run back into the past and hide. We want to pretend that we didn't hear the summons in the first place. The princess wants her ball, and the frog fetches it, but she is not willing to honor the bargain she has made with him, for she finds him repulsive and only wants to get away. The hero now becomes a reluctant hero. The greatest fear that any of us ever have is fear of the unknown. And what lies ahead is completely unknown. So we try to pretend that everything is all right, we try to hold things together, we go and have a face lift, or go on another of those slimming diets. Or maybe we work even harder and start to lean heavily on our emotional crutches and addictions. At the beginning of any hero's journey, the world sings sweet seductive songs and sends up countless distractions to bewitch us so we go no further.

In detective novels, the private eye tries to refuse the case being offered him, only later to accept it, although he would rather not. Somehow he gets a little push over the edge, and the tale begins to unfold. The frog follows the princess, refusing to take no for an answer. In *Star Wars*, Luke Skywalker turns away from Obi Wan Kenobi's call to adventure to run home to his aunt and uncle, only to find that the farm has been destroyed by the Emperor's stormtroopers. His hesitation is overcome by the evil that has been perpetrated on his ordinary world. Now he begins his personal quest.

Gritting our teeth and battening down the hatches is one way of refusing the call. So is being a servant to social niceties. Women who have forced themselves to live by such rules never have the rich relationships they long for because they cannot share their soul. This, in turn, creates a wasteland and loneliness—the loneliness of a soul that has been banished to the dungeon lest it challenge the rules. When the call comes, a woman is being asked to enter into the loneliness she feels and to walk forth into her wasteland with eyes wide open. If the loneliness we experience cannot be brought into the ordinary world and shared with others, then probably we are spending time with the wrong people. We also may need to do something on our own.

At this point in the journey, a mentor usually arrives to help us out. The mentor is often a Merlin-type character, a book, or an older woman who knows more than we do and who can help us find out what we don't yet know. The mentor's purpose is to help make the hero ready to face the unknown. He or she represents the tie between mother and child, goddess and woman, healer and the healed. The helpful crone and the fairy godmother are common mentor figures in European folklore. They provide the hero with the talisman she will need against the unknown forces she will have to meet. Glenda, the good witch in *The Wizard of Oz*, gives Dorothy her wisdom and a pair of ruby slippers for her journey. Then she sends her on her way. The adventure has begun in earnest, and the presence of a mentor helps to push the hero forward.

Guardians of the Threshold

Now, armed with the powers of destiny bestowed upon her by her mentor, our hero approaches her first passage. Here she meets the guardians of the threshold whose purpose is to prevent the fainthearted from entering the magical realms that lie beyond. Before she leaves New York, in *Romancing the Stone*, Joan Wilder has to face her publisher, who scathingly warns her not to go to Colombia to rescue her sister because she is not strong enough to handle the challenge. Like a nasty old witch, she even portends that something disastrous will certainly happen.

As women approach menopause, their lives are suddenly full of guardians of the threshold. Often these are well-meaning people who prey upon our worst fears—fears of inadequacy, of failure, of hopelessness, of illness, and of death. Whatever these fears are, they need to be faced before we can go on. Confront them head on and you pass through the gate. Now, at last, you are committed to finding out who you are and what your life is about. Crossing the threshold is the first step we take into the sacred realm of the Dark Goddess's world—gateway to the universal source. As Joseph Campbell says in *The Hero with a Thousand Faces*: "The adventure is always and everywhere a passage beyond the veil of the known into the unknown; the powers that watch at the boundary are dangerous; to deal with them is risky; yet for anyone with competence and courage, the danger fades."

Tests, Allies, and Enemies

Now comes the exciting stuff. Now it is time for the hero to deal with the tests, allies, and enemies she will meet along the road. Obstacles to change are always in our way: insufficient money, physical problems, and fears that we have no possibility of ever fulfilling our dreams. New challenges arrive; new things need to be learned. Yet each obstacle overcome, each puzzle solved, each difficulty embraced, brings us more power for what lies ahead. And we meet new people, new ideas, or make new relationships with nature, with animals, and with the unseen world. In *Star Wars*, Obi Wan develops Luke's skill in using The Force by insisting that he fight blindfolded. Before long, Luke faces minor battles that serve to hone his abilities further and help to prepare him for the supreme ordeal that is to come.

Joan Wilder—the timid little lady from New York—is forced to face gunfire, sinister men in black gloves, the loss of her belongings and threats to her life. Along the way, she picks up an ally—Jack—who will be her companion for most of the remainder of her journey. Dorothy picks up her friends the lion, the tinman, and the scarecrow while passing her tests. She oils the tinman's joints. She coaxes the lion to face his fear. She unhooks the scarecrow, who has been unable to move. With each challenge she meets, the hero develops her strength and collects more support from companions, both in the seen and the unseen world. They will turn out to be very useful to her purpose as she approaches the innermost cave.

The Innermost Cave

Now she approaches the entrance to the most dangerous place of all. Here the goal of her journey awaits her. It is the innermost cave. In Arthurian stories, this is the Chapel Perilous—the dangerous room wherein the Grail is hidden. For every woman, her innermost cave is the inner sanctum of the Dark Goddess. The hero entering the cave comes prepared. If he is a man, he knows that this is where the dragon will eventually need to be fought if he is to win the treasure. The same can be true for a woman, too. But more often than not, instead of having to slay a dragon, a woman will need to remain in solitude in this inner Goddess realm, enduring what seems to be unendurable silence. She will listen and need to learn before she can find her treasure. In stories with male heroes, the central image for what is sought is often a gem or a radiant jewel. For a woman, it is frequently the image of a child—the offspring of her spiritual birth.

It is now on the hero's journey that a woman makes her descent into the underworld. The journey a woman makes at menopause is usually fraught with confusion and grief and filled with loneliness and anger. In this place of bone-chilling darkness within the earth, she may feel turned inside out, naked and exposed. All the things she thought she knew don't seem to apply here. Far away from the comfort and companionship of the outside world—which by now she may only vaguely remember, anyway—have gone. Silence pervades. Endless tears without name can be shed. There is no place of comfort, nowhere to turn.

When a woman enters her innermost cave, she may not even have the strength to get dressed, let alone cook or clean or buy food. To her friends and family, she often seems like a creature lost. She may go to bed and stay there. She may forget things, she may dig in her garden or wander in the woods. All these things are wise work. For the route that will eventually lead her out of the underworld and return her in a transformed state to the land above is not the same as that of a man. He may need to move up *away* from himself out into the light. But to find her treasure, a woman is asked to lay aside any fascination she has with culture or games of the mind and turn within—to come instead to know her body, her sexuality, her dreams, her images, and her desires. She moves down even further into her depths to reclaim the parts of her that have been lost. It is here that she will face her supreme ordeal, confront her greatest fears, and undergo the psychological life-or-death moment that is the central crisis of her hero's journey. She tastes death and faces the shadow of herself. When at last it is all over, the Dark Goddess awaits to bless her and bestow upon her the greatest treasure of all—her soul.

The Road Home

Yet this is not the end of the hero's tale. Once she has made her descent, and won her treasure in a life-or-death struggle, she has the task of bringing it back. It is a job easier said than done. Dorothy escapes from the castle of the wicked witch, Luke rescues Princess Leia and gets the plans of the Death Star, the princess throws her frog against the wall and he turns into the beautiful prince. But the game is far from over. Having survived the ordeal, withstood the pressure, slain the monster, and taken possession of the treasure, a hero now has to make her way home. The underworld is not a place where anyone should remain for too long, for when Persephone is raped by Pluto and dragged kicking and screaming into the underworld, where she remains for a seemingly endless period, the crops on the earth above fail, the flowers wither, and the land becomes barren and desolate. Only when she returns will her mother Demeter allow the crops to grow again and the birds to sing.

Further difficulties invariably appear. Dorothy finds that the hot-air balloon that the Wizard has provided to take her back to Kansas is not the sure-fire form of transport she had hoped it would be. Toto runs off after a cat, and in trying to bring him back, the balloon takes off without her and we fear she may be trapped forever in the underworld. Luke Sky-walker and Princess Leia are pursued by Darth Vader as they make their escape from the Death Star. Joan Wilder, having defeated the evil men who wanted to kill her and steal the stone, returns to New York where she faces the arduous task of turning what has happened into her next romantic novel.

It is not easy for any hero to pass back and forth between ordinary and non-ordinary reality. Much energy has been spent during the supreme ordeal, and the hero may not have finished off the enemy completely. There still may be shadows lurking—old ideas, old ways of doing things. But the game has changed now. There, in the inner sanctum, some kind of alchemical process has taken place in us. We are no longer the women that we were. So we need to learn new ways of living and new methods of returning to the surface, since most of the rules we lived by before no longer apply. Sometimes on the road home, the hero can experience a sudden reversal of fortune just when it seemed that the worst was over. Here, too, the hero has the chance of testing out her newfound powers.

Resurrection and Elixirs

In primitive societies, whenever a woman had entered the moon lodge for a few days or whenever a man had returned from a hunt, he or she was required to be washed and purified before they could reenter the community, for they had visited the underworld of non-ordinary reality; they had walked in the land of the dead. The blood that had stained their hands and the mud that remained on their bodies needed to be washed away. The woman's soul that has taken birth is ready to emerge from the womb reborn a new creature. But first it must be blessed with water. So on her return from the underworld of menopause, a woman will often feel the need to regenerate herself using a diet that can spring-clean her body. She may also want to listen to music for hours on end or awaken at dawn and take long walks or carry out some ritual or meditation that can help restore her energies and refocus her life as she returns to the ordinary world.

At last, the hero arrives back with her elixir: the treasure, wisdom, or knowledge that the non-ordinary world exists and that trials can be faced and overcome. She has made her connection with her soul. Dorothy gets back to Kansas, having learned that she is loved and finds that after all is said and done, "there's no place like home." Luke Skywalker destroys the Death Star so peace and order can return to the galaxy. Joan Wilder writes her book, keeps the faith and gets her Jack complete with alligator boots and a boat in which she can sail around the world. The hero's journey has come full circle. She has returned to the place where she started. Yet somehow it is not the *same* place for her, for having carried her elixir intact from the special realm of numinous power all the way home, she is reborn. The world has been renewed.

The woman who completes her passage into the underworld and returns finds within the darkness and confusion and loneliness a new joy, a new sense of meaning, a knowledge that the world that once seemed fragmented all fits together. She also discovers her own power and freedom—that she no longer has to live by other people's rules. Indeed, chances are that it is no longer even possible for her. She is no longer "seducible" by those who would make her feel inadequate so they can sell her another body, another prestigious car, or another love affair just to fill up the emptiness that was once there. She has been released from it all to learn the new art of living as mistress of her own life.

And so the hero's tale ends. Yet one big question remains for every woman who has made her journey: What will she do with the treasure she has brought back? In most of the male myths, there are said to be two choices. Either he takes his treasure into his castle and lives happily ever after, or, like Percival, having found the Grail, he shares it so that the Fisher King's wounding is healed, and the land devastated by barrenness becomes fertile again.

It's My Nature

It is my observation that, having completed her journey, the female hero has no such choice. A woman by her very nature is so much more connected with fostering the energies of life and the powers of the earth, and so much more aware of the inner relationship of all things, that sooner or later she has no choice but to share the boon of her wisdom. She has experienced the power of the Dark Goddess, been given back her soul, and come face to face with the crone—the most essential and generous, wise and powerful of all the faces of woman. Once the crone has touched your heart, something of her generosity seems to be imparted to you. She teaches you without words that you *are* the wisdom that men seek, the bounty that battles are won and lost for—and the power and the joy. Once a woman learns this truth, like the crone who helped her discover it, she must bring her elixir to the world, fostering both her own life and the lives of all other living things. She seems to have no choice. It is her nature to do so—something so deeply entrenched in her genetic material that it cannot be denied.

Once upon a time, there was a scorpion who needed to cross the river. She could not swim, and the river was wide and deep. Sunning himself on the bank was a beautiful red fox. That fox, the scorpion thought, could easily carry me across the river on its back. "Hey, Mr. Fox," said the scorpion, "what about giving me a ride across the river on your back?"

"What?" said the fox. "Do you think me a fool? You are a scorpion. If I were to carry you on my back, you might sting me."

"Oh, don't be ridiculous," replied the scorpion. "I am not going to sting you. If I did that, then we both would drown." The fox thought about this for a few moments; then raising himself to his feet, he replied, "Okay, friend scorpion, a swim in the cool water would be pleasant; hop on my back." And so they started off.

Halfway across the river, the scorpion stung the fox. Stunned, and in terror for his life, for everybody knows that a scorpion's sting means death, the fox cried out, "You fool. Why on earth did you do that?"

"I don't know," replied the scorpion. "I guess it's just my nature."

Doing what somebody else wants you to do is living by a slave mentality. It is the perfect way to encourage physical degeneration and to lose one's soul. Doing what you do because the desire to do it springs forth from your soul is living with the crone's generosity. It is living with enthusiasm.

Enthusiasm is central to living in power. The word *entheos* means "god-filled." When you reach out for whatever fills you with enthusiasm—a sense of the divine—then what you do flows freely from your being without effort. You not only can help transform the world around you, but you have set yourself free.

SOUL LOSS

Regaining Identity and Reclaiming Life Essence

hen a woman takes up the challenge of her own passage to power and commits herself to her own journey, often the first message from her depths to surface is a sense that, quite simply, there is no one there. This is the experience of *soul loss*. And it is a common one. Women have throughout history been schooled in self-denial. Take a look at every acceptable female image in patriarchal societies—the mother, the coquette, the devoted employee. You will find that they all have one thing in common: All put the needs of others before their own. Most of us, regardless of how emancipated we think we are, fit into this way of being all too easily. It is almost as though self-sacrifice has been encoded so deeply in our flesh that it becomes automatic. Often the first inkling that a woman has that she has misplaced part of her soul comes when she stops serving others just long enough to ask herself the question: "But what do *I* want?" Not only is it a difficult question to answer, but for many women it seems difficult even to locate an "I" at all.

Soul loss occurs in each and every one of us to some degree or another. It is the sense that we cannot see who we are, that somehow we have lost a crucial part of ourselves that provides us with creativity, with vitality, or with a sense of meaning in our lives. Primitive people have long lists of experiences that can cause soul loss. They consider it a spiritual illness that in turn can produce physical disease. In tribal cultures, it is believed that soul loss can occur from all sorts of causes: meeting a particular animal in the woods, or entering a house where someone has died but the whole house has not been reblessed for life. In modern times, soul loss occurs in what is called in psychology "disassociation," which in its minor forms is where one part of a woman feels split off from the rest, and in its major forms includes the true multiple-personality experience.

The word *soul* is one that most primitive people have no trouble understanding. Yet it is a word that in our materialistic culture is easily misunderstood or dismissed as a figment of the imagination. Look the word up in *The Shorter Oxford English Dictionary*. It will tell you that "the soul is the principle of life...the spiritual part of man in contrast to the purely physical ...the seat of emotions, feelings or sentiment" and, perhaps most important of all, "...the essential part or quality of a material thing."

There is a belief in classical Jungian psychiatry that soul loss becomes conscious in or around the time of menopause, somewhere between the age of 35 and 50. "Soul loss can be observed today as a psychological phenomenon in the everyday lives of beings around us," writes Jungian analyst Marie von Franz in *Projection and Recollection in Jungian Psychology*. "Loss of soul appears in the form of a sudden onset of apathy and listlessness; the joy has gone out of life, initiative is crippled, one feels empty, everything seems pointless." A woman continues to do her duty, to carry out the obligations of her life from day to day while putting off her own inner desires so successfully that in time she no longer hears the inner voice that says that she would rather dance or dream or build bridges or wander through the woods. When a woman has ignored her soul voice long enough, it can grow very small—so small that it takes a lot of patience and stillness to make out the words that are being whispered.

There are many different experiences of soul loss that can surface as a woman approaches menopause. But whenever soul loss has appeared and in whatever guise, the challenge facing a woman is always the same: She is being called upon to heal the internal split that has occurred between herself and her own feminine nature.

Gilded Cage

A woman marries, and her husband provides her with a home and material possessions. They have a family. She is allowed to do pretty much whatever she wants to do provided the family is well fed and she continues to be a pleasant, decorative addition to the husband's life. From the outside, such a woman appears to have everything. She is often a source of envy to other women who face material struggles—rather like a bird in a gilded cage. The years go by, then one day, around the time of menopause, she begins to realize that she has become disconnected from her own sense of meaning, her soulfulness, and her passion. She has allowed herself to be swept away and seduced by material possessions, or by the promise that someone will love her, and she has embraced ideas supported by the patriarchal society she grew up in. This society would have her believe that woman's fulfillment should come from being a good woman and good mother. For some women, it mostly does. For others, such an imperative only strangles the very life out of them.

My mother was such a woman. An archetypally beautiful California blonde, she was a *prize* for any man. She also happened to have a passion for life, a belief that anything was possible if only you put your mind to it, and a great deal of talent. But, like a lot of women of her time, and for that matter, like many women of our own time, she never really questioned the cultural assumptions about women or the sacrifices they were asked to make in an attempt to live up to them.

My father was a piano player. Like my mother, he came from a poor family but had big dreams. They were married when she was 20 years old and he 23. Since he could only eke out the barest of livings in the early days of their marriage—at one point they had only 25 cents a day to spend on food and ate baked beans every day for weeks—my mother went to work for a tailor. Before long, thanks to her ingenuity and energy, the tailor's business had quadrupled. He offered her a partnership in the business. She loved what she was doing and wanted to take him up on the offer, but my father insisted it would be too much for her. He needed her, he said, and so she put aside her own wishes to support him—both emotionally and in his career. In fact, she put all the energy she had into making my father a success, day after day, year after year. She encouraged him when he felt hopeless, looked after him when he fell ill, did his books for him when he began to make a bit of money, as well as doing his publicity. And she stood by his side. Successful he became.

Not only was my father able, with my mother's support, to start up his own band, within a few years he had become one of the most well-known jazz musicians in America. Yet when anything went wrong or he was scared, he ran to my mother. She wiped the sweat from his brow and bound his wounds. While all of this was going on, there was never any time in my mother's life to even consider what she wanted to do. Before long, she gave birth to her first child so that now she had *two* people to sacrifice herself for—two people who needed her support and care and encouragement, which by now she knew superbly well how to give—that is, to everybody but herself.

Fair Rapunzel

Finally, her marriage to my father ended because she desperately wanted a husband who would stay at home and help her raise a family. Having gotten to the top in his career, all he really wanted was to stay there. At the age of 35, she married a man who she believed would give her the home and stability she had always longed for. He did, but at a price. The price was her soul. Like the golden-haired Rapunzel, he locked her up within a magnificent house that was built, it must be said, with the money she brought to the marriage, and he indulged her wishes to do yoga or to go to this or that restaurant. Yet he never really took her desires seriously, nor by now did she—when she could still hear what they were clearly enough to follow them. And before long, she had another child, another person to serve and care for.

Every so often, my mother would drink a little too much and verbally abuse her husband or children, but that was generally dealt with by all concerned as one of "Mother's little spells." Meanwhile, not fully understanding what was happening to this woman who by now had given everything she had to those she loved, I saw my mother show more and more signs of severe stress. It was very much like the stress an imprisoned animal demonstrates by pacing up and down in its cage, tearing at its fur and spending long hours staring emptily into space.

When her call to adventure came at menopause, she began to have fainting spells. Her mouth would fill up with water, and then she would black out. Her family dealt with them, as most upper-middle-class American families would, by calling in the doctors, who could find nothing physically wrong. They decided it must be "all in her head." She also suffered, as she had periodically throughout her life, from bouts of irrational fear.

Then an opportunity presented itself for her to work in a shop owned by her best friend from childhood. She took it, working a few days a week, despite her husband's disapproval. He said that he would rather that she be at home. Before long, his "need" for her wore my mother down, and she gave up work. She had also developed a passion for painting, and although she had no confidence in herself, she began to attend a weekly class. She discovered there that others, including her teacher, believed she painted rather well, and she loved it. But before long, subtle pressures from the family, coupled with new symptoms she had developed that gave her difficulty in breathing, forced her to cut down on the painting. Again, she was sent to the doctor. This time she was told she had emphysema and was put on medication.

It took four and a half years, with one drug prescribed to combat the side effects of a previous drug, before her strong body and magnificent spirit succumbed to death. Yet even then she seemed to have made a deliberate choice to sacrifice herself so her husband could live. The final 18 months of her life were full of terror for her and were extremely demanding in terms of the care she needed. It took its toll on my stepfather, so much so that he had a heart attack. Soon afterwards, my mother was told by the doctor that everyone needed to be careful not to put too much strain on him. Within 36 hours, she was dead. So far had my mother become separated from her own feminine nature that the call of her soul could only be heard in the form of physical illness. And by then it had been too late to heed it.

The Madness of Woman

Her story is not so extreme or so unusual. Fine novels have been written about such women, such as *The Madness of the Seduced Woman,* by Susan Fromberg Schaeffer. They describe what happens when women of passion have become so separated from their wild nature that the only possible triumph left to them is a triumph of spirit that ends in death or at the very least destroys them. This is an extreme example of soul loss. It is also, in my view, an inexcusable waste of a woman's life, as well as something that no amount of ranting and raving against the male world for what it may or may not have done to women is going to change. The only thing that can change it is each one of us coming to an increasing personal inner awareness of how soul loss may be operating in our own lives and then taking steps to correct it.

I was young and did not understand what was going on with my mother at the time, but I remember sitting for long hours and listening to her speak in confusion about herself. I was aware that she never really appreciated her own strength, and I know that she was forever giving the power that she had away to others. I also watched her at the age of 50 become increasingly embittered. Without ever realizing it, she had made an unspoken "devil's bargain" with the world. It was this: If only she were good enough, if only she gave enough, if only she cared enough for those around her, then life would reward her. Of course it didn't; it never does. And when she realized it didn't, the agonized fury of the soul that had become separated from her turned against her and eventually destroyed her. I don't think she ever even realized what had happened. All she had was a sense that somehow she must be the one who was at fault and that whatever she had done, she had not done it well enough.

Into the Desert

With the experience of soul loss, no matter what its cause, comes a sense of desiccation—a feeling that there is nothing inside you, or that whatever is inside you is likely to be of no real value. Living in such a barren landscape, it is virtually impossible for a woman to create anything other than frustration and fear. For other women, their sense of soul loss comes as a sense that it has gone into hiding, because there is too much pressure from the outside world and there is no place for the soul to live. This is often connected to the idea that a woman is basically on the earth for the purpose of serving others. So deeply ingrained is this notion in the female character that one of the few alternatives a woman has available to protect herself is for her soul to be "absent without leave."

Someone Else's Dreams

For women who have rebelled against the idea that a woman's place is in the service of others, the experience of soul loss comes differently. Yet it still brings with it a sense of emptiness, sterility, and dismemberment. Every culture has its own set of underlying myths and values within which its society functions. In our Western world, these myths are almost entirely male-defined. We value accomplishment, success, winning authority, worldly power, glamour, and prestige. Daughters of the father, unwilling to become the all-serving females, opt instead to play by the masculine rules of the game, and although they are usually not fully aware of it, do all they can to win masculine approval. Daughters of the father have bought into the stereotyped male values lock, stock, and barrel. They tend to spend their lives seeking (and often attaining) power in the world, financial success, or artistic or academic achievements. Sometimes they wake up somewhere between the age of 35 and 50 to find that the dream that they have been dreaming is not their dream but someone else's—that is, the values of the male culture in which they have been raised. *Why do I have this sense of emptiness, betrayal, or dislocation?* a woman asks. The answer is simple— because in her effort to succeed, to get things done, she has not had time to listen to her *own* instincts or followed her *own* dreams. As a result, she has lost touch with the deep relationship to her own wild female nature, which is the only thing that can feed her at the deepest levels. And she is hungry.

Any woman experiencing soul loss, whether she has lived in a golden cage, has become a successful daughter of the father, or has gone into hiding, finds herself living in a world that has lost its moisture—a desert known too well by any captive creature. However soul loss has occurred, once a woman crosses the threshold to begin her hero's journey, like the princess with the golden ball, she is faced with a reflection of herself that is inevitably fragmented, distorted, or simply not there.

Way of the Shaman

The group of people who understand most about soul loss are not the psychologists or the priests, but the shamans. Shamanism is a tradition of healing that has been practiced for tens of thousands of years by tribal communities throughout the world—in Africa, China, Australia, North and South America, Lapland, and Europe. The word *shaman* means "healer," or "one who sees in the dark." It is a Tungus word that originated in Siberia and Mongolia. It describes someone who, through drumming, dance, or some other meditational technique, places him- or herself in an altered state of consciousness and who then, by leaving the body, travels to a parallel universe that is outside time and space in non-ordinary reality in order to heal, to gain wisdom for the tribe, or locate and bring back a lost or stolen part of the human soul.

A shaman is a healer who him- or herself has been profoundly wounded. In fact, it is through the experience of wounding that a shaman develops the power to journey into the unseen world for the benefit of others. A shaman believes that—as a result of trauma or difficult life circumstances—a part of a person's essential nature will leave the body and move into a non-ordinary reality, usually as a means of protection so that the person is able to survive an otherwise devastating or life-threatening experience. This is soul loss. It is the shaman's job to retrieve that lost essence or soul and bring it back to the person who lost it. It is also the shaman's job to heal both the living and the dead. To accomplish this, he or she works with helping spirits in non-ordinary reality. Some of them are what are known as power animals. They are the shaman's constant companions on his or her journeys into the unseen world.

What makes the shaman different from the priest, psychologist, witch doctor, or other healers is the fact that he or she makes a journey in the non-ordinary world in order to discover both the cause of a person's illness and also to retrieve the parts of someone's soul that need to be brought back into that human being for healing to take place. Such splits can occur as a result of trauma, and in their most exaggerated forms appear to be the underlying cause of the multiple-personality phenomenon, where the basic integrity of a person's being is literally split open so that not only does soul loss occur, but the person can even be inhabited by spirits from other dimensions. Or, it happens because a person is forced to live in circumstances either as a child or an adult that literally create no space for the soul to be in, so fragments of it leave in a bid for survival.

American shaman Sandra Ingerman has written a compassionate and wise book called *Soul Retrieval*, in which she describes what the shamanic journey looks like, as well as the various causes of soul loss and the experience of having one's soul fragments returned:

> One can return only a certain number of soul parts at one time. The reason for this is simple. When the soul returns, it comes back with all the pain it experiences on leaving. The memories surrounding the trauma often take awhile to return. I don't want to overwhelm a person with too many memories of physical and/or emotional pain. The way I know how many parts to bring back is by following directions from my power animal, whose judgment I trust implicitly. When he says, "That's enough for now," my search ends. Integration of the returned soul parts takes some time.

So widespread is shamanism in primitive cultures, so long has it been practiced—thousands upon thousands of years—that it is believed to be the oldest and most widely used system of healing in the world. In our Western culture, shamanism was for many centuries suppressed by a materialistic culture that sought, despite its rhetoric to the contrary, not to free people so that they could live from the soul, but rather to make use of them to maintain the structures of social, political, and economic control, regardless of the cost to the soul. In recent years, however, shamanism has undergone a considerable revival. It is becoming a useful part of a holistic approach to healing and growth that respects human individuality and nurtures creativity.

In the hands of a developed and highly trained shaman, the process of soul retrieval can be a tremendously important part of a woman's journey at menopause. Shamans also concern themselves with retrieving the soul energy lost from forests, mountains, houses, and cities as part of a wider intention to bring healing to the planet, for soul loss is a spiritual illness that can result in a physical disease. What impresses me about shamanic journeying for soul retrieval is that it is so simple, yet so effective. It can often do in a couple of hours what years of psychotherapy has been unable to accomplish, probably because it cuts quickly through concepts and intellectual ideas and goes to the core of a person in a way that is nonthreatening and respectful of human life.

You may think of soul loss in a metaphoric sense, the way many psychologists do—as parts of oneself that are not accessible for use because they are repressed in unconscious material. Or, you might prefer to think of soul loss (as primitive cultures do) in a more literal sense—as fragments of the soul (in the case of someone in a coma, the entire soul actually leaves the body to dwell in other dimensions that are more comfortable for it). It makes little difference. After years of exploring the soul-loss phenomenon, I have come to believe that both points of view are valid—like two sides of the same coin. The important thing is that soul loss occurs regularly.

And how does one retrieve lost fragments of oneself? The first step is by being aware that they are not there. American shaman Sandra Ingerman lists a number of factors in someone's life that are thought to indicate possible soul loss. They include addictions, chronic illness during childhood, gaps in memory, chronic depression, a feeling of numbness or deadness, a difficulty in staying "present" in your body or a feeling that you are sometimes outside your body, a longing for something to fill up a sense of emptiness in your life, multiple-personality syndrome, a sense of possibly having blocked out traumas, or simple difficulty moving on with one's life. All of these experiences can be an indication of soul loss. The menopausal hero's journey is one of the means by which the missing pieces can be found.

———⟫●⟪———

CHAPTER NINETEEN

GIRL WITHOUT HANDS

Transforming Creative Impotence into Personal Power

The soul of a woman gets wounded in a very different way than that of a man. Where soul wounds in a man interfere with his ability to *feel*, those of a woman most often render her unable to *do*. She can feel, she can dream her dreams, she can have great visions, yet somehow, generations of soul imprisonment may render her unable to act on those feelings, unable to trust her instincts and desires. She is like a girl without hands.

There are many wonderful tales of the female hero's journey to inspire and comfort, to encourage and guide a woman who has heard her call. The myth of the ancient Sumerian goddess of heaven and earth, Inanna, is one. Inanna makes her descent to attend the funeral of her dark sister Erishkigal's husband in the underworld and has to remove her every adornment in the process. But Erishkigal, jealous of her sister's beauty, tries to kill her and hangs her from a meat hook to rot. The tale of how Inanna is finally rescued by humble creatures fashioned from the parings of the nails of a lesser god holds many secrets to be learned. So does the story of Demeter whose daughter Persephone is raped and dragged into the underworld by Pluto. Demeter wanders in the wasteland until she finds a means of reclaiming Persephone and restoring fertility to the earth. Of them all, there is one tale that I like the best. I suppose it is because it seems most relevant to women now. It is called "Silverhands" or "The Handless Maiden."

Told by the Brothers Grimm and hundreds of others in one form or another, this is a story of a girl whose father makes a bargain with the devil. It addresses the soul wounding of the woman who at menopause cries out in pain, "I feel so useless. Who am I? What can I *do*?" It also speaks of the damage done to the human spirit in both men and women by the mechanical world that we have created out of the Industrial Revolution. Like all good myths, it also points the way toward healing.

❀ ❀ ❀

The Handless Maiden

Once a miller lived with his wife and his lovely daughter deep in the forest. A good and honest man, the miller had been grinding grain to make bread for the villagers for 40 years with the help of his faithful ox and by the sweat of his brow. But grinding corn was hard work, and the miller had grown weary of the toil. One afternoon, as he was chopping wood at the end of a long day, a dark stranger appeared and said, "Why do you waste your time with all this chopping and grinding? Give me what stands behind your little cottage, and I will turn your grindstone for you and chop your wood by magic. I will also change your humble house into a great mansion."

It all sounded like a great idea to the miller. After all, the only thing that stood behind his cottage was an old apple tree. Who in their right mind would not trade that for a life of luxury and the freedom to spend his time as he chooses? So he agreed.

"Good," said the dark stranger, "then you shall have your riches and your freedom from toil. And I? I shall return in three years to claim what is mine." Then he disappeared as mysteriously as he arrived.

The miller picked up his shining axe and began to make his way back through the woods to his cottage. But who was this running toward him? It was his wife, except her simple housemaid's apron was gone. In its place was the finest velvet dress of crimson that he had ever seen. "Husband, you should see what has happened," she cried. "Our house is gone. In its place stands a great mansion with glittering turrets and an herb garden woven like a braid into the meadow."

Pleased with how shrewd he had been to do his deal, the miller told his wife of the bargain with the dark stranger. "But what did you promise him in return?" she wanted to know.

"Only that which stands behind our cottage—the gnarled old apple tree that I should most certainly have cut down soon anyway." The woman threw up her hands in horror. She wailed. She shrieked. "Oh, husband, what have you done," she screamed. "It is our daughter who stood behind the cottage this afternoon sweeping the path. You fool, you have sealed her fate forever." [Alas, terrible things happen when in his thirst for mechanical devices and in his lust for gold, a man is willing to win at the expense of the feminine.]

The miller and his wife returned home weeping despite their finery. They told their daughter what would become of her in three years' time. The girl took the news with patience and in silence. And for three years she awaited her fate. Then one day, sure enough, the Evil One appeared to claim his due. The girl washed herself, dressed in white linen, and drew a circle around her body with chalk. But when the stranger reached out to take her by the arm, he could not bear her purity. "Keep her away from water," he ordered, "or I shall have no power over her. I will return tomorrow." The miller does as the stranger bid him to do for he was terrified of the Dark One's power and could only tremble in his presence.

The next morning, when the stranger came back, he found that the girl had shed tears all through the night. Because she was clean and pure again, he could not approach her. By now he was furious. "Chop off her hands," he ordered the miller.

Horrified, the miller refused. How could he chop off the hands of his only daughter? "If you do not do exactly as I say," hissed the Evil One, "then I shall take you away with me forever." So, in tears, the miller approached his daughter.

"My child," he said, "the devil will take me far away unless I chop off both your hands with my ax. Forgive me the injury that I will do to you."

"Father," replied the girl, "I am your child. Do what you will." And she held out her hands. One swift slash with the ax, and they lay bleeding in the soil. Now the stranger arrived for the third time to find her stumps all bandaged in gauze. But again, the girl had wept so long and freely that they too were washed pure with her tears. Defeated, the Evil One knew he had lost all right to her and so he left.

The miller tried to make up to his daughter what he had done. After all, he was rich now and could offer the girl anything she wanted. She would be able to live in comfort for the rest of her life. He would feed her and take care of her and she would want for nothing. But the girl replied, "I cannot stay, father. I must go away. The kindness of people will provide for me." So her mother tied her maimed arms in fresh gauze and the girl set out on her journey— but to where and for what she did not know.

All day she walked. At dusk she came to an orchard full of trees heavy with wonderful-smelling fruit. Oh, how hungry she was. "If only I could get some of that fruit," she thought. But she could not enter the orchard. It was surrounded by a moat that was filled with water. She knelt upon the ground and said a prayer to the earth, her mother, "I shall die, sweet mother, if I do not taste of that fruit." Suddenly, an angel appeared and cleared the water. The moat went dry, the girl crossed, and reaching out with the gauze-bound stumps, she plucked a pear from the tree, held it, and ate it.

The orchard belonged to a king. He was a good man but somewhat miserly. He had his servants number every piece of fruit and keep a gardener on constant watch to make sure none was stolen. Of course, the gardener saw the girl. But he also saw the angel and so he was afraid that the girl might be a spirit. He decided not to report the loss to the king. The next morning when the king came to count his pears, however, he discovered that one was missing. "Your Highness," said the gardener, "I saw it go, but I know not if it was taken by a maid or by a spirit with no hands."

"And how did this spirit cross the moat?" the king wanted to know. The gardener had no answer. "Where did it go?" the king asked.

"Why, it disappeared into the thicket," said the gardener.

"Then I shall watch myself to see if it returns tonight," said the king.

So that evening the king and his magician concealed themselves behind an old wall and waited. Sure enough, a figure dressed in white came creeping from the thicket, approached the tree, took another pear, and started to eat it. The magician revealed himself. "Are you of this world or another?" he questioned the girl.

"I was once of the world, yet I am not of *this* world," replied the girl. "It has forsaken me." The beauty of the girl's face and the strange simplicity of her manner touched the heart of the king, who fell in love with her and rushed forward.

"Sweet maiden, you may be forsaken by the whole world, but I will not forsake you." So he led her to his palace, and there he married her and commanded his craftsman to fashion silver hands to replace the ones she had lost. But what good are silver hands to a woman who longs to make use of them?

A year went by. The king was called to war. The maiden, who was now the queen, awaited her first child. So the king went to his mother and asked her to care for Silverhands while he was away. When Silverhands was brought to bed, he told the mother she must send him word of his wife's state of health and of the child. Not long after, the queen gave birth to a boy. True to her word, the king's mother sent a letter saying that both were well and wonderful. But the messenger carrying it was waylaid. He grew tired at the bank of a river, stopped to rest, and fell asleep. This was the work of the Evil One, who had come to substitute the letter with another announcing that the queen had given birth to a child, half-man half-beast.

When the king read the forgery, he was much distressed. Yet he wrote back to say that his mother should care for them both until his return. On his way back to the castle, once again the messenger is overcome by drowsiness. The devil came, took the king's letter from his hand, and switched it for another, telling the mother she must kill the queen and her child. Horrified, his mother read the letter. She wrote back, sure that there must be some mistake. But yet again, the letters were switched. Finally, the last forged letter arrived from the king, insisting that his mother must kill the queen, then cut out her eyes and tongue for him to see on his return.

The queen could not bring herself to carry out his orders. So she packed up Silverhands and the babe and sent them out into the world and said, "I cannot kill you, but you must go far away and never return." She tied the child to the queen's back—for the queen's useless silver hands could not perform even a simple task like carrying her own child. In tears, poor Silverhands wandered away and went deep into the woods. Now in despair for the second time, she fell upon her knees and prayed. Once again, the angel appeared.

"You are welcome, fine queen," the angel said, leading her into a lovely cottage. There she untied the child from Silverhands' back, and it began to nurse. "How did you know that I was the queen?" asked Silverhands.

"I am a handmaiden of the Dark Goddess," the angel replied. "I have been sent to care for you and your child." So Silverhands stayed in that little house and was happy with her child and with her life. Gradually her hands grew back. In the beginning, they looked like baby hands, then like the hands of a child. Finally, they grew into the beautiful hands of a woman.

Not long after Silverhands left the castle, the king returned, having won his war to find his wife gone and the eyes and tongue of a deer in their place. His mother told him of the letters and admonished him for his cruelty. But no, it was not he who sent them. "How could you kill my wife and child?" he insisted, trembling with grief and rage.

"I could not kill them either," his mother confessed. "I killed a deer and sent them far away."

So for seven years the king wandered in search of his family. In all that time, he neither ate nor drank. His hair grew long, and his beard became tangled with brambles. Then one day he arrived at the cottage in the woods. The angel greeted him at the door and invited him in. He was so tired after his wandering that he fell immediately into a deep sleep, and the angel placed a fine linen handkerchief over his face. But the child—his very own child—came into the room. Finding a man lying on the bed, he lifted the piece of linen to see what was beneath. The king awakened and found this beautiful child and his own lovely wife gazing down on him.

"I am your wife," said the queen, "and this is your son."

"Alas, that cannot be," said the king. "My wife is called Silverhands, for she has no hands of her own."

"I was once she," his wife replied. "Through my dreams, my silence, and my care, these hands have grown back. I am no longer the handless maiden you once knew." She who had once been Silverhands now went to fetch the same silver hands and showed them to the king. Brimming with joy after his long years of wandering, the king embraced his family. They returned from the forest that very day while all the angels and the people of the forest celebrated with a great feast. When the king and his family arrived back at the castle, another wedding was arranged. The queen mother rejoiced. They had many more children and all was well.

❀ ❀ ❀

I love this story. It holds within it so many of our secrets. It tells of the terrible bargains we women blunder into, like the miller who trades his apple tree in a bargain with the devil, then finds he has sacrificed his daughter's hands. Similar to those in our Western world, he is seduced by wealth and the technology of magic, so he gives away what he loves most.

The miller betrays his daughter as we in all innocence betray ourselves—bargaining away our freedom and our wildness for what we think will bring us safety or for some bauble that catches our eye. We marry when we should not. We force ourselves to live lives that do not feed us. All such trades are devil's bargains. In making them, we lose our hands, our claws, our ability to do and make what deep within we want most to do and make—and our ability to protect ourselves. Meanwhile, the simplicity of human life has lost its flavor, and the devil stands forever by—ready to offer us another bargain we cannot afford to refuse.

The light of a young woman's soul that slumbers invariably attracts a predator. No evil creature can resist such sweetness. The girl's initiation, like our own, comes with the loss of her hands. She has given up dominion over her own soul. Yet in her innocence—knowing not what she has done, her tears of grief wash her clean so the devil cannot take her. And her loss, tragic though it is, is also her salvation, for it is the beginning of a hero's journey, which, after many trials and tribulations, will lead her deep into the forest where in silence and in the presence of an angel sent by the Dark Goddess, she will regrow her hands, regain her power, and her wholeness. It is the first betrayal that sends us on a journey that will awaken us. And when our soul no longer slumbers, then the dark stranger has no power. Evil cannot touch us.

The girl is lovely. Her beauty draws pity from the king and a certain kind of love. He will, he promises, look after her forever. Some would say a girl in such a condition is lucky to have the offer. Yet what woman can live her life, what woman can nurture her child, or paint her picture, or move her mountain with a useless pair of decorative hands bestowed upon her by her husband? There has to be another way if only we wait long enough, if only we can find somewhere deep within the woods where we can rest and listen and let our hands grow back—if only we can pray for that. And in those darkest times and in the deepest forest, prayers can be answered. We find our place. It is a place of stillness deep within the forest. There a woman is safest. It is her realm. Here she is happy amidst the ancient trees and amongst the beasts, amongst the flowers. There is no devil who can touch her here with his sinister bargains and his thieving ways.

Like all women, Silverhands has several initiations in her life. Each brings its lessons and its comforts until at last she finds her place and rests. Then, in time, she rises from the underworld of her magic forest peopled with sacred trees and beasts, both wild and tame. She returns to the world no longer crippled, but with soul intact and hands ready to do whatever she may ask of them. At last, she has reclaimed her wildness.

CHAPTER TWENTY

CRONE'S RETREAT

Entering the Cocoon of Transformation

he first step in any initiation is isolation, some kind of withdrawal from our ordinary lives so that we can confront the changes taking place in our bodies and the transformations in our lives, and so that we can come to terms with what within us is dying and make way for something else to be born. In primitive societies, when the signs of menopause arrived to herald the dark phase of the moon in a woman's life, she was allowed to leave the tribe and go away for a time. Rather like a modern sabbatical, this year away was known as the crone's retreat. It is an important ritual. Although few women these days can take off for a year's holiday all expenses paid, it is always necessary that a woman initiate some form of retreat in her own life around the time of menopause. It may mean giving up certain responsibilities, or arranging your life so that for at least two or three hours a day you are left alone simply to *be*. Like many ancient rituals, the crone's retreat developed out of a need that is universal in menopausal women: When menopause arrives, every woman needs the time and space to turn around and discover what is stalking her. Women who refuse to honor their inner demands for time alone often get sick and have it forced upon them.

When my own perimenopausal years arrived, I had never heard of the crone's retreat. I had hardly ever heard the word *crone*—except to refer to some terrible old witch on a children's television program. But what I did hear loud and clear from within was a demand that I turn away from the out-side world. I could not silence it. The call to retreat can come in as many different guises as there are women to hear it. In my own life, it came as a demand from somewhere deep inside that I stop everything I was doing and sit down to write a serious novel. This was something I hardly dared to dream was possible. It was responding to that demand—and I had little choice of not responding to it, so insistent had it become—that led me into my own crone's retreat, taught me firsthand about the nature of the hero's journey, and took me through my own initiation of the dark moon. What-ever else it was, it wasn't easy.

To anyone who has never done one, the idea of going on a retreat can conjure up visions of saffron robes and jasmine flowers or medieval clois-ters filled with pious nuns in black habits gently wending their way to even-song. To some, the idea of retreating from day-to-day communications for a time may seem like an extended holiday during which life's stresses are sloughed off. The reality, to say the least, is somewhat different. Crone's time away does something quite different than simply lift you out of your ordinary world and transport you into a comfortable realm of spiritual peace. It brings you face to face with the deepest layers of your own being. This is never a comfortable prospect. It always makes me laugh when someone at a dinner party begins to criticize recluses, monks, and nuns, saying that they should have the courage to live in the world. In my experience, living in the world can be an easy task next to entering the realms of the soul.

Charnel Ground

In the 20 years before menopause, I had carried out a number of short retreats, including one of several weeks in a Tibetan monastery in the Himalayas where (among other things) I learned that my greatest attach-ment was to porcelain lavatories, and my worst karma was with fleas. Each of them was some preparation for my lengthy crone's retreat, during which I gave up all my connections to the outside world to wrestle with the ques-tion of whether or not I could find new meaning in my life by writing my first novel. The task took me deep into the recesses of my own psyche. It was an experience which—only now that the period of withdrawal has come to an end—I realize had echoes of the cold, dark isolation that St. John described and the bleakness of wandering in Vajragini's (one of the great goddesses in the Tibetan tradition) charnel ground.

It is a funny thing how a crone's retreat usually comes about. It is quite different from setting aside a long weekend or a couple of weeks to go to a meditation center as a means of breaking out of your routine and deepening your spiritual insight. You do not choose it. It chooses you. In the beginning, you are rarely aware that this is what is going on. All you know is that something inside is demanding that you listen to it. It is a demand that often comes with ruthless insistence, even if listening to it means turning away from a life that on most levels seemed to be working well.

Ancient Dreams

My own retreat began when I was perimenopausal. It was to last more than three and a half years and only came to an end the same month I had my last period. Strangely enough, the first inkling of what it would be about had come 20 years before in a dream. I dreamed I was standing in the midst of a magnificent garden. It was like a garden in one of those Persian miniature paintings, filled with masses of flowers in luminous colors and trees all covered with fruits. There was a great pond in the midst of the garden, and Beethoven's music was playing. It was nothing of Beethoven's I had heard before, and yet I knew that it was by him. I stood in the center of this garden entranced by the colors, the sounds, and the beauty around me. As the music reached a crescendo, suddenly the trees and flowers, the fruits and the sky became transfigured with light. Then the hand of God—it looked like Michelangelo's God who reaches out to Adam on the ceiling of the Sistine Chapel—came down from the heavens. Its index finger touched the center of the pond sending ever-increasing circles outwards. This was more than I could bear. I closed my eyes and put my hands over my ears. Moments later, as the music began to descend from its climax, when I removed my hands and opened my eyes, I saw that the garden was returning to its previous colors and state. A voice within me said, "It is all right— the next time such beauty comes, you will be able to bear it."

That was all. The dream had occurred in my mid-20s. I had no idea what it "meant." All I knew was that it felt like some kind of a blessing had been offered or something fundamental had shifted in my life—at least in my *inner* life, for my outer life was full of trying to care for three children on my own and earning a living for all of us. I suppose that I learned something pretty fundamental about myself from the dream. It was strange, and I could make little sense of it: I learned that the thing that frightens me most is not the horror of pain, deprivation, or loneliness, but rather the intensity of a profound experience of beauty. Real beauty, like great joy, carries with it a devastating quality of truth. This, I learned from the dream, was what I have always feared most.

Then for many years I forgot about it. I immersed myself in earning a living, writing books, making television programs, and doing all the things we women do every day in the middle period of our lives when the responsibilities of a householder sit heavily on our shoulders. Some 15 years later, the dream came back to me, and with it this strange imperative: *You must put everything aside to write a novel about Beethoven.* I had never written fiction. I had never dared to dream I could. I fought the inner command with the vehemence of a trapped animal. It terrified me. At first I thought the fear was a fear of failure. Like many women, I have never suffered from an abundance of self-confidence. It was only much later that I was to realize it had another—far deeper—cause as well.

Into the Silence

My retreat began by withdrawing from my outside work. Having raised four children (by then I had had another child), I had been forced to spend quite a lot of my time earning a living—in fact, virtually all of the time not spent being with my children. Early on in the years of my research for the novel, I began to see that there was no way in which I could write it unless I could give up my work in the media and not have to earn a living until it was finished. I began to pray that this would be possible, although I saw no way in which it was going to happen given my financial responsibilities.

The trouble with prayer is that it can be dangerous. Often you end up getting what you pray for—which means that it is a good idea to be very careful about what you ask for. Many of us would like to convince ourselves that the only thing that is stopping us from doing what we want is money. It is only when such a prayer is answered that you realize the impediments to your moving ahead do not lie in a lack of money as you have always assumed, but rather in an unwillingness to embrace the absolute freedom of choice each of us has. This is exactly what happened to me. Until then, I had been able to see myself as a conscientious and caring mother—if somewhat long-suffering—who was willing to sacrifice her own desires to earn a living and care for her children. Suddenly I found this was no longer necessary. In my 40s, to my surprise, I found myself with all the material resources I needed to do exactly what I had been saying for several years I wanted to do, and just as the beauty in my dream had over-whelmed me all those years before, this newfound freedom terrified me. So began my crone's time away, for which I was ill prepared. The short retreats I had done before had been well structured within religious traditions: You went into meditation, you kept silent, you ate one meal a day, and so forth. All of that had been easy compared with what I now faced.

Wild Energy

In the Hindu and Buddhist tradition, there is an unusual spiritual path known as *left-handed tantra*. There is, I think, something decidedly *female* about the energy connected with it. It is *wild* energy—the energy of nature that refuses to fit into the shapes we would impose on it. Left-handed tantra is not much written or spoken about, and it is not much practiced. It differs from other spiritual pathways in that the empowerment that is believed to come to the individual from the divine (an intense energy that is highly volatile) in most religious traditions comes carefully packaged and struc-tured within ethical and meditational rituals. Usually they are carried out under the wise gaze of a teacher who has already trodden the path. In the case of left-handed tantra, all this numinous energy suddenly pours through you with no conceptual framework, no spiritual guidance, and no useful practices designed to render it more bearable. It was only after my lengthy retreat had finally come to an end—as had the novel that engendered it—that I realized I had unwittingly been thrown into the seemingly chaotic energies of left-handed tantra.

Somehow, a wild spirit—a ruthless manifestation of my own life force—had arisen from within, demanding that I follow it no matter how difficult or frightening that might become. It seemed to have an almost total disregard for my personal comfort or for the wishes of my ego. Like a dis-ciple who attaches himself to the guru and follows his master's every whim, I found myself in the service of creating this book. At each moment during the years that it took to complete, I had a choice to make—either to honor my commitment or to run away. The experience turned out to be nothing like what I had assumed the writing of a novel would be about. For one thing, it was not at all a question of "making it all up." It was more a process of uncovering layer after layer of truth and meaning as though the form and shape of the book was already there and it was my job to uncover it. In the process, layer after layer of my own psyche became uncovered, although an awareness of what was going on remained mostly hidden from me until after the process was all over.

To Be or Not to Be

I began the writing of *Ludwig* the way I have begun every other project—with a reasonable sense of organization and the intention that I would produce 2,000 words a day until the book was finished. My naïveté in assuming I would be able to do this still stuns me. When I look back to how I was then, I see myself as a callow youth with little understanding of the processes involved in creation. I was pig-ignorant—ignorant enough not even to have an inkling of how truly ignorant I really was. I found the writing very difficult. I would have to stop for weeks at a time. At one point, I discovered that I could not work at all in the light. I would pull down all the blinds in my studio and sit for hours on end in front of my computer screen in the dark. Every day I would get up and run for an hour along the cliffs where I live in West Wales, then I would swim in the sea, as I had been doing for years. Afterwards, I would return to my darkened room to write.

Before long, the whole process had brought me to my knees. Everything I had learned before about writing simply did not apply. I could not, as I had rather arrogantly assumed, write this book from the same practical, matter-of-fact framework that had worked for all my other books. This novel demanded something different. In short, it demanded *everything*. Then one morning as I ran into the sea at dawn, I realized that I was so filled with despair and frustration at what I perceived to be the impossibility of the task I had taken on that I wanted to swim out into the Irish Sea and never return. What was happening to me? I knew only one thing: that I had a choice, do I live or do I die? There in the white foam as the sun rose over the sea that morning, I made my choice. I cried out defiantly to whoever or whatever might be listening, "Okay, if you want to destroy me, that is your business, but I am not going to help you do it!"

Back on Home Ground

I could not understand what was happening to me. Where was all this anger and despair coming from? I wondered if I was ill. I went to have my endocrine system checked out only to find that most of it—the pituitary, the adrenals, the thyroid, the ovaries—were badly out of order. Instead of worrying me, this news delighted me. Now, at least I was on familiar territory; I could fall back on what I knew from my many years of working in health. I knew what to do to help my body. The knowing brought me the only feelings of security I had felt ever since I had entered this new world. So I went on a seven-week juice fast. The practitioner who had examined me and voiced deep concern over how imbalanced my hormone system had become was amazed. He had never seen anyone recover so quickly. Yet, despite my rapid recovery, the book had to be laid aside for almost six months. I felt as though I had fallen into a great luminous sea—a sea in which all things were possible and anything could be brought into being—which so completely dissolved the boundaries of who I thought I was that I felt I could not function.

The years of my crone's retreat were spent in learning patience and humility—that I was nothing, am nothing, and can do nothing by myself; yet that in my nothingness, and out of it, all things may be born. So many internal events occurred that it would be impossible to speak of them all. So deeply did my research into Beethoven's life and music take me, and so immersed did I become in the spirit of the book, that in time I began to experience his symptoms. I had the same deafness in the ears, the same pain in the liver and upsets in the colon that are described in his medical reports. My research for the novel took me into two other areas outside Beethoven's life, which, although I did not know it at the time, were to change my view of the human psyche and of worlds—both seen and unseen—beyond all recognition. The first was the phenomenon of the multiple personality. The second area was the whole question of the nature of human freedom and the political and economic forces that stifle it. Before my retreat began, I had voiced only the vaguest interest in either subject.

Some of what I experienced during those years went into the novel itself. In the process of creating it, I was forced to make my own descent. I learned firsthand about the archetypal nature of the hero's journey, about the vast nature of the human psyche, and about the quality of the wasteland. Until then, these were nothing more than ideas that I had read about with detached curiosity. I was to learn that a woman's experience of the descent is very different indeed from the rather facile description of it that you can find in many books on psychology. I learned that myth is the only language one can legitimately use to speak of it. I discovered, too, that a woman's inner world and outer one are but reflections of one another—as within, so without. And, in a messy piecemeal way, I made my passages. They were not passages of my own choosing; from some deep inner place within, they had been chosen for me. My teacher and guide was the task I had chosen. My challenge was to use my crone's retreat to complete it. I followed this imperative, never knowing from one day to the next if that would happen.

The first two-thirds of the book took me three and a half years to write. During most of that time, making words was like squeezing blood from a stone. Like many women, I was riddled with self-criticism and hardly dared to think that I might succeed. Even to contemplate such an action went against all my conditioning. I discovered that all my life I had been carrying around a notion that a woman should sacrifice her needs for others. It is an idea that now seems ancient history. During the last three months, I wrote the final third of the novel—mostly in a frenzy. Suddenly words began to spill forth in such profusion and intensity that I could hardly get them down. I would get up at three in the morning to begin work, my body stiff with pain, because, although most days I still ran along my cliffs, I had become so completely immersed in the mythic world out of which the novel grew that I badly neglected the needs of my body. I would say to it, "Just support me for a few weeks more, and then I will take care of you."

Caterpillars and Butterflies

One day the novel was finished. Six hours later, I left for New Zealand to do a series of lectures and workshops for International Green Month. When I arrived there, I felt like someone who had come back from the dead—a caterpillar who, bound inside its cocoon, had watched while its body dissolved into a white gel in the hopes that one day it might be reformed as a butterfly. Now, three years later, it feels as though I may be just beginning to emerge from that cocoon. My wings are very stiff and very wet. My menopausal passage is over. The world is different. I have had to learn all sorts of brand-new languages to live in it. What did I gain from all of this? Only the absolute knowing that there is an incredible natural order that regulates our lives even when we perceive ourselves to be in total chaos. Within this order is to be found a quality of love and compassion that goes far beyond anything I could ever have imagined. It continually asks that we venture deep into the realm of wisdom, and it knows exactly what is right and necessary from one moment to the next in our lives. Now I am in the process of having to learn to trust it with all of my being. This is all

I know, except perhaps for one thing more: that something fundamental has changed in me. I have walked through a door, and I can never return. Soon there may be other doors to be opened, other descents to be made, and new treasures to be found. For now, I am trying to learn to use my new wings to fly, to where or how is anybody's guess.

———⟶⟵———

CHAPTER TWENTY-ONE

THE RETURN

New Life, New Freedom, New Joy

After any hero's journey has been completed, there are certain issues that arise. One of them is the issue of boundaries—where you end and others begin. Being fosterers of life, women often give their souls away to those they love or those who are in need of care, believing that this is the best way to help. One of the important revelations that begins to develop during the return part of the journey is the awareness of how important it is to decide that you will not allow other people to live off your energy, nor will you live off theirs.

Sealing the Self

There are several things that can help one to accomplish the above. First, allow yourself to become aware of energetic shifts that take place, and, without passing any judgment, become conscious of situations in which either you feel yourself giving away your energy or being drained of energy by others. Once a woman is aware of this, it is a relatively easy matter to stop it from happening. This is very important on a physical level, too, for energy boundaries work very closely together with the immune system, and if you allow your boundaries to be breached on an energetic level, you are also opening the immune system to compromise. This increases your susceptibility to illness and to degeneration.

Another thing that can be helpful when you sense that an energy drain is happening is something I learned from Sandra Ingerman. She suggests that women in any situation in which we feel vulnerable to energy loss or leakage envisage themselves—their whole body—surrounded by a translucent blue egg, and then say silently, "I will not give up my soul to you." It takes a bit of practice to get the hang of it, but this little exercise can bring a remarkable sense of wholeness and integration and help break through years of habitual energy loss.

Something else we usually need to learn on the return—something that many women who lead busy, dedicated lives forget to do—is to continually set aside enough time to restore yourself. Go into the garden and sit, go for walks by yourself, take time to listen to music, learn to honor and care for yourself, and take your needs seriously. It can also be helpful to learn the practice of transmuting negative emotion, both your own and those of others. Anger, grief, sorrow, resentment—all these are nothing more than energy, whether they are feelings that are being felt by you or feelings of others that have been directed toward you. Once you become aware of them, without making any judgments about them, you can choose to transmute them into healing energy for yourself and for the planet by simply asking internally that this be done.

Living Now

A woman returns from her journey with a new understanding of who she is and what she needs. Week by week, this becomes clearer as an awareness of one's own identity begins to emerge. When you begin to experience the freedom that follows, some conscious decisions need to be made. You might decide, for instance, to no longer put your energy into worrying about what is going to happen next and how you are going to survive, choosing instead to use your newfound freedom as creatively as possible in your life. This usually involves searching to find out what brings you the greatest joy and the greatest sense of meaning, then immersing yourself more and more in doing it as the days go on. The more you do, the more physical energy is likely to be available to you. Following one's passion and feeling one's joy releases all sorts of energy that before may have been wrapped up in worry, frustration, and negative feelings toward yourself or others. Women who in earlier years have suffered chronic fatigue are often surprised how it is replaced by a new vitality, for so much of our energy gets locked up. I think this must be what anthropologist Margaret Mead was talking about when she spoke of "postmenopausal zest."

All energy is neutral, and unless it is directed toward the positive, we are always in danger of finding that it creates even more entanglements, frustration, and negativity. It becomes important to ask the question, "How can I express my core energy in my life?" You don't have to be an artist to do this, neither do you have to have big ambitions. Quite the contrary. In fact, it is best to take things one step at a time. Think of one single thing that you enjoy doing, and then promise yourself that you will do it, whether it be dancing, tapestry, taking long walks, doing some sort of public service, or learning about a subject that intrigues you for the sake of learning itself. Then the more you direct your creative energy, the more energy there seems to be to direct. Once it starts to flow steadily, you will find that other outlets suggest themselves. When these impulses arise, follow them until gradually the flow of energy, rather like the flow of water in a river, grows larger and larger and can be directed into any number of activities or concentrated to be experienced in whatever you choose.

Joseph Campbell used to urge people to "follow your bliss," and "participate joyously in the sorrows of the world." It is good advice. By following your bliss, he does not mean going out of your way to have a good time or chasing rainbows. Far from it. He means coming in touch with whatever is your particular individual passion and then pursuing it for its own sake, simply because it brings you joy. For women, this may be gardening or going back to college or traveling. The whole point about following one's bliss and honoring one's passions is that doing so leads step by step down a road toward the kind of fulfillment that has nothing to do with striving for success or the approval of society. It is rather like rediscovering the joy of being a child, when for hours one could sit and perform a particular act or work with a particular skill—all the while experiencing the joy of living in the moment.

Not long ago, I discovered what brings me bliss. What I like doing best in the world is making beautiful things—anything beautiful—from a salad to a piece of sculpture or a painting, although I have no training and no particular gifts for either.

Nine months ago, a close friend gave me a dreamcatcher—a circular mandala-type wall hanging that comes out of the Native American tradition. Dreamcatchers are made from leather thong, chamois, beads, and feathers. They consist of a circle inside which is woven a weblike structure, from which is hung long pieces of beaded chamois and feathers. A dreamcatcher is hung above the bed and is designed to catch your dreams. It is said to eat the bad dreams, the way the spider eats the fly. Your good dreams get caught by the web, and when the web grows fat enough with them, they will spill over it, making their way down the beaded chamois, leather, beads, and feathers intensified, the way water flows faster as it spills over a waterfall. So, the good dreams are given back to you in abundance.

I had seen one or two dreamcatchers, found them interesting, and had evidently mentioned this to my friend. She decided to gather together what was necessary and make me one. I was fascinated by the gift. I hung it above my bed. A few nights later, I became aware that what I wanted most to do was to make a dreamcatcher of my own. I asked her to show me how to weave the beautiful web that forms the net. It turned out to be very easy, and I began to make dreamcatcher after dreamcatcher. To my surprise, I rediscovered a sense of joy and excitement in what I was doing that I had not experienced since childhood. This is something I have rarely experienced as a writer. I am a woman who, after I have created something, no longer has any interest in it. I have always tended to feel little satisfaction from anything that I have made. I found that working with dreamcatchers was completely different. I would sit in the middle of my studio surrounded by a total chaos of beads and stones, shells and chamois, small pieces of wood and dried flowers, and spend hours at a time twisting things and building upon the webs to create dreamcatchers of great diversity. Each one seemed to be a universe in itself.

To Catch a Dream

My experience of making dreamcatchers was so intense that at times I would feel I was running a fever while working on one. For the first time in my life, I was able to work without thinking—that is to say, without making any rational judgments or having to control what I was doing. I would begin by weaving a web, a repetitive process that I found stilling to my mind, and satisfying. Once the web was woven, then I would allow my instincts to direct me toward putting together whatever objects, beads, or forms I wanted to add next. At first, I experienced some of the same fear I often do when I am beginning a writing project—a fear that I don't know how to do anything, and that I need to see the overall picture to make it work. But in my dreamcatcher making, I was conscious that there *was* no way I could see the overall picture. So I would just begin anywhere, putting together different forms and objects. I found out that I don't have to know where I am going with each dreamcatcher to get there. Each dreamcatcher has a soul of its own, and all I have to do is work in a dedicated, intuitive way, letting myself put together one thing after another to discover it. If something didn't work, I simply ripped it apart and began again. The delight I felt working with very ordinary physical objects such as stones and feathers and beads was such that for the time I was working on a dreamcatcher it could totally absorb me.

Each time I finished a dreamcatcher, I would stand back to look at it and feel a sense of awe at the richness of the form that had somehow come through me into this object. It was for me very much an experience of following my bliss. From it, I have learned that one does not have to know exactly where one is going when one begins a task or takes up a challenge. You need only work with clear intention from one step to the next. And there is great joy in this, because it means that you are living in the moment, and most important of all you love what you do. Meanwhile, somehow, the dreamcatchers made themselves simply by my carrying out my intention and trusting that it would happen.

Rituals of Intention

Freeing ourselves from beliefs and attitudes that have been blocking us creates a great open space ahead. What we need to fill it is just two things—intention and trust. This trust is not only in life to support your intentions and help you fulfill them, but trust in yourself. At some point near the end of the journey, a woman is being asked to stretch her visions beyond what she used to be capable of doing and to let go of any roles or attitudes that may be in her way. In directing creative energies and living a life that has meaning, it is enormously helpful to be clear about what you intend. Rituals can help a lot here. One ritual that I like very much is to sit and write down three, four, even half a dozen things that are important to me that I want to be or feel or accomplish. They can be internal things, such as "I want to feel at peace," or external things, such as "I want to create a home for myself at such and such a place."

Write each of them down on a separate piece of paper, writing before each one, the words "I intend," followed by the things that you want. Each morning, sit quietly during a time of meditation or recollection, and, holding your intention in your hand, read through it three times before going on to

the next. Let your mind play on the words. Then, give thanks for its fulfillment even before it is fulfilled. In the non-ordinary world, there is no such
thing as time or space, and the sense of gratitude that is created out of experiencing a fulfilled intention is a powerful ally in bringing it about. Then go
on to the next intention. Such intentions repeated every morning and evening
can be a useful way to gather one's energy and to draw upon our unseen
helpers, allies, spirits, and ancestors, who can help us to fulfill them.

Powers of the Circle

When one has made a journey to the core, retrieved pieces of one's own
soul that have not previously been lived out, and discovered other treasures
from the underworld, these treasures have to be brought back and lived out
within the community. Community, a sense of connectedness with others,
begins to take on a new meaning. Many women find that during menopause and
afterwards, their relationships with other women deepen dramatically, especially women who have followed the pathway of daughters of the father and have
sometimes experienced a considerable sense of loneliness in doing so. There is
something remarkable about relationships between women. Unlike male relationships that tend to be hierarchical—between a dominant and subordinate
male—relationships between women tend to be egalitarian, circular rather than
linear. There is no hierarchy, only a sense that each woman brings to the circle
or community what she has to bring and takes away what she needs. The circle
is the simplest and most profound shape in all of life. It has no top and no bottom, no start and no finish. It excludes nothing and embraces all.

I discovered this for myself many years ago when I decided to have a
large circular table made for our home while my children were growing up.
I had some vague idea, although I couldn't explain it, that a circular table
might create an atmosphere of unity and equality between everyone in the
family and enable each person to express more easily and more fully eye-to-
eye whatever it was that he or she thought or felt. When the table was finished, we brought it to the house and had a bit of a celebration sitting round
at dinner that night. I was amazed at the effect the shape seemed to exert on
all of us. There was much livelier conversation than there had been before,
a closer sense of connection between us, and lots more laughter. I figured
that Arthur must have known what he was doing in creating the round table
for his knights. Because a circle has no beginning and no end, everyone who
sits around it feels him- or herself to be an equal part of the whole.

Like women's menstrual cycles and the cycles of the moon, all transformation takes place in a circle. The interconnectedness that women experience in a circle or community—most especially one of other women—can bring us much closer to an understanding of our own individual nature and how we fit in with life around us. To a woman who has never experienced real community, it can be a revelation around the time of menopause—when one can begin to share dreams, hopes, disappointments, and experiences with other women in an open and unguarded way. It can also bring about a sense of self-acceptance that is hard to come by via any other means. Such community both encourages and inspires. It fires women with a desire to walk, talk, and live from their soul.

One of the wonderful things about egalitarian female energy is the way it helps women celebrate the successes of other women rather than feeling threatened, as men so often do. After menopause, many women find that they come together to celebrate the cycles of life and to give thanks for their connections with each other, to help each other overcome their personal fears, and to encourage each other in the expression of individual creative energies, whatever form they take. Such community helps a woman develop courage, compassion, humility, and patience. It can also help her accept the parts of her that have remained unloved or that have exercised tyrannical influences over her.

Such community does not have to be experienced only through people, of course. It can also come through animal friends—dogs, cats, horses, birds. It can even be experienced through objects, when you create a special place in your home to keep the things you find or have been given that have particular meaning for you. They, too, remind you of your power and restore your center when periodically you seem to lose it.

My own experience of menopause and new community continues to make me clear about what I think and what my values are. I believe:

- that each woman is born unique and gifted with great creativity of soul. This, which I call her *seedpower*, is wrapped in the cloak of her soul. A woman's purpose on the earth is to live out that seedpower fully—in effect, to live out the truth of her own being.

- that creativity is wild and free and female in nature even when found in a man.

- that too often a woman's creativity is stillborn. Her seedpower has been crushed, and her soul has been silenced by her culture or by her own lack of self-belief. Unless she takes action herself, it tends to remain imprisoned.

- that every woman has a right to walk her own path and speak with her own voice. More than a right, it is essential that she does so if her creativity is to come to fruition.

- that all life, art, sexuality, wishes, and dreams move in cycles, as do the flow and ebb of a woman's hormones and the changes of the seasons on the earth.

- that as women we have tended to allow our own imprisonment and to treat it as normal. It is as though we seem to volunteer to remain caged even though from a logical point of view we should be able to break free. Imprisoned creatures, women among them, who have been held captive for too long, suffer deep injuries to their instinctual nature so that they no longer feel able to defend themselves. I believe it is important that this damage to instinct be brought to light and healed.

- that making a hero's journey at some time in a woman's life is essential for her to find her freedom.

- that a woman must above all honor her instincts.

- that a woman's wild spirit, energy, and creativity is best fed when she surrounds herself with what she loves and does the things she likes doing best.

Our cultural conditioning has taught us to undervalue the wild feminine within us—that part which is instinctual, irrational, nonmoral, and full of passion. The male-dominated linear society in which we live is so frightened of these things that we ourselves have been taught to fear the feminine within us and judge it harshly. Too often, we swallow our anger even when it is righteous. We put our needs and wants below those of others. We crush our wild nature. We judge ourselves wrongly and we see ourselves as ugly. Doing so dissipates our power and fragments our soul. Only when we learn to embrace the irrational feminine and honor her can any of us—man or woman—fully complete the hero's journey and return in wholeness. The most difficult task any woman comes up against is that of accepting the part of herself that she finds most ugly and loathsome. Yet, locked within what we most hate and fear lies the greatest power for our transformation. Let the tale be told in myth.

One Christmastide, Arthur rode out with his knights to hunt. By chance he became separated from his companions and found himself at the edge of a great brackish pond. There, a knight in black armor emerged from the shadows and challenged him to a fight. Arthur reached to draw his sword Excalibur and call on its power to protect him from all harm. Alas, he had come away from court without it. He could feel every ounce of strength drain away from his body in the presence of the dark and evil stranger who raised his sword and threatened to kill him. Being a responsible king, of course, Arthur told the dark knight he didn't think that killing him was a good idea—he had a country to rule, after all, and knights to look after. Where would *they* be without him? The stranger, bored at the thought of such an easy kill, relented, and replied, "I won't kill you so long as you return to this place in three days with the answer to a riddle I shall give you. If you fail, I shall remove your head in one full sweep."

Arthur agreed. He reckoned that, given half a chance and a mug or two of fancy mead, his pals back at the castle would be sure to come up with something. The riddle the stranger posed was this: What does every woman want?" So Arthur headed home to ask all his knights and wise men to give him the answer. Everyone from Merlin to a goose girl he met along the road had a go at it. Each gave him a different answer. "A woman wants beauty," said one. "A woman wants power," said another, or fame, or jewels, or sanctity. None could agree.

Time was running out. Finally, although he had done his best to hide from his beloved Guinevere the seriousness of the situation, the third morning arrived. Bound by his word of honor to the Black Knight, Arthur had to return as promised. Along the road to the meeting at the brackish waters, Arthur came upon an old woman. She sat on a tree stump by the side of the road calling his name. Arthur dismounted and approached her with all the courtesy he could muster. The closer he came, the more ghastly this old hag appeared. Although she was dressed in fine silk and wore magnificent jewels on her gnarled and twisted hands, she was unquestionably the most hideous thing he had ever seen, or dreamed of for that matter. Her nose was like a pig's, her mouth was huge, toothless and dribbling. What hair remained on her head was greasy, and the skin all over her misshapen and bloated body was covered in oozing sores.

Arthur swallowed hard, forcing himself not to have to look away. "My lord," she said in a surprisingly gentle voice, "why look you so dismayed?" Summoning up all his chivalrous training, Arthur apologized for his manner, trying to explain it away by telling her he was most unsettled at the prospect of returning to meet his death at the hand of an evil knight because he could not tell him the answer to the riddle, "What does every woman want?"

"Ah," said the hag. "I can tell you that. But such knowledge cannot be given without payment."

Arthur, hoping once again for a reprieve from death, replied, "Of course, madam, anything you desire shall be yours for the answer—even half my kingdom."

The Loathly Lady made Arthur bend down while she whispered a few words in his ear. The moment Arthur heard them, he knew his life and his kingdom had been saved. He was about to leap on his horse again and ride off to meet the stranger, when she tugged on his cloak and said, "Now I want my reward."

"Of course, madam, what is it that you want?" he asked. "I want to be the wife of your bravest knight and live at your court." Arthur, who only a moment before had felt his spirits soar, was plunged into the deepest despair. How could he possibly expect any knight to consent to marry such a hideous hag? And what would it be like to have to endure such ugliness every day at court?

"But, madam, that is impossible!" he said. The words slipped through his lips before he could catch them. Aghast at his own lack of courtesy and agonized by having to ask any of his knights, Arthur said, "I beg your pardon, madam. You are quite right. Come to court tomorrow. There waiting for you will be your future husband." So saying, he mounted his horse and rode off to meet the Black Knight to convey to him the answer to the riddle.

When he got back to the castle, Arthur was distraught. The knights questioned him. He confessed that he had won his life from the Black Knight, but then told them at what cost and reported his promise to the Loathly Lady. "My very honor is at stake," said Arthur, wringing his hands, "unless one of you will agree to wed her."

His knights were horrified at the prospect and tried to avoid his gaze. But one, the youngest knight of all, Sir Gawain, the most courageous and purest of heart, stood up. "Worry not, my liege," Gawain said, "I shall save you. I will marry the woman no matter what her mien."

Gawain did not have long to rue his offer. The marriage was planned for the following morning, and the hag arrived at court. When he looked upon her, even Gawain, with all his chivalry, did not know how he could go through with the ceremony. It demanded every ounce of his courage. Somehow he managed it. But things got worse. When the festivities were over, the couple were obliged to retire to their chamber for the night. Gawain, unable to face the hideousness of his wife, sat for long hours in their bedchamber with his back to the lady, writing at his desk and praying she would go to sleep without him. Was he to spend the rest of his life shackled to such a hideous monster?

Long past midnight, as the candle burnt low, he felt a hand come to rest upon his shoulder. "Will you not come to bed now, my lord?" a voice whispered from behind him. Shuddering with horror, Gawain mustered his courage to look at her. To his astonishment, there stood not the ugly hag he had married, but the most beautiful woman he had ever seen. She had golden hair and ivory skin. "Why do you seem so surprised, my lord?" she said to him. "I am indeed your wife. I was enchanted by a wicked magician. But now the enchantment is half broken by your having consented to marry me and so you see, I stand before you now in my true form." Gawain could not believe his luck.

"Half broken?" he asked.

"Yes, my lord," was the reply. "Sadly, I am only allowed to spend half the time in my true form. For the rest I must return to the shape of the same hag that this afternoon you married. And now you must choose, my lord. Would you have me be my true self at night when we are alone together, and the hag during daylight hours?" Gawain, whose mind was flooded with passion at the thought of her beauty in his bed each night, replied eagerly, "Yes, that is certainly how it must be."

In the eye of his beautiful lady appeared a tear. "But sir," she said, "would you then have me suffer the humiliation of the court who cannot conceal their horror at my ugliness?" Now Gawain, if he was nothing else, was compassionate. He could not bear to cause this beautiful woman a tear of sorrow.

"No, of course not," he replied. "It shall be the other way round, of course. You shall be my beautiful wife for the court during daylight hours and the hag at night." But this only made the lady weep the more.

"Oh, sir, would you then deny me forever the joy and pleasure of your embrace?" she asked.

Poor Gawain, who after all was but a man (and man has never found it easy to deal with woman's grief), did not know what to do. After much thought, he replied, "My lady, whatever choice I make will be the wrong one. It is therefore for *you* to choose which you prefer."

At the sound of his words, the lady threw herself into his arms in glorious laughter. "In so saying, my lord, you have given the right answer. You have bestowed upon me what every woman wants—*her own way*. The spell at last is broken. You will never have to look upon the hideous hag again. I am my true self, and it belongs to you forever."

⚛ ⚛ ⚛

Such is the power of accepting that which to ourselves is most loathsome. And such is the power of myth in reminding us of it.

PART III

RITES AND RITUALS

ANGELS IN THE ARCHITECTURE
Osteoporosis Can Be a Simple Challenge

Osteoporosis is characterized by a decrease in bone mass and a deterioration in bone tissue that makes bones fragile and creates a high risk of fracture. Osteoporotic fractures create disability and can lead to death. In the United Kingdom alone, the total cost of osteoporotic fractures is estimated at over a billion dollars each year. However, osteoporosis is not a normal part of menopause, is in no way inevitable, and as a growing number of doctors working with natural methods have discovered, can be healed even in women long past menopausal age.

How do you know if you have osteoporosis? The simple answer is that you don't, because of its insidious nature. A woman often does not know that she has it until a bone breaks. Osteoporosis used to be called *menopausal* osteoporosis since nobody ever thought of it occurring before menopause. A woman may have lost a quarter of her bone by the time menopause arrives and be totally unaware of it until a fracture appears two years later. There is a simple test that you can carry out for yourself to give you some idea of what your bone status is. Have your husband or a friend mark your height against a wall every couple of months. If your height drops as much as three inches in a year, you have osteoporosis and need to take action. Bone shrinkage cannot be reversed by anything except serious changes in eating and lifestyle habits, including regular weight-bearing exercise, as well as natural progesterone and nutritional supplements.

Common Tests

There are various medical techniques used to measure bone density. The original way was by taking x-rays. Although still used in many places, it is a relatively useless method of measurement since x-rays cannot reliably measure bone mass loss or gain until there has been a change of about 30 percent. Even if you were to have an x-ray taken at 40 years of age and then another at 45, the radiologist—no matter how good—cannot tell you whether you have gained or lost bone until the change has exceeded the 30 percent mark.

Now, with the advent of better methods, some tests are so good they can measure bone density at 96 to 98 percent accuracy. This means they can detect a change of anything over 2 percent. That change is real—you can count on it. One of these methods is dual-energy x-ray absorptiometry (DXA), where low-dose x-rays are used. This is the most widely practiced method. Measurements can be made of the spine, femoral neck, forearm, and total body skeleton. Recently, measurements have also been made of the lateral lumbar spine by DXA. DXA is accurate, as is computerized tomography (CT), but both involve radiation (especially high doses in the case of CT), which many doctors concerned with natural menopause would rather not subject a woman to. Other methods, such as single-photon absorptiometry (SPA) and dual-photon absorptiometry (DPA), are safer, since they do not rely on radiation but rather on passing light through the skin. They work rather the way a flashlight held against the palm of the hand in a darkened room enables you to see the shape of bones as the light shines through. Photons are passed through the skin of the body. They bounce off the minerals of the bones, instead of passing straight through, and therefore cast a shadow. The energy that is lost when photon beams are sent through the body is then calculated by a machine to give an accurate reading of bone density.

Drug Treatments

There are a number of common drug interventions officially touted as useful in slowing bone loss and preventing fractures. Most have little to offer. They include calcitonin, the biphosphonates, anabolic steroids, and, the most commonly prescribed of all, sodium fluoride. All can have serious side effects, and none are truly effective. Be wary.

Fluoride supplements are frequently touted as a treatment for osteoporosis since initial research showed that fluoride does increase bone mass. But follow-up studies have shown that, although bone mass does increase slightly when fluoride is given, the new bone has a very poor structural quality, is highly brittle, and actually makes bones *more* prone to breakage. Stay away from fluoride.

Risk Factors

- Poor calcium metabolism as a result of inadequate vitamins and minerals, including vitamin C, vitamin D, zinc, and magnesium during the menstruating years, often from years of living on a diet of processed foods.

- Excessive phosphorus intake from colas or processed meats, which leaches calcium from bones.

- Excess alcohol, which renders your blood acidic. Acidosis destroys bones because the body has to steal alkalizing minerals (calcium) from them to keep blood pH from dropping into the acid range where it can damage cells.

- Physical inactivity and lack of weight-bearing exercise.

- Smoking.

- High-protein diet. Excess protein also creates a negative calcium balance, leaching calcium from bones and causing more to be lost in the urine than is taken in through food.

- Malabsorption of nutrients, either from low levels of hydrochloric acid in the stomach or as a result of using antibiotics.

- Antacids that contain aluminum. They disrupt normal calcium/phosphorus interactions on which the maintenance of good bone depends.

- The regular use of drugs such as cortisone, thyroid hormones, barbiturate anticonvulsants, and heparin.

- Progesterone deficiency. Inadequate bone building results from anovulatory menstruation, especially in the five to eight years before menopause where, although periods appear normal, inadequate progesterone is being produced. This reduces the activity of osteoblast cells so that more resorption of old bone is taking place than building of new bone.

- In a *few* women there is a risk of inadequate estrogen after menopause. This results in increased osteoclast bone resorption. Estrogen supplementation can slow resorption, but its use carries serious potential health risks (unless you use estriol, E3). It will only help as long as you continue to take it. Estrogen can do nothing to *reverse* bone loss.

Wise Woman Ways

- *Horsetail*—Drink horsetail tea regularly. Steep one teaspoon of the dried herb in a cup of boiling water. It is rich in silicon. Other herbs that go well with horsetail are sage, alfalfa, uva ursi leaves, and nettle, which you can mix together and use as a tea.

Exercise

Probably the most neglected of all the actions a woman can take to prevent and to treat osteoporosis is exercise. It needs to be *weight-bearing* exercise. But it has taken until very recently for official bodies such as the United States Academy of Sciences to come out with the statement that weight-bearing exercise is essential to build and maintain bone strength. A lot of the "official-line" booklets such as those sent out by the National Osteoporosis Society in Britain make only vague references to it, saying that women should not be inactive or suggesting that "walking, dancing, playing tennis, and keeping fit are ideal," as though any old exercise will do.

The fact is that although walking, running, cycling, and aerobics might be great for your heart and lungs, they will not get the job done when it comes to strengthening your bones because they stress only the long bones of the legs and don't supply enough load. You need weight training—whether the weights be tins of beans held in each hand, dumb-bells, or barbells. The simpler they are, the better. Moving weights around in a way that stresses the muscles and bones all over the body is what builds strong bones. Weight training also builds muscle tissue and enhances your Lean Body Mass to fat ratio (see chapter 12). This is particularly important for women as they get older, since a shrinkage in lean tissue depletes the body of hormones and energy and makes the body and the face look older. So important is weight training for overall well-being that the American College of Sports Medicine recently altered its standard advice on using exercise to retain fitness and health to include exercise with weights. Thirty to 45 minutes of this kind of regime three times a week will have your bones brimming with the piezoelectric energy that builds them beautifully.

Diet

For the prevention and treatment of osteoporosis, diet is the first order of the day—low in fat and moderate in protein, with plenty of green leafy vegetables, no colas or processed soft drinks, and little meat and alcohol. Official World Health Organization figures calculate that we need no more than half a gram of good-quality protein for each pound of body weight. So if you weigh 150 pounds, that means about 35 g of protein a day. The average Western diet serves up between 60 and 150 g of protein a day—far more than we need.

The countries with the highest consumption of protein per capita and the highest consumption of dairy products are where you find the highest incidence of hip fractures and osteoporosis. To prevent acidosis of the blood, which is not only a major factor in osteoporosis but also in chronic fatigue, depression and many other negative conditions that women are frequently faced with, it can be useful to be aware of the foods that tend to be acid-forming, those that are relatively neutral, and those which are alkaline-forming. Then you can choose your menus, leaning heavily on the neutral and alkaline-forming foods.

Acid-forming	**Neutral Foods**	**Alkaline-forming**
alcohol	apples	bicarbonate of soda
artificial sweeteners	apricots	blackberries
beef	aubergines	broccoli
butter	bananas	celery
carob	beans—fresh and dried	chicory
casein	blueberries	cinnamon
cheese	buckwheat	daikon radish
chicken	cauliflower	garlic
chickpeas	carrots	ginseng
chocolate	cherries	grapefruit
cocoa	courgettes	kale
coffee	dates	kohlrabi
corn	eggs—chicken, duck	lentils
fried foods	figs	limes
jam	fish	mangoes
ice cream	goats' cheese	melon
lard	grapes	mineral water
lobster	honey	miso
most medication	lemons	molasses
nuts	lettuce	mushrooms
oat bran	maple syrup	mustard greens
oils—hydrogenated	milk—cow, goat	nectarines
pasta	oatmeal	onions
peas	organic flax seed oil	papayas
pork	organic olive oil	peppers
rye	oranges	potatoes
soy beans	peaches	raspberries
soya milk	pears	sea salt
sugar	pineapple	sea vegetables
veal	plums	shitake mushrooms
vinegar	pumpkin	soy sauce
	raisins	sweet potatoes
	rice—wild, brown	tangerines
	strawberries	turnips
	turkey	watermelon
		yams

- *Eat More:*

  — Fresh fruits eaten raw.

  — Fresh green leafy vegetables, at least 50 percent of which are eaten raw: broccoli, collards, kale, cabbage, mustard greens, Swiss chard, lambs' lettuce, rocket.

  — Fresh green herbs.

  — Legumes such as beans, peas, lentils, chick peas, etc.

  — Whole grain breads, cereals, pasta, and noodles—preferably two different varieties of grain a day, together with one legume, which will give you all the essential amino acids you need, even without meat. Steer clear of wheat if you suspect any sensitivity to it.

  — Nuts, tofu, soya milk, and other soya products including soy beans, free-range eggs, fish, free-range chicken, and game, and seeds in moderation. Remember that it is not necessary to eat any animal products if you don't want to.

- *Eat Less:*

  — Dairy products, except for butter in small quantities, including milk, cheese, cream, and anything containing them. Natural live yogurt is something everyone needs to experiment with to find out if they are better off without it. Cut it out for two weeks, along with all other dairy products or anything containing them, and examine how you feel.

  — Refined foods such as white bread, white rice, white pasta, and most breakfast cereals that are not only refined, but riddled with sugar.

  — Sugar

  — Soy-based ersatz meat substitutes.

— Margarines, golden oils.

— Fried foods. Use only cold-pressed extra virgin olive oil or soya oil.

— Drink less coffee, tea, or colas—and avoid cigarettes.

Bone Makers	**Bone Breakers**
Adequate magnesium	Processed convenience foods, junk fats
Alfalfa and barley high in minerals and trace elements	Diuretics and antibiotics
Boron	Crash dieting
Calcium in moderation (best from food sources)	Deficiencies in minerals and trace elements
Leafy green vegetables	Smoking
Moderate protein diet	Soft drinks including diet colas
Organically grown whole foods	Salt
Progesterone	High-protein diet
Sea plants and green supplements—spirulina, green algae, and Chlorella	High-fat diet
Silicon	Sedentary lifestyle
Soya-based foods	Coffee
Sunlight and vitamin D	Antacids that contain aluminum
Vegetarian diet	Sugar
Vitamin C, which improves calcium absorption	Fluoride and chlorine in drinking water
Weight training	Too many dairy products
Whole grains	Alcohol
Zinc	

Nutritional Support

Calcium—The best source of calcium is not in supplements, but in foods. Rarely is it necessary to take calcium supplements, and you should never take calcium on its own. Instead, change your diet so that you are getting calcium in foods, preferably not milk products. The ratio of calcium to magnesium is 8 to 1 in milk—far too high. When magnesium isn't absorbed in proper relation to calcium, then the calcium does not end up in your bones. It is more likely to end up in inflammatory areas, causing tendinitis, carpal tunnel syndrome, arthritic spurs, and extra calcium deposits around tendons. Doctors will be likely to call it arthritis or rheumatism and—because they have not been trained in nutrition—will not have the slightest clue that it is a calcium/magnesium imbalance.

Get your calcium instead from plants—whole grains and vegetables, especially sea vegetables. Calcium is not in the roots; it is in the structure of a plant—the leaves, the stems, and the stalks—and it is not at all difficult to get 600 to 800 milligrams of calcium a day from plant sources. Research suggests that the megadoses of calcium supplements that many women take may actually decrease bone strength and in animal studies has been shown to induce internal bleeding. A vegetarian or someone on a good moderate-in-protein diet needs only 500 to 600 mg of calcium a day. Eating unprocessed foods makes it easy to get this amount, especially if you include sea plants in your menus. Calcium is found in good quantities in whole grains such as rye, wheat, millet, brown rice, and quinoa, as well as legumes. These foods are also rich in magnesium. The thing to remember about calcium is that once you get it out of the stomach and into the bloodstream, you have to get it into the bones. This is where exercise comes in, as well as adequate progesterone (or testosterone in the case of men). I have given a list of common foods and the amount of calcium each contains.

CALCIUM CONTENT OF FOOD AND DRINK

<u>Vegetables</u>	<u>Calcium Per Cupful</u>
beet greens	165 mg
broccoli	175 mg
Chinese leaves	125 mg
kale	180 mg
mustard greens	100 mg

bok choy	200 mg
parsley	122 mg
spinach	300 mg
turnip greens	250 mg
wild greens	350 mg

Legumes	**Calcium Per Cupful (Cooked)**
black beans	135 mg
chickpeas	150 mg
pinto beans	130 mg
soy beans	130 mg

Sea Vegetables	**Calcium Per Cupful (Cooked)**
agar agar (dry flakes)	400 mg
dulse	570 mg
hiziki	610 mg
kelp (kombu)	300 mg
wakame	520 mg

Mineral Water	**Calcium Per Liter**
Contrexeville	450 mg
Perrier	140 mg
San Pellegrino	200 mg

Nuts	**Calcium Per Cup**
almonds	300 mg
brazil nuts	260 mg
hazelnuts	282 mg

Soya Products	**Calcium in 4 oz. (112 grams)**
tempeh	170 mg
tofu precipitated with calcium salts	300 mg
tofu soybean curd	100 mg

Other Foods	**Calcium**
blackstrap molasses	140 mg per tablespoon
spirulina	30 mg
tahini	120 mg per 1/2 oz. (14 g)

In comparison:

Dairy Products	Calcium
cheese	200 mg per 1 oz. (25 grams)
low-fat cheese	150 mg per cup
milk	300 mg per cup
nonfat yogurt	295 mg per cup
skimmed milk	285 mg per cup

While spinach also contains a good quantity of calcium, it is high in oxalic acid which decreases calcium absorption and should not be relied on as a calcium source. If, for any reason, you decide to take some form of calcium supplement, choose a food-state calcium, chelated calcium or calcium citrate rather than the usual calcium carbonate or one of the other cheap versions that are not well absorbed. Also consider using betaine hydrochloride.

Hydrochloric acid—One of the major factors in ensuring you get enough calcium is adequate hydrochloric acid in the stomach. The plants containing calcium go into the stomach; to get the minerals from there into the bloodstream you need two things—plenty of hydrochloric acid and adequate B vitamins. If either is missing, then this will stop the absorption of calcium, making it pass on through the colon and out of your body. This is important to know because many women as they get older don't produce enough hydrochloric acid in their stomachs to absorb calcium. An important question to ask yourself is: "Are there foods that I used to be able to eat but now I can't?" If there is even the slightest indication that this may apply to you, it can be useful to take a supplement of hydrochloric acid—usually in the form of betaine hydrochloride. What many women don't realize is that a lot of indigestion comes not, as the advertisements would have us believe, from "over-acidity," but rather from the lack of hydrochloric acid. John Lee tells an interesting story that illustrates this situation:

> One of the first patients I had with osteoporosis was in her seventies. She had come from a clinic, and she wanted to be treated for osteoporosis because it was bad. They wanted to give her fluoride, and she didn't want that. I tried the progesterone cream and the diet, but in six months' time I could see no improvement. Then she said, "I don't think I am absorbing the calcium." I said, "Why do you think that?" She said, "I've been tak-

ing those calcium pills and when I go to the bathroom, I can see them in the toilet." I said, "Right, I don't think you're absorbing the calcium." She said, "Maybe if I took it as a liquid?" I said, "No, that doesn't help, you're not absorbing it because you are lacking either vitamin B or hydrochloric acid." She was already taking vitamin B, so I said, "You have to take the hydrochloric acid." She said, "Oh, they're treating me for indigestion by giving me Tagamet and antacids." They said her indigestion was from too much acid. I said, "How old are you?" She said, "74." I said, "No, your indigestion is from *not enough* acid, and you are not going to absorb the calcium unless you get some." So I gave her some betaine hydrochloride and lo and behold, those calcium flakes did not show up in the toilet anymore. Her indigestion went away, and her bone mineral density took off. Within three years, she had gained 48 percent new bone. I discovered then that, provided a woman has enough hydrochloric acid and eats a good diet, she will get all the calcium she needs from her foods.

Supplementing main meals with hydrochloric acid also improves the digestion of proteins and helps many people avoid indigestion and food sensitivities by protein foods not being broken down adequately in the stomach (see Resources).

Magnesium—Sixty percent of the body's magnesium is contained within the bone. Although it makes up only 0.1 percent of bone (compared to calcium's 20 percent), magnesium is vital to good bone formation, as it both increases the absorption of calcium from the foods we eat and also enhances its role in mineralizing bones. Magnesium helps convert vitamin D into its active form in the body, and it also helps fix calcium into the bone tissue. There are over 300 enzymes known to require magnesium.

Foods high in magnesium include black-eyed peas, curry, almonds, whole grains and legumes, eggs, liver, and green vegetables.

Vitamin D—This vitamin is necessary in good quantity for the transportation of calcium and phosphorus into bone tissue. It also helps prevent too much calcium being lost in the urine. The best sources of vitamin D are natural sunlight, which enables the body to synthesize the vitamin from exposure to sunlight, and natural vitamin D found in fish oils.

Zinc—This mineral is also essential in the formation of new bone, and like magnesium, it is processed out of our foods. Zinc deficiencies have now become so widespread that supplementing the diet with zinc appears to be important for many people. Zinc tends to be low in women with osteoporosis and in women who take calcium supplements. A co-catalyst for enzymes that change beta-carotene into vitamin A in the body's cells, zinc is essential for the formation of the collagen matrix on which both strong bones and healthy skin depend.

Vitamin C—Another important player in the bone formation game, vitamin C is essential since the matrix to build bone with calcium cannot be made without vitamin C being present. Vitamin C levels decline as women age. They are also drastically reduced by exposure to pollutants in the air, including cigarette smoke. A couple of extra grams of vitamin C each day can protect bones.

Silicon—An important trace element in the formation of connective tissue, bone, cartilage, hair, and nails, silicon also helps protect the body from some of the damage caused by aluminum in the system. Concentrated in sites of active calcification in the bones of the young, silicon is an unusual element. It is the second most widespread element in nature after oxygen. Silicon is enormously hard and has the ability to bind into tissues other minerals that are needed there. Silica is readily available in unprocessed vegetables, but hard to come by when eating processed foods or foods grown chemically. This is why supplements of silicon can be useful. It can also be taken in the form of horsetail tea (the plant that has the highest content of the trace element) and can do wonders for improving the state of nails, hair, and skin.

Boron—Only recently has boron, another trace element, been thought to be important as a nutrient. During the 1980s, a number of studies indicated that boron may affect calcium, markedly reducing its urinary excretion (as well as that of magnesium). The presence of boron reduces calcium loss and increases the level of some of the estrogens in the body. In one study of 12 postmenopausal women on a low-boron diet for 119 days, 3 mg of boron daily reduced their calcium excretion by an average 44 percent and also increased their production of estrogen. Boron also affects hormone levels in women and appears to help normalize them. Boron has been shown to improve the metabolism of calcium, phosphorus, and magnesium, and aid the manufacture of vitamin D by the body. Alfalfa and kelp are good sources of boron as are some of the other seaweed foods.

Vitamin B6—Working together with magnesium, this member of the B complex vitamins is a co-catalyst for such a variety of enzymes in the body that it would be tedious to list them all. It supports the production of progesterone and helps minimize inflammatory reactions in connective tissue, as well as encouraging the formation of important new collagen. A number of studies indicate that women with osteoporosis have low levels of this vitamin.

Typical Supplementation for Osteoporosis

- **Magnesium**—300–600 mg a day in divided doses as magnesium citrate or chelated magnesium.
- **Vitamin D**—350–400 IU a day.
- **Zinc**—15–20 mg a day as zinc citrate or picolinate.
- **Vitamin C**—2,000–4,000 mg a day in divided doses.
- **Silicon**—Take as horsetail tea.
- **Boron**—2–8 mg a day.
- **Vitamin B6**—50 mg a day before bed.

Dr. John Lee's Typical Osteoporosis Treatment Program

Diet	Leafy green and other vegetables emphasized. Avoid all sodas, and limit red meat to 3 or fewer times per week. Limit alcohol use.
Vitamin D	350–400 IU daily.
Vitamin C	2,000 mg per day in divided doses.
Beta-carotene	15 mg per day (equivalent to 25,000 IU of vitamin A).
Zinc	15–30 mg per day.
Calcium	800–1,000 mg per day by diet and/or supplements.
Magnesium	300 mg per day.
Estrogen	Use in minimum doses 3 weeks/months only if needed for vaginal dryness. Do not use if contraindicated for any reason.
Progesterone	Natural progesterone cream applied daily during the last two weeks of estrogen use or 3 weeks/months if estrogen not used. Use one jar per month initially for 3

months. Later, half the amount per month may suffice, as determined by serial BMD tests.

Exercise   12–20 minutes daily, or one-half hour 3 times a week.

No cigarettes

Report any occurrence of vaginal bleeding

From *Natural Progesterone,* by John R. Lee, M.D., BLL Publishing, Sebastopol, CA, USA, 1993.

In addition to Dr. Lee's program, other experts in natural menopause suggest using 50 mg of B6 once or twice a day, spirulina either taken in tablet form (see Resources) or in powder form stirred into a glass of juice or a cup of vegetable broth, and a cup of horsetail tea each day. Also, eat plenty of seaweeds in salads, soups, and vegetable dishes, since sea plants are rich in boron and trace elements and other micronutrients vital for flexibility and strength of bones. So are organically grown grains and vegetables, and many sprouts, including alfalfa.

Progesterone

Progesterone helps spur the osteoblasts to make new bone. The message that progesterone carries is "make new bone." Some pretty remarkable results have been reported in the last 15 years from doctors who have used progesterone creams. It has brought clinical relief of osteoporotic pain, stabilization of height loss, reduction in fracture incidence, and improved density *regardless of age*, even in women who already have osteoporosis—in both women who have used progesterone cream alone and in those who have used small doses of estrogen as well. When height has been lost as a result of crush fractures in the vertebrae, the pressure on the nerves is often alleviated with the use of progesterone cream and exercise. When you put a woman into a warm swimming pool up to her chest and let her walk, the buoyancy of the water takes the weight off the spine. Exercise like this can help the bones relocate themselves the micromillimeter distance it takes to relieve pain. The nerves in the spine are very tough and hard to kill, and space created where they arise can compensate for the pressure that has occurred. John Lee reports having seen women, with what looked on an x-ray like a total obliteration of the parameter where nerves emerge from the spine, who in time were restored to pain-free normal states.

Because natural progesterone applied in cream form has so many other benefits and virtually no side effects, it would seem unwise for a woman who has any indication of bone loss or who is concerned about preventing osteoporosis not to use it. (See chapter 30 for protocols.) The nutrients listed in this section are important for progesterone to be efficiently used by the body. It generally takes about three months for women who begin progesterone treatment to begin to experience the sense of well-being that generally accompanies it. If you have been diagnosed as osteoporotic, then it is wise to have serial vertebral bone density studies done at intervals of six months to a year to monitor progress.

BAD BLOOD

*PMS, Endometriosis, Fibroids, and Other Female
Challenges Yield to Natural Treatment*

ounting xenoestrogenic pollution in our environment and widespread use of artificial hormones for birth control and HRT have produced an epidemic of female problems that develop out of a state of estrogen dominance in a woman's body. It is this that is creating a need for progesterone supplementation. They have set the stage for the development of the *bad blood* plague of the late 20th century that we are experiencing. Here are some of the most common bad blood conditions now appearing in ever greater numbers.

ENDOMETRIOSIS

Endometriosis is a mysterious and rapidly increasing condition of modern times in the Westernized world. The normal endometrium or uterine lining that develops each month during the follicle phase of the menstrual cycle, instead of breaking down and being shed fully with menstruation, proliferates inside the uterine cavity. Tiny islets of endometrial tissue can arise in or migrate to other areas of the pelvis, the fallopian tubes, the surface of the ovaries—even beyond, occasionally—to the sides of the pelvic wall and occasionally on to the bowel. Endometriosis can be accompanied by pelvic pain, cramps, infertility, and disturbed menstrual cycles. Pain is often worse at ovulation and during menstruation or just before a period begins.

Although many women can experience endometrial buildup without apparent symptoms, in others it results in painful intercourse because of the pressure, or pain when moving your bowels. The only sure way to diagnose the condition is via laparoscopy, although sometimes endometrial lesions can be seen during a pelvic examination on the vagina, vulva, or cervix. Often endometriosis and fibroids are found together. Because these endometrial islets are of the same endometrial tissue as found in the womb, they swell and diminish with the ebb and flow of monthly hormones, then are shed at menstrual time, bringing pain in their wake. The incidence of endometriosis has increased dramatically in recent years, partly because women are giving birth later and having fewer children, and most probably because of widespread estrogen dominance. Estrogen is the hormone of proliferation—responsible for the buildup of endometrial tissue. When it gets out of hand, endometriosis can be one of the results.

Common Treatment

The standard medical treatments for endometriosis include giving birth control pills in an attempt to artificially cycle the buildup and sloughing of the womb lining, using a progestogen to suppress menstruation, prescribing analgesics and narcotics to kill the pain, or giving a GnRH agonist drug that acts directly on the pituitary to stop its cyclic hormonal secretions altogether—in effect rendering a woman menopausal so long as the drug continues to be given. Although they can relieve pain so long as you take them, GnRH agonists in common use do carry a number of potentially unpleasant side effects, including the thinning of vaginal walls, hot flashes, and osteoporosis. Other drugs such as danocrine sulphate, which is also commonly used for the treatment of endometriosis, can bring masculinization, such as facial hair growth. None of these treatments have been shown to be very successful. Surgery is another standard treatment for endometriosis—either for the removal of the endometrial lesions themselves or, more radically, a complete hysterectomy as well as ovary removal. Since adequate progesterone inhibits the secretion of LH and FSH and therefore the proliferation of endometrial tissue, it is not surprising that a growing number of doctors, nutritionists, and naturopaths prefer to recommend the cyclic use of natural progesterone so that the pain and menstrual flow are adequately reduced and the need for surgery eliminated.

Soul Searching

There are always complex interactions and imbalances between thoughts and feelings that affect a woman's immune system when endometriosis is present. Many women with the condition also show autoimmune characteristics such as having developed antibodies toward their own tissues, which in turn disrupts reproduction.

Endometriosis is often called the "career woman's" ailment. It is a way in which a woman's female power can be demanding her attention through pain or abnormal menstrual cycles—asking her to turn back from total absorption in the externals of her life and become more self-nurturing, self-examining, and self-honoring. Listening to the symptoms you are experiencing is important, as is writing down whatever comes to you as you do so. This works best if it is done without paying much attention to what you are writing—just letting the words pour out of you. You may be surprised by some of the impulses and desires that get expressed. Honor what comes. Do you need more time alone? Do you need to allow yourself more freedom of self-expression in your work? Your relationships? Are you in need of self-care? Time off? Are you resting enough? What changes would you like to see in your life if anything were possible? Are you in any way living somebody else's values—your parents', your boss's, your family's—rather than your own? Do you feel helpless—a victim of your condition and your pain, or do you conceive of the possibility that you can change your life?

Castor Oil Packs

Castor oil packs are an age-old remedy traditionally used to treat everything from colitis and peptic ulcers; to arthritis and female problems; to back pains and fibroids, PMS, and endometriosis. They work. Preliminary research at the George Washington School of Medicine has shown that they are likely to improve the functioning of the immune system. They are an excellent helper for endometriosis—not only to alleviate discomfort, but also to help speed recovery. Use them at least three times a week, preferably every day.

What You Need

- Cotton or wool flannel cloth (can be a piece of an old sheet if necessary, but make sure there are no synthetics in the fabric).
- Plastic freezer bag or plastic sheet.
- Hot water bottle or electric heat pad.
- 2 safety pins.
- 6 oz. (150 g) castor oil.
- Bath towel.

Prepare the flannel cloth by tearing and folding so that it is 2 to 4 thicknesses and, when folded, turns out to be about 10 inches (25 cm) wide and 12 inches (30 cm) long. Pour castor oil into the cloth so that it is saturated with the oil but not dripping. While lying down, apply to the abdomen, then lay the plastic bag or sheet over the soaked flannel. Put the hot water bottle or heating pad on top of that as warm as you can manage, then cover with the towel folded lengthwise over the whole area. You can leave a castor oil pack on all night if you can manage it. One hour is the minimum. While using the pack, let your mind gently wander over questions such as those above, and see what comes to you. Afterwards, cleanse the skin using water to which a teaspoon of baking soda has been added. Provided it is kept clean, the soaked flannel can be used many times.

Wise Woman Ways

Two herbs are traditionally used with success in the treatment of endometriosis by wise women: raspberry leaves and Chastetree, or *Vitex agnus castus* (Chinese variation is Man Jing Zi—*Vitex rotundifolia* or *Vitex trifolia*). They work well together.

Raspberry leaves—Raspberry leaf tea is easy to make. Simply steep a tablespoon of the dried herb in a pint of hot (not quite boiling) water for five minutes, and drink hot or cold throughout the day with a little honey if you like.

Chastetree—*Vitex agnus castus* can be taken in the form of fresh powdered berries (three to four capsules a day with food), made in tea form from the powdered berries or, easiest of all, taken in tincture form (15 drops in a little water two to three times a day).

Vitex, which has been used for two millennia, has a reputation for being virtually free of side effects. It is rich in flavonoids and micronutrients. Although it contains no phytosterols itself, it is an enormously useful natural remedy for severe hot flashes that occur as a result of low levels of estrogen. It can help eliminate flooding, spotting, irregular cycles, fibroids, and endometriosis; while balancing emotions, making skin clearer, and improving vaginal dryness. It is also a great remedy for relieving hormonally related digestive distress from constipation to poor digestion. It also counters most of the usual PMS problems from headaches and depression to water retention and breast tenderness. *Agnus castus* is slow acting, but profound in its effects, thanks to its ability to enhance certain hormones such as progesterone and leutotropic hormone and inhibit others such as follicle-stimulating hormone and prolactin. It can also increase your sense of emotional well-being, as it has been shown to increase the production of the brain hormone dopamine. I first learned the virtues of *agnus castus* from Dr. Dagmar Leichti von Brasch (see chapter 9).

Important to remember*: Agnus castus* is slow acting. Results begin to show in two or three months of daily use and can become permanent after a year—a botanic well worth persevering with.

Diet

Throw out the coffee, sugar, colas, and dairy products. Cut out all milk and milk products. Throw out anything containing hydrogenated oils such as margarines, junk fats, cooking oils, and convenience foods. Eliminate shellfish. Eat 50 percent of your foods raw (see *The New Raw Energy* by Susannah and Leslie Kenton), especially fruits and vegetables; also, make sure you eat plenty of high-fiber whole grains, lentils, and beans. Avoid red meat, and use organic tofu as a protein food. Use a green drink of Chlorella, spirulina, green barley, or wheatgrass in water or fresh vegetable juice daily.

Nutritional Support

- **Natural iron tonic**—such as Floradix.
- **Good B-complex vitamin**.

- **Vitamin B$_6$**—50 mg three times a day for three to six weeks, then 50 mg a day taken in the evening.
- **Pantothenic acid**—100 mg three times a day.
- **Vitamin C** in buffered form (calcium ascorbate)—2,000 mg three times a day.
- **Bioflavonoid complex** once a day.
- **GLA** (gamma linolenic acid)—2 x 500 mg capsules three times a day.
- **Magnesium Citrate or Chelated Magnesium**—at least 200 mg three times a day.

Progesterone

Used in the form of a cream rubbed on the skin twice a day or in oil or pellet form either sublingually or intravaginally from day 10 or 12 to day 26 of your menstrual cycle (see chapter 30 for additional information). Says John Lee, "I recommend that a woman increase the dose of the cream until she is satisfied her pelvic pains are decreasing. Once that dose is reached, a woman can continue for three to five years before gradually lowering it." Lee finds that this regime decreases menstrual flow and gives the body time to heal the endometrial lesions. If the pains recur, he advises women to continue the treatment until menopause. Lee has treated patients with mild to moderate endometriosis in this manner for the past 13 years, and none of them has ever had to resort to surgery.

Vary the sites to which you apply the cream—breasts, back, belly, face, neck, and thighs. Progesterone oil can be useful when symptoms are severe, since it contains more progesterone. To use the oil, put four or five drops under the tongue, and keep it in the mouth for at least five minutes without swallowing (this takes a bit of practice). Vaginally, you can drop the oil on your finger and then apply it to the walls of the vagina from where it is readily absorbed. Vaginal absorption is more efficient than sublingual. Increase or decrease the dosage of the oil or cream depending upon the severity of the symptoms and on how rapidly the cream is absorbed. Oral progesterone can also be prescribed by your doctor, usually in doses of between 50 and 200 mg a day. However, much of the hormone is wasted when taken orally because of first-pass liver actions.

FIBROID TUMORS

Fibroids are benign (noncancerous) tumors of the uterus. They are whorls of tissue, very much like the tissue of the womb itself, that grow into unusual shapes that either lace the lining of the womb or are attached by a stump to its outer walls. Probably 50 percent of women in the West have fibroids, although most never know they are there. They are more common in black women than in white, and if you are going to get them, they usually develop in the eight to ten years before menopause when anovulatory menstruation and lowered progesterone levels occur. Fibroids can be tiny or can weigh as much as a newborn baby or more. (The biggest reported in medical history weighed 80 pounds!)

Only if fibroids cause trouble do doctors usually consider that they need to be removed. Many women with fibroids have no symptoms at all. Others experience menstrual cramps, pelvic pains, pressure on the bladder or rectum, a swollen belly, or extremely heavy periods, which can result in long-term fatigue and anemia. When a woman's hormones are fluctuating wildly, as they can do in the years just before menopause or when she is under a lot of stress, fibroids can grow quickly, sometimes even causing hemorrhaging. Fibroids are responsible for a third of women's gynecological problems and are the most common reason that hysterectomies are performed, for they can often be hard to remove without taking out the womb. Occasionally, fibroids are removed without taking out the uterus through an operation called a myomectomy, but this is generally only done when there is a single large fibroid present or when a woman wants to become pregnant, since the operation is difficult. Fibroids are *very* rarely cancerous.

Fibroids have a tendency to grow and shrink in size as a woman's hormone levels shift during monthly cycles. They are highly estrogen dependent, so they are most prevalent in estrogen-dominant women, particularly women who have not had children early on in life and are in their late 30s or 40s. The good news is that once menopause arrives and estrogen levels diminish sharply, fibroids shrink so small that often they can no longer be detected by pelvic examination. The presence of fibroids in a woman is usually confirmed by a sonogram or ultrasound, since it can be difficult for a doctor to distinguish between an ovarian growth and a fibroid through pelvic examination alone.

Common Treatment

Until recently, the best treatment for most fibroids—provided they are not creating too much discomfort in a woman—has been to watch and wait for menopause when they would go away, provided, of course, that a woman was not given estrogen replacement. Now, doctors at the forefront of the natural menopause revolution urge women to make dietary changes and recommend the use of progesterone cream or oil. Sadly, the majority of doctors and surgeons, even those considered to be "experts" in the gynecological field, continue, unnecessarily, to remove women's wombs.

Soul Searching

Many transpersonal psychologists and clairvoyant healers insist that fibroids are directly related to frustrated creative energy. In some women, they almost seem to be a physical manifestation of plans, projects, or dreams that have either outlived their usefulness or have not yet been brought to birth. Fibroids tend to develop when powerful creative energies have been truncated in some way or have been dissipated. Sometimes fibroids are linked with conflicts over whether or not to have a child or an intimate relationship. Sometimes they can appear to be the physical manifestation of hard, immovable anger or deep frustration.

Energy Medicine

Don't use an electric blanket. Help pelvic energy to flow via meditation for ten minutes twice a day. Visualize drawing life force down from the head and chest into the pelvis and vagina and flooding it with warmth and gentle light. Some women report benefits from spiritual healing, the laying on of hands healing, or Reiki. Investigate energy medicine treatments from scalar wave generators or magnetic field therapy.

Take long epsom salts baths regularly. Take two cups of household-grade epsom salts (available from a pharmacist), pour it into the bath, and fill the bath with hot water. Then immerse yourself for 20 to 30 minutes, topping off with warm water when necessary to maintain a comfortable temperature. Afterwards, lie down for 15 minutes, or, better still, have an epsom salts bath just before you go to bed.

Castor Oil Packs

Use three times a week or more when there is any discomfort, heavy bleeding, abdominal pressure, or other symptoms. See previous section, under *Endometriosis*, on castor oil.

Wise Woman Ways

Lady's mantle (*Alchemilla vulgaris*) tincture has long been used as a natural treatment for fibroids among herbalists. Also called lion's foot, this is one of the sacred plants among wise women. *Agnus castus* is also useful, as is a combination of mistletoe and butterbur.

Lady's mantle—Lady's mantle is said to carry magical properties, offering support to any woman either entering the role of motherhood or leaving it. It is also good for excessive menstrual flow and flooding taken as a tea— 1 oz. (28 g) of the herb to one pint (570 ml) of boiling water or, in tincture form, 10 to 25 drops several times a day. Lady's mantle is excellent for relieving headaches, too.

Agnus castus (*Vitex agnus castus*)—Chastetree berries are also good in tincture form: 10 to 20 drops two to three times a day. Both of these herbs are anti-estrogenic in their actions. They can be profitably used together.

Mistletoe and butterbur—A combination of mistletoe (*Viscus album*) and butterbur (*Petesites hybridus*) is also one of the best herbal remedies for shrinking fibroids. It was developed by the Swiss physician Dr. A. Vogel. When American pharmacist Lynne Walker gave it to six women with fibroid tumors in 1991, she found that within a week, all the women reported that bleeding and other painful symptoms had decreased significantly. Before long, two of the women found that their fibroids had reduced from the size of a grapefruit to that of a walnut. Soon after, the combination that Walker was using was taken off the market in the United States. The FDA refused to let it be sold, because apparently it was not listed among its "accepted" herbs. Other doctors, naturopaths, and wise women who have tried the combination are delighted with the results. It is available in most countries in the form of Petasan tincture, made by Bioforce. Normal dosage is 10 to 20 drops, three times a day.

Diet

Whole grains are full of lignins (compounds that are anti-estrogenic in their effects on the body). Eat plenty of rye, millet, soya products, oats, buckwheat, barley, corn, and brown rice. In a coffee grinder, grind two tablespoons of fresh flaxseed and sprinkle over porridge in the morning or over a salad. Reduce your fat intake to 15 to 20 percent of your calories. Try to take 50 percent of your foods raw (see *The New Raw Energy* by Susannah and Leslie Kenton). Avoid coffee, cocoa, chocolate, or sugar; and stay away from junk fats such as margarines, golden cooking oils, and anything that contains transfatty acids. And, of course, eliminate junk foods and fried foods from your diet (see chapter 11).

Nutritional Support

- **High potency B complex**.
- **Beta-carotene**—50,000 to 300,000 IU a day.
- **Zinc Picolinate or Zinc citrate**—22–25 mg a day.
- **Vitamin C**—2,000 mg a day minimum.
- **Flaxseed oil**—3 capsules a day.
- **Vitamin E**—600 IU of d-alpha tocopherol a day.
- **Vitamin B6**—50 mg three times a day for a month, then twice a day for two weeks, then once a day.

Caution—The Chinese herb Dong Quai or Tang Kuei (*Angelica sinensis*), which in general is excellent for many female problems, should not be used if you have fibroids since it has been shown to increase their size in some women. Avoid estrogen replacement, since this, too, increases their growth.

Progesterone

Provided dietary changes are also made, when enough progesterone is supplied, fibroid growth is arrested and frequently reversed. Good herbal support (see above) works well in tandem. Progesterone cream should be rubbed on different areas of the skin twice a day. It can also be used in oil form either sublingually or intravaginally from day 12 to day 26 of your menstrual cycle. Use enough cream so that you get through a jar during this two-week period, varying the sites to which you apply the cream—breasts, back, belly, face, neck, and thighs. Progesterone oil can be particularly useful when symptoms are severe, since it contains more progesterone (see chapter 30).

Progesterone plays an important psychological-cum-spiritual role for women with fibroids by helping to soften the frustration or anger often associated with them so that these feelings can then be examined and life change more easily instigated. This is thanks to progesterone's role as a precursor to important brain chemicals and stress hormones.

My sister, Christi, is 41 years old. She suffered from fibroids and heavy bleeding for several years, and spent a fortune in New York going from doctor to doctor and test to test in an attempt to do something about them. She started using progesterone cream and then, after a month, added the oil, too. She discovered that her fibroids shrank progressively so that in two months she was completely free of the pain that she'd had for two years, as well as of the heavy bleeding. Delighted though she was to be free of both, in many ways the psychological and energetic effects of the natural progesterone meant even more to her. Not only did she experience a return of energy and enthusiasm for life that had been missing for years, but she also reported: "For five years I have felt oppressed by the universe. Now I feel as though the universe is supporting me. At least I am no longer a victim. I feel I can do whatever I want." Her experience is a good example of how physical change through diet, herbal supplements, and natural progesterone can help shift long-standing psychological or spiritual blockages as well. It is always worthwhile to have your doctor monitor the results of such natural treatment by way of regular ultrasound scans or sonogram tests three or four times a year to verify shrinkage.

VAGINAL IRRITATION, DRYNESS, AND THINNING

Some women at menopause experience a thinning of the vaginal tissues that can lead to irritation, and in a few cases, to repeated urinary infections. The lining of the vagina is a cornified epithelium, which makes it strong and resilient. After menopause, some women shed the outer layers of this cornified epithelium so that their vagina walls become thinner, have less protection, and can more easily become irritated, causing dryness, itching, and pain during intercourse. In some women, an increase in the normally low pH of the vagina makes it more susceptible to bacterial infection. This thinning of the walls of the vagina and the things that can accompany it—referred to by the medical experts as *atrophic vaginitis* or *vulval dystrophy*—is by no means inevitable. Many women, especially those who are physically active and have active sex lives of any sort, which brings regular stimulation to genital tissues, never experience it at all. Others have had to handle a tendency toward dryness since their 20s.

Soul Searching

Forget the feeling that you are somehow odd or incapable of enjoying intercourse or that this is the inevitable consequence of growing old. Vaginal thinning, which is a natural part of lowered estrogen levels in menopausal women, can be simple to counter without ever having to resort to potentially dangerous hormone drugs. So just in case you have been feeling bad about yourself or timid, lay those feelings aside and do something about it. Your body will thank you for the renewed sense of comfort. If you have been leading a celibate life and suddenly find yourself in the embrace of a lover, it is important to be gentle with your body. It has been in a kind of sexual hibernation, so give it time to thaw out. Also, make sure that you never force intercourse before your vagina is ready for it—and this means before your soul is ready for it. Vaginal moistness and receptivity depend on arousal, and despite what all those Hollywood movies with people continually surrendering themselves to passionate embraces would have us believe, arousal is a soul-centered activity, not a mechanical response to external stimuli. Regular sex itself keeps the vagina plump and healthy.

Wise Woman Ways

Stay away from soaps, bubble baths, shower gels, and nylon tights or underwear, since all of these things can worsen the condition of vaginal irritation, dryness, and thinning. There are several botanicals that are great to treat it: motherwort and chastetree taken internally; and calendula, aloe vera, and comfrey used externally. They can also help prevent recurrent vaginal and bladder infections.

Motherwort—Taken as a tincture, 15 to 20 drops in a glass of water several times a day, motherwort is an excellent way of restoring thickness to vaginal tissues when it has been lost and of remoisturizing the vagina (see chapter 25).

Chastetree—A tincture of this berry enhances many hormones in a woman's body, including progesterone and luteinizing hormone. Although it was used in the Middle Ages to calm the lascivious thoughts of celibate monks (hence, its name), it has a powerful stimulating effect on women's libido taken over a few months. It is also excellent for bringing moisture and circulation to vaginal tissues when they are hungry for them.

Calendula—This herb in a good cream base (see Resources) can help soften yet toughen vaginal tissues and tissues of the vulva. It can also relieve itching when applied three times a day and help protect against infection.

Comfrey—In a cream base (see Resources), comfrey is the best soother of all for itchy vaginal tissue. It can be applied both externally and internally to foster the growth of healthy new epithelial cells in the vagina. It can also be used as a lubricant instead of the usual Vaseline or KY jelly during intercourse. Use it three times a day for three months, and you may never need to use it again.

Aloe vera—Pure aloe vera juice is useful when vaginal tissues have become hot, dry, and uncomfortable. Simply wipe it on several times a day.

Cesium gel—This is the *pièce de résistance* when it comes to rejuvenating vaginal tissues. In 1975, when Dr. Zhen Lin at Jishuitan Hospital in Beijing made an important discovery about acupuncture, little did he know it would have powerful implications for regenerating tissue. This esteemed Chinese surgeon discovered that stimulation of acupuncture points by needle, finger pressure, magnetic fields, or the burning of a traditional herb (moxabustion) had a positive effect on the body because they triggered activity of one particular enzyme at the point treated—acetylcholinesterase. This enzyme acts on the neurotransmitter acetylcholine, creating a stimulation through the nervous system—in effect, heightening "aliveness" in that area at a molecular level.

A year later, Zhen began his hunt for a completely safe-to-use substance that would have a strong acetylcholinesterase-releasing effect that could be put directly on skin. He found it in cesium salts. He began treating various diseases with solutions, creams, and plasters soaked in these mineral salts and found that many were either cured or dramatically improved—everything from sprains and stuffy noses to primary hypertension, asthmatic bronchitis, and trigeminal neuralgia. He even used cesium plasters to prevent the pain of cervical dilatation during abortion. A light, colorless gel containing cesium salts was developed by Beth Jacobs. You can apply it to encourage the healing of cuts, acne, sores, burns, and other skin problems (as well as banishing the pain of injuries and muscles in spasm); and it has remarkable skin-rejuvenating properties when you put it on clean skin twice a day before applying moisturizers or treatment creams. It is also excellent rubbed on the vulva and in the vagina three times a day as an energy treatment for vaginal thinning. It affects not only superficial tissue on which it is applied, but at a much deeper level as well. Cesium gel is also useful during intercourse when extra lubrication is needed, or to heighten pleasure.

Natural Estrogen Cream

There is a very good natural estrogen cream that you can order (see Resources). High in the safe natural estrogen estriol (E3), it can be used sparingly on vaginal tissues and tissues of the vulva. Usually an application of as little as one-quarter of a teaspoon two times a week is enough to remoisturize and thicken vaginal walls.

PREMENSTRUAL SYNDROME (PMS)

PMS is a very big problem. Today, somewhere between 40 and 60 percent of menstruating women in the Western world suffer to some degree from premenstrual syndrome. There are no specific laboratory tests for PMS. Neither are there specific clinical signs for the condition, which is why it is called a *syndrome*—a symptom complex appearing to have one specific cause. Each month, PMS usually comes on after ovulation and before menses. Women with PMS can experience symptoms (from bloating and depression to mood swings, headaches, weight gain, irritability, fatigue, and lack of interest in sex), which begin a week or more before a period starts and usually decline dramatically within 24 hours of menstrual onset. The common symptoms associated with PMS are included in the chart that follows.

COMMON SYMPTOMS ASSOCIATED WITH PMS

Psychoenergetic	Neurological-Digestive	Respiratory-Skin	Edema-Reproductive
chronic fatigue	migraine	sinusitis	weight gain
irritability	dizziness	chest infections	swollen extremities
mood swings	diarrhea	runny/blocked nose	tender breasts
weeping	fainting spells	bronchitis	abdominal bloating
sudden anger	headaches	asthma	period pains
depression	flatulence	skin rashes	lowered libido
drug abuse	poor digestion	acne	joint/muscle pain
alcohol abuse	constipation	conjunctivitis	
attempted suicide	backache	thinning hair	
lethargy	palpitations	soft/brittle nails	
insomnia		tonsillitis	
cravings		dry skin	
food binges			

Dr. Guy Abraham, former Clinical Professor of Obstetrics and Gynecology at the University of California in Los Angeles, has done more to study the physical causes and treatments of premenstrual syndrome than anyone else in the English-speaking world. He categorizes premenstrual syndrome into four types. Type A, he says, is accompanied by anxiety, mood swings, and irritability. Type C is accompanied by sugar cravings, headaches, and fatigue; type H by bloating, breast tenderness, and weight-gain; type D by depression, memory loss, and confusion. Other experts such as Dr. Susan Lark, author of *Premenstrual Syndrome Self-Help Book*, have identified two other common subgroups: the first in which women experience acne, pimples, and oily skin and hair; and the second in which women experience dysmenorrhoea with cramps, low back pain, and nausea.

Soul Searching

The causes of PMS are many: some nutritional, some psychological or stress related. Even a woman's attitude toward menstruation has a part to play in the development of PMS. In our culture, menstruation has long been associated with the work of the devil. It is often called the "curse." The whole cycling in a woman's body involving the buildup and flow of blood has been treated as humiliating, rather than inspiring a sense of awe at the magnificence of its complexity and power for bringing new life to birth. This has created a situation where literally millions of women have never experienced the miracle of inheriting a female body, with its finely balanced hormonal system. They grow up fearing that there is something diseased and unclean about their body, or even that somehow they are being punished by God. Instead of the period of menstruation itself being an exciting time of heightened emotion, creativity, and personal drive, it turns into a period of suffering. In the last 50 years, women have been stuffed with thyroid supplements, prescribed tranquilizers, and given psychiatric counseling, all in an attempt to help them handle PMS.

Exercise is important for PMS—not only because of the biochemical and physiological benefits that regular exercise bring a woman's body, but also because regular exercise can enhance self-esteem and help a woman experience a sense of *living in her body*, thereby erasing the old patterns of feeling a victim who goes through monthly suffering. Menstruation is a woman's time to celebrate mysterious female power—the dark moon phase of a woman's monthly life during which she is said to be able to touch the greatest mystery of all. Nothing should be allowed to interfere with that.

Wise Woman Ways

There are a number of botanicals and herbs that bring potent medicine to a woman wrestling with PMS. Some of the best botanicals are motherwort, wild yam (either *Dioscorea villosa* or *Dioscorea mexicana*), black cohosh, and Dong Quai (see chapter 25).

Motherwort—My favorite plant of all for PMS—particularly for the emotional ups and downs—is motherwort. Ten to 25 drops of tincture of motherwort works wonders when you are feeling unsettled. Alternatively, you can take 5 to 15 drops of the tincture every day for a month or two to stabilize emotions long term. Motherwort is the most comforting herb I have ever come across. It brings a sense of inner security and calm strength. It is also strengthening to the heart and tends to enhance courage and self-esteem.

Wild yam—The most effective single botanical for PMS for most women is wild yam, from which so many hormones are derived. Taking three grams of powdered wild yam a day, split into two doses, works so well on many women that, unless they are seriously estrogen dominant and anovulatory, this course of action—together with changes in diet and lifestyle—is often enough to banish the condition permanently. And the nice thing about using wild yam is that after taking it for three to six months, many women find they can stop using it altogether without a return of symptoms (see chapter 25).

Dandelion root—Ten to 20 drops of tincture of dandelion root three times a day with meals usually works for eliminating water retention.

St. John's wort—Oil of St. John's wort rubbed on sore breasts relieves pain, thanks to its action on nerve endings.

Yellow dock root—Tincture of yellow dock root—five to ten drops, two or three times a day—can help counter indigestion, constipation, and intestinal gas.

Sage—Drinking sage tea or taking tincture of sage (10 to 20 drops three times a day), which is rich in phytosterols, can help counteract PMS.

The Light Factor

Full-spectrum lighting, such as that which you get in broad sunlight, is important in the treatment and avoidance of PMS, as it is in a woman's hormonal health after menopause. Some experts in light therapy suggest that sleeping with a 100-watt bulb in a bedside lamp from day 14 to day 17 of a woman's menstrual cycle for six months can help regulate periods. Many studies show that exposure to lighting in the form of overhead lights or light boxes that emit full-spectrum light can vastly improve PMS, as well as lift depression and aid a woman's hormonal functions in menopause and beyond. I have used full-spectrum lights and light boxes for the past two years with excellent results. I find I can work far longer without fatigue than I could before, and I find that I no longer suffer from "February Blues" as a result of long, dark winter nights. It works through the stimulating effect that full-spectrum light has on the pineal gland, stimulating the production of melatonin during the hours of darkness that follow. This kind of lighting equipment, which was originally developed to counteract Seasonal Affective Disorder, or SAD, needs to be used for only an hour or two a day to work its magic (see Resources).

Diet

Excessive consumption of animal fat, which triggers an increase in the hormone prostaglandin, also increases estrogen levels and decreases progesterone levels, thus contributing to PMS. Vegetarians who live on a low-fat, high-fiber diet excrete two or three times more estrogen in their feces than meat eaters. They also have 50 percent less unconjugated estrogen in their blood than nonvegetarians and much less PMS as a consequence. Studies show that PMS patients consume on average 62 percent more refined carbohydrates, 275 percent more refined sugar, 78 percent more salt, 79 percent more dairy products, 53 percent less iron, 77 percent less manganese, and 52 percent less zinc than do women without PMS. They are also lower in B complex vitamins than normal women.

When it comes to eliminating PMS, initiating the dietary changes suggested in previous chapters is instrumental in making deep shifts in metabolism and energy that help make it a thing of the past. Dr. Tori Hudson, Academic Dean at the Natural College of Naturopathic Medicine in Portland, Oregon, recommends that a diet to protect women from PMS should include fresh vegetables and fruit, whole grains, legumes, nuts, seeds, and fish. Also, one should avoid all refined sugars, large quantities of protein, dairy products, free fats, salt, caffeine, and tobacco. Another major item to avoid at all costs is junk fats—salad oils, margarines, and convenience foods filled with processed transfatty acids. These, more than any other single dietary item, interfere with hormonal functions (see chapter 11).

Causes of PMS

- Poor nutrition.
- High-fat diet.
- Too much calcium and too little magnesium.
- Deficiency of some vitamins such as B_6.
- Low levels of progesterone.
- High levels of estrogen.
- Poor thyroid function.
- Poor adrenal functions.
- Diet high in junk fats.

Using a simple detoxification program based on fresh foods every four to six months, such as my *10-Day Clean-Up Plan*, or the Miso Detox and Rebuild (see chapter 26), can clear away the accumulation of wastes that builds up to interfere with enzyme actions and metabolic processes, which are responsible for the proper functioning of the reproductive system. Even a day or two a month on miso broth and seaweed in the premenstrual period helps to cleanse the system and remineralize the body.

Nutritional Support

No nutritional supplement is going to replace a proper diet and lifestyle. However, certain supplements, especially magnesium, zinc, vitamin B6, and the other B vitamins that play important parts in enzyme reactions related to the production, metabolism, and elimination of hormones, can be instrumental in clearing PMS and need to be looked at. In an uncontrolled study where women with PMS were given a multivitamin and mineral supplement containing high doses of magnesium and B6, 70 percent of them showed a reduction in symptoms (see chapter 28).

Magnesium—This is an essential catalyst in many enzyme reactions, particularly those involved in energy production and sugar metabolism. A deficiency in magnesium appears to be a strong causative factor in the development of PMS. Low magnesium often produces symptoms of aches and pains, as well as nervousness, lowered immunity, breast pain, and weight gain.

Vitamin B6—The liver needs B complex vitamins, especially B6, to break down and deactivate estrogen in the body. Many studies have shown that vitamin B6 supplements are useful in treating PMS. In one double-blind crossover study, 84 percent of women reported a lowering of symptoms during the period of treatment with B6. In another study, the incidence of acne was reduced by 72 percent when women were given a supplement of 50 mg of B6 daily for a week before and during the menstrual period. Vitamin B6 is best taken with a high B complex supplement.

Zinc—Zinc is another important cofactor in many enzyme reactions related to reproduction, fetal development, sexual functions, fertility, and mental alertness. Zinc deficiencies are common in women who have taken synthetic hormones in oral contraceptives and HRT. Coffee and tea drinking interfere with zinc absorption.

Vitamin E—The fat-soluble vitamin E oxygenates tissue and protects unsaturated fatty acids, sex hormones, and other fat-soluble vitamins from oxidation. Most of the research into the beneficial effects of vitamin E on PMS has centered around mastalgia. However, double-blind studies show that women given vitamin E supplements experience significant improvement in other PMS symptoms as well, including headaches, tiredness, depression, insomnia, and nervous tension.

Beta-carotene—Precursor to vitamin A, beta-carotene is a safe alternative to vitamin A. But it is best not to take common synthetic supplements. Look for naturally derived beta-carotene. In doses of 100,000 to 300,000 IU per day, it has been shown to reduce PMS symptoms in the luteal phase of the menstrual cycle. In animal studies, vitamin A has been shown to support the activities of the corpus luteum, which produces progesterone. Beta-carotene is believed to be converted into vitamin A when needed by the corpus luteum.

Vitamin B complex—B complex deficiencies result in depressed liver functions. Much PMS develops out of an excess of estrogen in the blood that results from the liver's inability to clear estrogen from the system. As far back as the 1940s, researchers remarked that there is a relationship between B complex deficiency and menorrhagia, cystic mastitis, and menorrhagia, as well as PMS. Supplements of B complex vitamins have been shown to help clear these problems.

Bioflavonoids—Substances such as quercetin and apigenin act in the body to inhibit estrogen synthesis and have been shown to be useful in eliminating many symptoms of PMS.

Essential fatty acids—To manufacture and metabolize hormones properly, essential fatty acids—especially linoleic acid and gamma linolenic acid (GLA)—are necessary. The proper metabolism of essential fatty acids demands adequate magnesium, vitamin C, zinc, vitamin B_6, and vitamin B_3. This is a major reason why all of these nutrients are so important in the treatment of PMS. When the body's enzymes are working properly and the diet is not full of transfatty acids from junk fats, it can convert linolenic acid into GLA. In many women with PMS, because of poor diet usually over many years, this conversion is difficult if not impossible for their bodies to carry out. Using borage oil, starflower oil, blackcurrant oil, or evening primrose oil supplements, which are all high in GLA, will bypass this conversion and can be very helpful for PMS in many women.

Typical Supplementation for PMS

- **Vitamin B complex**—25–50 mg of major B complex vitamins a day.
- **Vitamin C**—one to two grams a day.
- **Vitamin E**—200–400 IU a day.
- **Bioflavonoids**—Mixed flavonoids—1,000 mg a day.
- **Beta-carotene**—Equivalent of 50,000 IU a day.
- **Magnesium**—400–800 mg chelated magnesium a day in split doses.
- **Zinc**—18–22 mg chelated zinc or zinc picolinate a day, preferably at night.
- **Linseed or flaxseed oil**—one to 2 tablespoons of cold-pressed refrigerated oil a day on salads or 4 capsules (see Resources).
- **GLA, borage oil, starflower oil, blackcurrant oil, or evening primrose oil**—500 mg, 3 to 4 times a day.

Progesterone

Underlying all PMS, whether primarily nutritional, emotional, or stress-related in origin, is an imbalance in hormones. In most PMS, the imbalance in hormones is a simple one—too much estrogen and too little progesterone. While this is not the case for *every* woman, it is certainly what happens in the vast majority of cases regardless of which PMS "group" her symptoms place her. Many of the common treatments for PMS, from the use of extra vitamin B6 to changes in diet, actually work because through one action or another, they are able to influence hormone balance. Levels of progesterone lower than they should be in the second half of the menstrual cycle—the luteal phase—can cause the hypothalamic center to become hyperactive, increasing the production of LH and FSH and creating many symptoms associated with PMS.

The swelling that occurs near a menstrual period is not simple extracel-lular edema. It is *intracellular,* where water actually gets blocked within cells. This can mean as much as a six- or eight-pound weight gain over the course of ten days just before menstruation. In women who experience such weight gain, the use of a progesterone cream for three months from day 12 to day 26 or day 27 of their menstrual cycle will almost invariably clear this up. After several weeks of using the cream, John Lee suggests that women weigh them-selves during the time of the month that the edema was always there.

"When a woman sees that the edema that has always been there is now gone," says Lee, "it proves to her that the progesterone is working." After using progesterone cream, Lee's patients reported that they felt much bet-ter, that they felt they had a handle on their life again, and that they could get on with things without the disturbing effects of their PMS. "Not all PMS is due to progesterone deficiency or estrogen dominance," says Lee, "but a large proportion of PMS women have estrogen dominance and are helped by progesterone."

Biochemist Ray Peat used transdermal progesterone therapy on 200 women who were suffering from a wide range of PMS symptoms from migraine, depression, and acne; to lethargy, mastalgia, and edema. He dis-covered that almost all the women treated were able to determine for them-selves the appropriate dose to control their symptoms. He also found that a few women needed thyroid supplementation to shed excess fat from their bodies, as well as using progesterone cream. British physician Barry Dur-rant-Peatfield frequently combines progesterone with thyroid treatment when appropriate, with good results. One of the interesting things Peat reported was that many women have difficulty at first grasping how a con-dition such as PMS, which is hormonal in nature, can be cleared up using a hormone.

Another expert in PMS is Joel Hargrove, M.D., director of the PMS and Menopause Clinic at Vanderbilt University. Hargrove, too, is an advocate of natural progesterone. Unlike Lee, he uses it orally, prescribing much high-er doses of the steroid, since progesterone taken by mouth is largely destroyed in the liver before it can reach the bloodstream. Hargrove gave progesterone in doses of 500 to 800 or 1,000 mg a day orally to several thousand women whom he studied for 12 years. He reported a 94 percent success rate. A jar of progesterone cream contains only about 900 mg of progesterone. If that is used over the course of the month, you are most like-ly to take in 30 to 60 mg a day and probably only absorb 15 to 25 mg. How-ever, that's usually sufficient to establish balance. If you are packing the use of the cream into a 10- to 12-day timetable, then you will be receiving some pretty good levels.

"This is magic stuff for PMS," says Lee. "I don't say 94 percent, maybe 80 or 90 percent. That is pretty darned good for PMS. And you don't have to use diuretics and tranquilizers and pep pills—which neither I nor my patients were ever happy with." Lee suggests that women using a progesterone cream can best monitor themselves. "If they feel the PMS getting worse on a certain day, they should just apply more," he says. "It is unnecessary to pick the dose exactly. It usually picks itself through the woman using it. It is also usually best rising progressively in the ten days before a period."

Here Are Some of John Lee's Protocols for PMS

Use a jar of cream in a ten-day period, ending just before expected menses. With experience, many women discover that the progesterone dose can be applied in a manner to produce a *crescendo* effect in the four to five days just before menstruation begins. In fact, some women prefer to add the use of sublingual drops during the last four to five days, in addition to the transdermal progesterone in the cream. Others find that additional cream can be applied several times a day close to a period, depending on their symptoms.

"The important thing to remember about dose," says Lee, "is that the right dose of progesterone for any particular woman is the dose that works." The way Lee achieves the crescendo dose is for a woman to use a full jar in 10 or 12 days from days 14 to 26, or days 12 to 28, aiming to have finished the jar two days before the period. In the last five days, Lee adds four drops of progesterone oil sublingually to create the crescendo effect. You can also use progesterone in the form of sublingual pellets or granules that most women find easier to manage. Taking progesterone sublingually is a little tricky to get used to, as the oil has to be held under the tongue for three to five minutes to allow it to be properly absorbed through the mucous membranes of the mouth. It often takes practice to hold the oil there for long enough without swallowing.

NEVER COME MORNING
Secrets of Blissful, Restful Sleep

INSOMNIA

*I*nsomnia is one of women's greatest fears. Eight times more women report sleep difficulties to their doctors throughout their lives than do men. Apart from the motherhood-induced insomnia that comes from having to feed a baby, if ever you are going to have trouble sleeping, it is most likely to be during the perimenopausal years, just before your periods stop, or much later on in your 70s and 80s. People sleep less as they get older for a number of reasons—not the least of which is a decrease in the production of a substance called melatonin, which regulates the body's circadian rhythms. Hot flashes and night sweats can interfere with sleep, too, and taking action to ease them (see chapter 25) is often enough to make you sleep blissfully through the night.

Sleep patterns vary tremendously from person to person. Some women need only four or five hours a night, while others need eight or nine. Short sleepers are often more outgoing, contented, and lively than their long-sleeping sisters, who may get as much as ten hours a night. Studies show that long sleepers tend to worry more, and be more introverted and anxious. How much sleep you need can change depending on your life circumstances. When you are pregnant, eat less wholesome foods, or are under stress or ill, you may need more sleep. You also need more sleep when you gain weight. When losing weight or during a detoxification regime, you will often sleep less.

The sleeplessness that occurs in women around the time of menopause and in the few years just before is most usually not a difficulty in going to sleep, but a tendency to awaken regularly at the same time each night (usually two or three in the morning) and to lie in bed wide awake. Because we are accustomed to sleeping through the night, we assume that there must be something wrong. Yet sleeplessness can sometimes bring new insights, if you are ready to receive them. Many artists, writers, and composers will tell you that they receive inspiration for new projects and discover ways of overcoming creative challenges on awakening during the night.

Common Treatment

That being said, when sleeplessness becomes chronic, it can leave you feeling exhausted, hopeless, and washed out. Sleeping pills are not the answer. Their side effects include digestive problems, poor concentration, disorders of the blood and respiration, high blood pressure, liver and kidney troubles, problems with vision, depression, dizziness, confusion, and damage to the central nervous system. Using them can even lead to worse insomnia. There are better ways.

Soul Searching

Native Americans refer to the unseen world of inspiration, myth, spirit helpers, animal helpers, and magic as *dreamtime*. They insist that once a woman claims her own right to the transformation of menopause by embracing her power and learning to hold her wise blood within her body, then the magic implicit in dreamtime becomes present to do her bidding, and sleep comes at her command. But this, they say, does not happen until she has passed through the energetic chaos that is part of the transformative journey—chaos that can manifest as flashes of hot and cold, surges of energy, waves of fatigue, and powerful emotions. These are all part of the transition from the ordinary world of the childbearing woman to the extraordinary realm of the young crone.

One of the most wonderful experiences for a menopausal woman is that of letting go of all time constraints and freewheeling. If you can manage it, take a weekend or even a week away from all responsibility, either by staying at home alone or by going on a retreat (see Resources), so you can sleep whenever you like. Freed from the bonds of time, you can nap at any time of the day or night and heed any creative impulses that arise. Forget your watch; don't watch television or listen to the radio. See what it is like to move away from the restrictions of outward time and to align yourself with the times of the earth, the sun, and the moon, as well as your own internal rhythms. It can have a remarkable effect, both on your creativity, and also on eliminating once and for all the feeling of being trapped in time and full of anxiety if you don't sleep as much as you think you should.

A Breath of Medicine

When sleeplessness arises out of anxiety or brings worries in its wake, it can be useful to shift the focus of your energy toward the breath, using one of the most simple yet powerful techniques I know from yogic breathing. Practice it first when you are relaxed so you know it well. Call on it during sleepless nights to transform your anxious energy into calm, and at any time during the day when you may feel worried, or when a sense of panic comes on about anything.

Sitting straight in a chair or with your legs crossed on a cushion on the floor—once you get the hang of it you can do this exercise lying down as well—place the tip of your tongue on the ridge on your pallet just behind your front teeth. Keep it there during the entirety of the exercise. Breathe out completely through your mouth, pursing your lips a bit if necessary, and letting the air move out around your tongue (it makes a soft whooshing sound). Now you are ready to begin.

- Close your mouth, and silently inhale through the nose to a count of four.
- Hold your breath to a count of seven.
- Now exhale fully through your mouth again, making a whoosh sound as you do so to a count of eight.
- Repeat all of the above four times.

The inbreath is taken silently through the nose with the mouth closed, and the outbreath, which takes twice as long, is made through the slightly opened mouth. How much time you spend on each phase of the breath is up to you. In the beginning, it is likely to be faster, and later on, when you have used the exercise a lot, it is likely to slow down a great deal. This really does not matter. What is important is that you maintain the same 4:7:8 ratio during the whole exercise and that your tongue remains on the ridge just behind your upper teeth. The reason for the tongue placement is that according to yogic theory, there are two kinds of energy in the human body—positive and negative nerve currents—one being solar and the other lunar. They begin and end at this spot behind the upper front teeth and at the tip of the tongue. By putting the two together, you are completing a circuit that enables you to hold the power of breath energy within your body, rather than letting it dissipate, thus restoring balance and serene well-being.

This is a marvelous exercise that brings about an instantaneous shift of consciousness after only four breaths. After you have learned it and used it for a few weeks, extend from four to eight breaths for even deeper calming effects. This is not a good idea until you know it well, since it might make you slightly lightheaded. Use it whenever anything disturbing happens in your life.

Wise Woman Ways

There are some excellent helpers from the "plant people" that various wise women have taught me to use. Each has its own spirit and character. Some will work better for you than others.

Valerian—This is the root of the plant *Valeriana officinalis,* which was the primary herbal sedative used on both sides of the Atlantic before the advent of barbiturate sleeping pills. It is a safe and well-tested herbal remedy with a smell like dirty old socks (the smell drives some people's cats wild). Don't let that put you off, since valerian is a powerful and useful tool for inducing safe sleep—more potent than most of the other natural tranquilizers, such as hops or skullcap or chamomile.

You can taken valerian in two ways, but I like the tincture best: 10 to 20 drops in a little water before bedtime or in the middle of the night when you awaken. Alternatively, you can use a couple of capsules of the dried root. Valerian in lower doses is also useful when your nerves feel "shot" during the day. Very infrequently, valerian will be too strong for a particular woman so that she awakens with the sense of a slight hangover in the morning. If this applies to you, either cut down on the dose, or try another milder remedy. In any case, it is a good idea to change remedies every so often so your body doesn't become accustomed to one, rendering it ineffectual.

Passion flower (*Passiflora incarnata*), also known as Maypops, is a climbing plant that boasts magnificent white flowers with a purple center. It has a wonderful sedative and mildly narcotic effect on the body. Passion flower is most useful for women who wrestle frequently with nervous tension, and particularly helpful when nerves seem to be edgy before and around the time of menopause. It is also useful for relieving pain, thanks to its mild analgesic and antispasmodic qualities, all of which have been well demonstrated in laboratory and clinical tests. Passion flower can also be useful for a woman troubled with PMS. It is not as strong as valerian in its actions, is more calming than sedating, and as such is a great alternative to tranquilizer drugs. Use 10 to 20 drops of the tincture or the same amount of the liquid extract in water. Alternatively, take two capsules of the dried extract up to four times a day as needed. Where you might take valerian at night just before going to bed, the best results from passion flower often come from taking it during the day to calm nerves and make everything easier and less stressful.

Chamomile tea (*Matricaria chamomilla*) was one of the nine herbs sacred to the Anglo-Saxon god Wotan. Chamomile was also much loved by the Romans. Its name *Matricaria* is derived either from the Latin word *mater,* meaning "mother"; or from *matrix,* meaning "womb." For thousands of years, it has been used as a woman's herb to help painful menstruation, to calm anxiety, and aid sleep—even to help build strong bones, since it contains a form of readily absorbed calcium. Chamomile is also a uterine tonic—something else that has been scientifically evaluated. It boasts many other therapeutic properties such as being antibacterial in its actions and good for skin. The easiest way to take chamomile is in the form of a tisane or tea. Infuse 5 to 10 grams of the dried flowers in hot water before bedtime, or whenever you need to relax. Chamomile works particularly well when taken together with passion flower.

Hops (*Humulus lupulus*)—The flowers from this British herb are often used together with other remedies to treat everything from indigestion to nerves. Like valerian, hops has a pronounced sedative effect, but is milder. Unlike valerian, hops smells sweet and can be used without concern about side effects. You can use hops in the form of a tincture, but particularly for women who are awakened in the middle of the night and have trouble going back to sleep, it is good to drink hop tea that you make before going to bed by steeping the flowers for ten minutes in hot water, then straining and allowing to cool. Put the tea, sweetened with honey if you like, by the side of your bed so you can drink it when you awaken in the night. Also wonderful is a little pillow stuffed with dried hops blossoms, which you put under your neck when you go to bed or if you awaken.

Oatstraw (*Avena sativa*)—The straw from oats has an ability to restore energy when nerves have been frayed, and it is useful for counteracting insomnia. It can help ease night sweats, calm anxiety, and even relieve headaches. Stuff a little pillow with oat husks, or infuse them in hot water as a drink (see "Hops" above).

Hormone Magic: Melatonin

Melatonin, a hormone from the pineal gland, decreases the time that a woman is awake before falling asleep again, as well as reducing the number of times she awakens. It also increases daytime alertness and energy levels. The dose generally recommended is between 3 and 15 mg, preferably taken on an empty stomach an hour before going to bed, although some people seem to need more. Melatonin is one of those compounds which, although it has often been given in much higher doses (between 40 and 80 mg), appears to be more effective for many women in low doses (see chapter 28).

Sleep Rituals

When it comes to getting ready for sleep each night, the body loves routines. They foster relaxation and let it know what to expect.

Routines—Make bedtime and rising time as regular as possible and go through the same routine each evening of putting the cat out, opening the window, reading a book, or whatever suits you.

Movement—Take plenty of aerobic exercise each week, preferably out of doors. Experiment with exercising at different times of the day to see which time works better for you in terms of relaxing you and making you ready for sleep at night.

Stay awake—Don't take on any new activities late in the day, and don't take a nap in the evening or late afternoon.

Eat early—Don't eat dinner late in the evening—the earlier the better. Make it the smallest meal of the day, and avoid snacks after dinner since they can interfere with sleep. Everybody sleeps better on an empty stomach despite what the hot-drink manufacturers would have you believe.

Midnight soak—Soak in a lukewarm (not hot) bath for 30 minutes. Blot your skin dry without friction, and go straight to bed, moving slowly. This can be a great thing to do in the middle of the night if you awaken. Use a candle instead of turning on the light, and let yourself relax the way you probably never can during the day when a telephone could ring or someone might demand something from you.

Sleep alone—Insist that you sleep in a room by yourself if you want to be alone. Many women stay in the same bed with their mate night after night, year after year, out of habit, insecurity, or a fear of upsetting the boat should they voice a need for solitude at night. It is every woman's right to sleep alone when she wishes. In fact, it is sometimes not so much a question of right, but of necessity if you are to make your own passage to power and come to know your emerging self.

The water margin—Drink plenty of water during the day. Sleep is induced by the brain, and brain cells need adequate hydration both to stay awake during the daylight hours and to trigger the dreamy relaxation that brings on sleep. Hardly anyone drinks as much water as they profitably could. I discovered this a couple of years ago and regularly consume at least $3\frac{1}{2}$ pints (2 liters) of mineral water a day now, in addition to whatever other drinks I may have.

Cut out stimulants—Eliminate all stimulants from your life—coffee, tea, colas, and chocolate, as well as some of the stimulating plants such as guarana (a caffeine source from South America), yerba mate (another one), and ma huang or Chinese ephedra, which is a natural source of ephedra. All of these stimulants work against a good night's sleep when they are in your system even if you have taken them many hours before bedtime.

Give thanks—Count your blessings and say your prayers. It is an old-fashioned idea, but it is a true key to deep relaxation and blissful sleep. Each night as you turn off the light, think of six things during the day that you have to be thankful for, regardless of your physical or emotional state or how difficult your life may be at any time. Give thanks for them, and surrender your body to the bed, asking that the love of sleep wash over you, cleansing and renewing you for tomorrow. It gradually trains the mind to dwell on pleasurable themes even when you are awake. It can even improve the quality of your dreams.

FIELD AND FOREST

The Wise Woman's Guide to Herbs and Plants

Using plants and herbs for health and healing offers many advantages. First, their powers for balancing an organism and restoring or enhancing health go far beyond their ability to alleviate symptoms. As living things, they are *supraphysical* in their ability to affect a woman's vital force. Besides all their chemical properties, botanicals carry to the body their own brand of ineffable life energy. Wise women often like to use the whole of a plant, rejecting the principles of allopathic medicine that choose to give isolated active ingredients or drugs.

In medicinal plants, there are two kinds of compounds, each of which has an important part to play in treatment. The first are the active ingredients. These are what capture the imagination of chemists and drug producers who often isolate them from a plant and then go on to chemically modify them and make molecular analogues that can be patented and sold as drugs. The second are the compounds and substances that drug manufacturers ignore altogether and seek to eliminate, but which wise women and good herbalists insist play a supportive role in the healing that a particular herb can bring to the body. These compounds work synergistically with the actives, making them more easily assimilable, or buffering the action of what are otherwise potent plant chemicals—helping to protect the body from side effects. Some even help protect from taking too much of a particular active ingredient by causing nausea if the body's safe level of tolerance is passed. It is the synergy of these primary active ingredients and their secondary helpers that make herbs work so well.

There are many different substances and compounds in plants and herbs that offer health-supporting abilities—the volatile oils, the mucilages, the tannins, alkaloids, bitters, glycosides, flavonoids, anthraquinones, and saponins. For the purposes of treating female problems and enhancing women's health, the most important are the steroidal saponins. The steroidal saponins fall into various categories. Some resemble cholesterol from which the body makes its own steroid hormones or cortisol—that is, the estrogen, progesterone, the androgens or vitamin D. Others (the triterpenoid saponins) give to the body a unique ability to regulate its own hormonal balance and activities, probably because they provide the raw materials out of which the body can make whatever hormones are needed to enhance health. These plants are known as adaptogens. They include many of the herbs long used by wise women to help menstrual and menopausal problems. Because of this balancing ability, unlike drugs or isolated ingredients, they are often used to treat two apparently completely opposite conditions. Ginseng, for instance, can be used to treat both high and low blood pressure. Wild yam is useful for progesterone insufficiency as well as low estrogen. Some of the adaptogens—wild yam and licorice, for instance— also act as anti-inflammatories.

PREPARATIONS

Herbs can be taken in many different ways—as infusions, decoctions, syrups, tinctures, suppositories, and in baths; or as ointments and creams, as well as in capsules to bypass the taste buds on the tongue. You can even grow your own herbs and then, using these or herbs you have bought in bulk, make up your own infusions. The dried plant is by far the cheapest way to use herbs, since you can buy 500 grams of most powdered herbs from a good supplier very cheaply and even encapsulate them yourself in capsules that you fill by hand. However, if you are a complete beginner, it is often easiest to rely on good-quality ready-made herbal products—whole herbs, herbs in capsules, and herbal extracts. Tinctures are quite concentrated extracts that employ both water and alcohol to draw out a plant's chemical constituents and preserve them. They are taken in a little water. They are best either bought ready made from a reputable supplier or left until you have mastered the use of herbs in other ways, as each herb demands a specific ratio of water and alcohol to plant material. This ratio can be found in a pharmacopoeia.

It is worth remembering that, just as plants have different personalities, so do people. One plant might work better than another for different individuals.

Infusions

These are made the way you would make a cup of tea, using the leaves, stems, or flowers of a plant, whichever is appropriate. Take a couple of teaspoons, or 1 oz. (25 g) of the dried herb or 2 oz. (50 g) of the fresh herb and put into a large teapot. Fill with boiling water (or water just off the boil for fresh herbs), cover immediately and steep for 10 to 15 minutes. Strain and drink immediately, or store for up to two days in a refrigerator and use as needed. Sometimes infusions are taken by the cupful, sometimes by the spoonful, depending upon the plant.

Tinctures

The part of the plant you are using can be fresh or dried, finely chopped or powdered. I prefer to use fresh plants in a ratio of 1:2, or one part of the plant to two parts of the fluid. If the plants are dried, the ratio becomes 1:5 as a general rule. In the case of chamomile, for instance, use 1/2 lb. (200 g) of the dried flowers and pour over it 1 3/4 pints (1 liter) of the alcohol, the correct ratio of alcohol for this flower being 45 percent. The best alcohol is vodka, but you can also use brandy, remembering that 90 proof is equal to 45 percent alcohol. Put the mixture in an airtight container, and allow it to macerate in a dark place away from direct sunlight for two to four weeks, shaking the jar thoroughly twice each day.

Now the mixture is ready for pressing. Using a muslin bag or clean cloth, press as much of the fluid as you can from the herb so you waste as little as possible. You can use a cheese or wine press for this if you like. Then, throw away the waste from the herb (it is great for making compost), and placing the tincture in a dark bottle, store in a cool place. Tinctures will keep almost indefinitely, although I would never use one more than two years old.

Herbal Vinegars

Take a bottle of organic cider vinegar. Fill a jar with the part of the fresh plant you are using—root, rhizome, leaves, berries, or flowers—then cover with the vinegar and allow it to sit for six weeks. Vinegar must never be allowed to come into contact with metal, for it will corrode it, so cap the jar with plastic or protect the top with a piece of cellophane before closing. Vinegars are particularly good for plants that have a high content of alkaloids, since they dissolve well in the medium. Vinegars can be taken by the spoonful, mixed into a glass of spring water.

THE PLANTS

Here is a small and simple repertoire of herbs for women. Get to know them. They are like making new friends. Each has its own personality and characteristics. All have been used for centuries for menstrual and menopausal treatments. The therapeutic actions of many have been scientifically validated.

Black Cohosh *(Cimicifuga racemosa)*

Also known as squaw root, black snake root, or Sheng Ma in Chinese herbal repertory, this pungent root comes from the hardwood forests of the New World. It has been used for hundreds of years by Native Americans for its ability to treat disorders of the womb; promote and restore healthy menstruation; soothe irritation and congestion in the cervix, womb, and vagina; relieve pains and promote a trouble-free delivery in childbirth—hence, the name they gave it: squaw root. It is one of the great plants for managing menopause well. Black cohosh contains phytoestrogens, and as an adaptogen, has the ability to balance hormones in a woman's body. It can be particularly useful when a woman has aches and pains to deal with; as well as anxiety, rheumatic problems, arthritis, or mental stress. In a German study carried out in 1988, it was shown to relieve hot flashes, sleep disturbances, and irritability as effectively as HRT but without dangerous side effects.

How to Use

By infusion: one teaspoon of the dried root in a cup of boiling water for 12 minutes, then allow to cool and take by the spoonful every few hours during the day. Tincture of the fresh root: 10 to 30 drops in a little water spread throughout the day.

What It Can Do

- **Calm hot flashes and decrease their frequency**—Rich in phytosterols and micronutrients, black cohosh helps the body produce the hormones it needs to rebalance itself, while reducing LH when you use it regularly over a few months.

- **Ease aches and pains**—The root contains natural salicylates that help relieve pain in the body.

- **Heighten energy and calm nerves**—As an adaptogen, the root can raise the body's vital energies and improve one's ability to handle stress; it is traditionally used to treat hysteria. It also alleviates water buildup in the tissues.

- **Help prevent prolapses**—The root has long been used in Oriental medicine to correct prolapses of the womb and bladder.

Caution—Black cohosh is never used to treat pregnant women or when there is menstrual flooding.

Sage *(Salvia officinalis)*

Also called garden sage, red sage, or Shu Wei T'aso in the Chinese pharmacopoeia, from Native Americans to the ancient Romans, sage was a sacred plant burned to clear negative energy from places and people. I use sage in its many forms all the time. I often burn dried sage to cleanse the atmosphere of a room, calm stress, and heighten awareness. The word *sage* means "to save." Sage is a plant with an affinity for female energy, which has a powerful force for deep cleansing and for drying out that which is too wet. This is one of the reasons it can be so helpful in the treatment of night sweats and the kind of hot flashes that produce copious perspiration. Sage is a plant rich in phytosterols and flavonoids. Like black cohosh, it can be as effective as the synthetic estrogens of HRT in banishing hot flashes. It is also used to treat infertility, is the best gargle for a sore throat you will find anywhere, and makes a great mouthwash. Sage is one of the easiest herbs to grow—it will grow just about anywhere. As the Latin saying goes, *cur moriatur homo cui salvia crescit in horto*—no man should die while sage grows in his garden.

How to Use

Make an infusion of one teaspoon of the dried leaves in a cup of water, let it sit for 10 minutes, then drink one tablespoon of the cooled mixture one to 8 times a day. Alternatively, use 10 to 25 drops of a tincture made from the fresh leaves every day. Also, use sage in cooking, sprinkled on steamed or wok-fried vegetables and salads; and in cooked grains, soups, and casseroles.

What It Can Do

- **Calm anxiety, banish depression, and balance mood**—A natural tranquilizer, sage helps calm the nerves and creates peaceful sleep, since it is rich in the calming minerals—magnesium, calcium, and zinc. It also helps balance emotions and banish emotional swings, in no small part because it helps replenish lost minerals from your system.

- **Reduce infection**—Sage is one of the best herbs in the world for helping the body overcome infections. Its essential oils concentrate in the urine, countering bacterial growth and helping to clear infections there; used as a mouthwash or a gargle, it counters a sore throat; and drunk as tea or taken as a tincture, it helps banish infections in the body as a whole.

- **Relieve headaches**—The herb supports the actions of the liver and encourages good circulation, while many of the saponins it contains help ease pain in the head.

- **Banish night sweats and hot flashes**—Often acting quickly to bring relief, sage can calm sweats day or night; half a cup of sage tea taken at bedtime can make all the difference to women who awaken drenched in sweat.

- **Balance hormones in the midst of change**—Sage has been used for thousands of years by wise women to help women at major times of change—to ease menarche, to increase fertility in childbearing years, and to make menopause a smooth transition, thanks to its ability to balance hormones regardless of whatever imbalances are present in a woman's body.

- **Improve digestion and strengthen the liver**—The volatile essential oil of sage contains both alpha and beta thujone with cineole, borneol and other chemicals. It helps both the stomach and the liver produce more enzymes, making digestion work better and eliminating nausea and gas.

- **Relieve flooding and menstrual cramps**—Sage's tannins and volatile oil relieve pain in the womb and help dry up menstrual excess.

- **De-age the body**—A natural anti-ager, sage is full of antioxidants, antiseptics that protect against bacteria, and minerals to act as co-factors for enzymic processes that decline with age. It has been used for generations by wise women to protect hair from graying and skin from wrinkling, and helps prevent cancer and other degenerative conditions.

- **Ease inflammation and clear joint pains**—Its phytohormones help oil the joints, dissolve mineral deposits in the joints, and ease aches and pains.

Caution—Sage is a drying herb, and, as such, should not be used by a woman who is experiencing vaginal dryness or a dry mouth. It is an herb to use frequently when needed but not continuously over long periods of time without a break, or it may lose its effectiveness.

Motherwort *(Leonurus cardiaca)*

Also called lion's tail or Yi Mu Cao in the Chinese pharmacopoeia, motherwort grows in waste places. It has gained its name from the ancient practice of using it to reduce anxiety during pregnancy. The plant has good sedative properties that have been well validated by scientific experiments and is able to calm the nervous system, while at the same time acting as a tonic to the body as a whole. Culpepper, who believed that motherwort belonged to the goddess Venus and to the astrological sign of Leo, wrote, "There is no better herb to drive melancholy vapors from the heart, to strengthen it and make the mind cheerful, blithe, and merry." I think this sums up the virtues of motherwort very well. Its leaves are full of mind-altering natural chemicals that studies in China have shown to decrease the levels of blood lipids and exert a regulating action on muscles such as the womb and the heart, bringing calm in its wake. This is one of the reasons why—in addition to being used by women to ease hot flashes, banish insomnia, and even restore elasticity to the walls of the vagina—it is an excellent herb for the treatment of many heart conditions. I find that it is the most physically and psychologically comforting plant I know.

How to Use

Motherwort is rich in alkaloids and bitter as an infusion. It is easier to take as a tincture or made into an herbal vinegar. Take 10 to 25 drops of the tincture made from the fresh plant every 2 to 6 hours, or one to 2 teaspoons of the herb vinegar as desired.

What It Can Do

- **Calm the nerves**—There is something so calming and balancing about motherwort that it is hard to describe to someone who has never used it; used frequently, it can relieve anxiety, nourish the nervous system, and relax tensions, while at the same time act as a tonic for energy; it is wonderful used just before confronting stressors of any kind.

- **Minimize hot flashes**—The herb can reduce the intensity, length, and frequency of hot flashes, even helping to calm the dizziness or faintness that can accompany them, thanks to its ability to oxygenate the blood, detoxify thyroid, liver, heart, and womb, and invigorate circulation. For best results, you need to use it regularly for 12 weeks or longer, but sometimes 10 drops or so of the tincture in a little spring water can ease a hot flash while it is happening.

- **Promote undisturbed sleep**—This herb is a wonderful help when you awaken in the night with sweats and have trouble dropping off again. Take 10 to 20 drops of the tincture (kept at the side of your bed with a glass of spring water), and swallow some each time you wake up. It will even help banish anxiety and bad dreams.

- **Eliminate waterlogging**—Take a little motherwort every few hours, and it acts as a natural diuretic, reducing water retention; this is useful after a flight when legs and feet can become swollen.

- **Tonify and elasticize womb and vagina**—Improving circulation and thickening tissues that have lost their elasticity and tone, the herb can rejuvenate the tissues of the bladder, womb, and vagina when you take it several times a day for two to four weeks (see chapter 23).

- **Relieve cramps**—Simply the best for clearing up menstrual and uterine cramps when the menstrual flow is absent or light to moderate. Use 5 to 10 drops of the tincture or one-half to one teaspoon of the vinegar every few minutes until the cramps have gone, and repeat as necessary; prolonged use strengthens the muscles of the womb and makes it resistant to cramping in the future.

Caution—Motherwort is not an herb to use when a woman is experiencing menstrual flooding, since it can aggravate this tendency.

Ginseng *(Panax ginseng)*

Oriental ginseng that is widely cultivated in China, Korea, Japan, and Russia is probably the most studied plant in modern times. It is more potent and effective than its American cousin *Panax quinquefolium* and best chosen carefully as there is a lot of relatively worthless ginseng on the market. It has been praised for centuries for its rejuvenating properties, its ability to protect against illness, to enhance the body's ability to handle stress—even to prolong life. The herb is a great ally—the most potent of all the plants for handling very severe symptoms in menopausal women. You should be aware that many of ginseng's benefits will be lost if you take more than two grams a day of vitamin C, while taking vitamin E will enhance ginseng's actions. The most effective ginseng is the dried root that you chew or a good tincture made from it. Extensive research has shown that for ginseng to work, it has to be replete with ginsenosides—the active compounds from the plant. Ginseng can heighten immunity, improve the functions of the heart and lungs, counter fatigue, and balance female hormones, thanks to its estrogenic effects.

How to Use

Always buy the best ginseng you can afford, and take it either as a fresh root tincture (5 to 20 drops one to three times a day), as an infusion or as a tea in which 1 oz. (25 g) of the dried root is taken in a cup of water each day, or by chewing on a piece of the root the size of the tip of your baby finger every day. The effects of ginseng are cumulative, so you need 6 to 8 weeks of taking the plant to feel its full benefits.

What It Can Do

- **Regulate hormones and banish menstrual flooding**—Rich in phytosterols, ginseng encourages the body to produce the quantities of estrogen and progesterone it needs, along with other steroid hormones, gradually making it possible for the body's endocrine system to completely rebalance itself. This can be particularly helpful in the years just before menopause when it can balance menstrual flow and prevent flooding.

- **Enhance the ability to handle stress**—Nothing compares with ginseng's adaptogenic abilities to strengthen the body's adrenals and support the functions of glands such as the thyroid, pituitary, and hypothalamus, which are involved in stress protection. Ginseng banishes fatigue and slowly rebuilds stamina and energy.

Echinacea *(Echinacea purpurea)*

Purple cone flower, or Black Sampson, is a plant native to the prairies of North America with unequaled properties to stimulate the immune system, heal wounds, enhance skin, counter infection, and calm inflammation. The Sioux used it for snake bites, blood poisoning, and wound healing. Until the 20th century, its roots and rhizomes were primary agents for the treatment of fever and infections from flu and colds; to serious conditions such as typhoid, meningitis, malaria, diphtheria, boils, and abscesses.

When drugs came into being in a big way, the beautiful Echinacea plant was almost forgotten—except in Germany. There researchers began to quantify its effects on the body, discovering that it has properties equal to and often greater than most antibiotics to prevent and heal infection. It offers cortisonelike anti-inflammatory activity, interferonlike activity to heighten immunity, an ability to stimulate T-cells—important mediators in the body's immune system—and can even help slow down the rate at which the body and skin ages. This latter property comes as a result of its ability to prevent the breakdown of one of the body's primary defense mechanisms—the so-called H-system of hyaluronic acid, which cements cells together and acts as an effective barrier against infection. Echinacea is a plant product I would never want to be without. I use it to protect from infection through the long, dark winters and to treat illness in myself and my family.

How to Use

By capsule of the ground herb: one to four capsules, three to four times a day, depending on whether it is being used as a prophylactic or treatment for illness. In the form of fresh plant tincture, it can be taken in a little water: 15 to 50 drops at a time once or twice a day for prevention; several times a day as treatment; up to two teaspoons an hour for a day or two at the onset of illness.

What It Can Do

- **Bring health insurance against illness and premature aging—**
  Used throughout periods of stress, Echinacea contains two poly-
  saccharides that reinforce the body's defense mechanisms and
  heighten immunity, making it easy to ward off colds, flu, and
  fungal infections by continually detoxifying the body and
  strengthening its vital powers to resist illness and degeneration.

- **Boost immunity when illness strikes—**The immunostimulatory
  activities of Echinacea make it a bold ally in fighting off viral or
  bacterial infections, including boils, abscesses, and carbuncles; as
  well as healing wounds. The plant's polysaccharide fractions activate macrophages and trigger an increase in interleukin I to
  enhance immune functions and help the body heal itself.

- **Protect skin and body from degeneration—**Hyaluronic acid is
  the intercellular cement that forms a barrier against infection
  and helps keep skin strong, resilient, and youthful. As the body
  ages, an enzyme attacks the hyaluronic acid so it loses its vis-
  cosity and changes from a firm jelly to a thin, watery fluid. Echinacea prevents the enzyme from dissolving, thereby inhibiting
  the spread of infection and maintaining good collagen and
  elastin in the skin.

Caution—Like many plants, Echinacea should not be used continuously,
since the body can become accustomed to it, and this may negate some of
its potent health-enhancing abilities.

Golden Seal *(Hydrastis canadensis)*

Favorite cure-all of the Cherokee Indians, golden seal has in recent
years won praise from scientists for its widespread benefits, which include
banishing morning sickness and nausea, calming digestive disturbances,
and banishing skin diseases and hemorrhoids. A potent nerve and endocrine
gland tonic, it includes among its active principles berberine and hydra-
stine, which are both potent antibiotics. It can be used as a douche in the

treatment of vaginal infections, as a mouthwash in the treatment of gum problems, and to fight off the infections of flu and fevers. One of the most generally effective of all remedies, this is something I would never want to be without.

How to Use

Use the powdered root in capsule form rather than as an infusion, since golden seal is very unpleasant tasting (one to four capsules three times a day). Tincture of fresh herb: 10 to 30 drops three to four times a day.

What It Can Do

- **Soothe digestion and ease liver problems**—A bitter tonic, golden seal was much used in the 19th century to soothe disorders of the stomach and heal the liver—good for gastritis, dyspepsia, peptic ulcerations, colitis, and a liverish feeling. The berberine alkaloids that the root contains stimulate bile production and secretion, destroy unhelpful bacteria in the gut, and increase the tone and movement of the gastrointestinal tract. The root has overall tonic actions on the nervous system, and is excellent applied topically (on the skin) in strong infusion or tincture against eczema and many other skin problems.

- **Counter infection**—Excellent for the treatment of all kinds of infection, including mucous membranes and body tissues, golden seal can banish catarrh in the head, throat and bronchial passages; and clear up infections of the teeth and gums when used as a mouthwash.

- **Calm uterine contractions**—Gently strengthening to muscle tone and circulation, it has a mildly sedative and muscle-relaxing effect on the body and helps stabilize blood sugar. It can be used for menstrual disorders, especially menorrhagia.

Caution—Do not use when pregnant.

Chastetree *(Vitex agnus castus)*

Also called Monks' Pepper, the equivalent in the Chinese pharma-copoeia is Man Jing Zi, *Vitex rotundifolia,* or *Vitex trifolia.* This plant gets its name because of its ability to calm the lascivious desires of men. For most women, however, it has the exact opposite effect—stimulating libido and energizing the whole system, while balancing emotions. Chastetree is the most helpful and far-reaching in its effects of all plants for perimenopausal, menopausal, and postmenopausal women. It works superbly whether hormones are deficient or in excess by acting on the pituitary to harmonize imbalances. What is wonderful about the berries is that it is hard to get too much of them since the herb never forces the body to make more of any particular hormone than it needs.

It is far better known in Europe and the Orient than in Britain and the Americas. There, its berries have been used for centuries to protect from and even to help cure cancers of the breast and womb, to reduce breast lumps and tenderness, banish edema, clear skin problems, moisten vaginal tissues that have dried, and banish hot flashes, as well as eliminating menstrual cramps and restoring emotional calm. Research shows that these remarkable berries used daily increase the production of the brain hormone dopamine. They also tend to enhance progesterone and LH, while they inhibit FSH and prolactin. Vitex is not a phytosterol rich plant; it relies on its glycosides, micronutrients, and flavonoids to work its wonders, so be patient. Chastetree goes deep in its effects on the body and psyche, but this takes time. Look for good results after daily use for 8 to 12 weeks. In about a year to 18 months, you will probably be able to stop using the plant and find that improvement has become permanent.

How to Use

As an infusion: Make one cup of tea from freshly ground berries each day. As fresh powdered berries in capsule form: one capsule three to four times a day. Fifteen drops to one teaspoon of the tincture one to three times a day.

What It Can Do

- **Eliminate hot flashes**—German research shows that the chaste berry can increase LH, stimulating progesterone synthesis and secretion, and balancing high FSH and excess estrogen, which can cause hot flashes in some women.

- **Regulate periods and banish cramping, endometriosis, and fibroids**—Whether the problem is spotting, flooding, or irregular periods, this plant can help, due to its action on the pituitary. Its anti-inflammatory properties can also help soothe the endometrium and shrink fibroids when used regularly for 12 to 36 months.

- **Keep vagina moist**—Thanks to its estrogen-balancing abilities, chastetree helps regulate vaginal secretions, while offering protection from estrogen-dominant illnesses such as cancer.

- **Strengthen bones**—Due to its ability to increase progesterone production, it is an important ally against osteoporosis and may even help reverse bone loss.

- **Ease constipation and digestive problems**—Sluggish digestion is no match for the chaste berry, which helps restore digestion easily and permanently, provided you take it long enough. It can also clear skin troubles that develop as a result of hormonal change, and banish waterlogging from the tissues with regular use.

- **Eliminate depression and balance mood**—Typical PMS problems from migraines and depression to ordinary headaches and anxiety can yield slowly but permanently to Vitex, which helps ground women. This usually takes about six months, and it is wise to continue with the plant for at least another six months, to make the benefits permanent.

Caution—None.

Dong Quai/Tang Kuei *(Angelica sinensis)*

This is the most prized of all the Oriental plant treatments for women's hormonal problems. Studies have shown that this root, which acts like a sister to ginseng in its actions, quickly clears the kind of hot flashes that are the result of too little or the wrong kinds of estrogen in your body, and it performs many other useful tasks as well. It will lower blood pressure; fight bacteria and viruses; get rid of water retention; improve the body's use of oxygen at a cellular level; calm menopausal anxiety; stimulate a sluggish metabolism; protect the cardiovascular system; and eliminate insomnia, nervousness, and depression. This remedy works fast—usually in a week or two. It is best used together with ginseng, since it is yin in nature to ginseng's yang, and they perfectly balance each other. Ginseng's yang chi (*chi* means energy) is toxifying, while dong quai's yin energy nourishes the blood deeply. Chinese teaching about menopause is that it is the yang or active expression of yin or wise blood. The Chinese often use dong quai together with other herbs such as peony root. Western wise women sometimes suggest taking dong quai for two weeks, then ginseng for the next two weeks to reap the greatest benefits from both.

How to Use

Like ginseng, a thin slice of dried root can be chewed three times a day. As an infusion, one-half to one cup a day. Fifteen to 30 drops of the fresh root tincture one to three times a day.

What It Can Do

- **Improve sleep**—Rich in calming minerals such as magnesium, cobalt, and phytosterols, dong quai can be a blessing when trying to handle the sleeplessness of menopause; it calms nerves and soothes mood swings in the daytime, too.

- **Moisten vagina**—Known for its ability to moisten a vagina that has become dry, dong quai soothes the whole of the pelvis, relieving cramps and aches and restoring warmth and vitality to the tissues.

- **Ease hot flashes**—Fast working, this root is excellent for treating hot flashes, particularly if by nature you tend to be cold; it is not the plant of choice for a woman who tends to be naturally very warm, since taking it can make you warmer.

- **De-age skin**—This plant's ability to nourish the energy—which in Chinese medicine is known as wise blood—improves circulation to the skin and brings a glow to the face, smoothing out fine lines and thickening skin that has thinned from age. It also thickens the walls of the vagina and bladder and relieves many rheumatic aches and pains.

Caution—Dong quai is not a remedy to use if you're bloated, have menstrual flooding, have diarrhea regularly, or if you have fibroids. Neither should it ever be used if you are on blood-thinning herbs or taking aspirin. Any tenderness or discomfort in the breasts while using it is a sign that it should be discontinued.

Wild Yam *(Dioscorea villosa)*

There are many related species of the dioscoriaceae family that have similar properties to *villosa*, including *Dioscorea Mexicana*. Root and rhizome found commonly in the United States and some tropical countries may hold the secret to natural birth control, although you will not find this attribute listed among its virtues in any herbal pharmacopoeia (see chapter 10). Wild yam was traditionally used to prevent miscarriage, as a natural tonic, and for natural birth control without side effects, as it does not interfere with normal periods. Then in 1936, Japanese scientists found that the glycoside saponins of a number of Mexican wild yam species yielded steroid saponins such as diosgenin, from which progesterone itself could be easily converted. Progesterone is an intermediate compound in the production of cortisone. Since then, wild yam has been used to produce steroid drugs derived from diosgenin including oral contraceptives, androgens, estrogens, and corticosteroids through a series of chemical steps. That is why it is now grown and used widely by pharmaceutical manufacturers. The whole plant, which supplies the raw materials for the body to make hormones, has much to offer perimenopausal, menopausal, and postmenopausal women. It is also useful for its anti-inflammatory properties; it calms joint and muscle aches and pains, it soothes the nerves, eases menstrual pains, and encourages the production of progesterone in a woman's body to counter estrogen dominance and the many conditions associated with it. It is useful to counter intestinal gas, colic, nausea, and calm nerves. It stimulates libido in many women. The root has also been shown to lower blood cholesterol and high blood pressure.

How to Use

As an infusion of the dried root: one-half to one cup once or twice a day; or as a tincture of the dried root, 10 to 30 drops three or four times a day. You can also take the ground root in capsules. According to midwife Willa Shaffer, wild yam can be used as a means of natural birth control provided it is taken for three months, along with some barrier form of birth control before relying on it alone. A maximum of 1,500 mg of the plant must be taken in capsule form *absolutely* regularly morning and night. In practice, this usually means four to five capsules morning and night daily (depending on the size of the capsules). Shaffer insists that high doses of vitamin C—above three or four tablets a day—invalidate its actions. You can also use wild yam on the body in the form of a cream, which contains converted natural progesterone as an antidote to osteoporosis, and helps to reverse bone loss after it has occurred (see chapter 30 for protocol).

What It Can Do

- **Ease joint and muscle pains and headaches**—The root is one of the best anti-inflammatory plants known to man.

- **Reverse osteoporosis**—Progesterone cream increases the rate of bone formation. As John Lee writes in *The Lancet* (November 24, 1990): "The signs and symptoms of osteoporosis cleared in every patient [using the wild yam cream] and the incidence of fractures dropped to zero."

- **Moisten vagina**—Due to its hormone-balancing capacities, when taken internally, wild yam helps calm itching and burning in the genitals of menopausal and postmenopausal women; wild yam cream with natural progesterone is also effective in doing so when applied directly to the vagina, labia, and whole genital area.

- **Banishing PMS and menstrual pain**—Because of its ability to stimulate the production of progesterone in a woman's body, wild yam is enormously helpful in soothing the nerves, easing menstrual pain, preventing flooding, and countering PMS in most women; some who also use it as natural birth control claim that it has changed their lives completely, making them feel content, balanced, and in control of their own destiny.

Big Note of Caution—Remember that all of the information on wild yam used for birth control is anecdotal. There have been no controlled studies done on it and probably never will, since no pharmaceutical company is likely to fund them. If you decide to use wild yam as natural birth control, be absolutely sure of the purity of the plant you are using and of the exact amount. Steer clear of prescription drugs and high doses of vitamin C (above two tablets a day), or Willa Shaffer warns that it will not work. Use some barrier form of birth control for three months before relying on it completely.

RESURRECTION

Regeneration and Rejuvenation of Body and Spirit

A time of death and rebirth, menopause offers a woman approaching it or passing through it an unequaled opportunity to regenerate and rejuvenate her body, and the ability to transform her life both physically and spiritually. It is as though the energies involved in the changes her body is experiencing at this time—energies that may have been dormant for years—are now rising to the surface and becoming accessible. Take advantage of them. Menopause is also a time to take stock of what works in your body and what does not, a time to begin listening to the rhythm of your body and your soul even if you, like many of us, seem to have forgotten how or wonder if there is any soul there to be heard. There are many techniques and compounds that can help a woman do this—from immune stimulants and green medicines, to nutritional supplements and brain enhancers (see chapter 28). Now is the time to explore what they can offer. But, first, for any woman to make the most of them, her body needs to be as clear and pollution-free as possible. For most of us, this calls for carrying out a simple program of detoxification that can eliminate body pollution that may have built up over the months and years, while at the same time helping to supply the body with a good quantity of minerals, vitamins, and micronutrients to support enzyme reactions and hormonal balance.

Such a program can be as useful to a menstruating woman who wants to minimize PMS as it can to a menopausal or postmenopausal woman wanting to regenerate her body. Deep cleansing the body can be done in a number of ways: by spending time at a clinic where the principles of nature-cure are put into practice with deep cleansing regimes, by carrying out a spring clean such as the one in my *10 Day Clean-Up Plan*, or—this is my favorite in midlife— by making periodic use of a Miso Detox and Rebuild. It is a program that is best used for at least a week at a time, but can be carried out for several weeks to great advantage. During the first week of the program, it is best to stop all supplements you may be taking except for a high-quality vitamin C supplement that can actually help in the detoxification process. After that, it can be useful to add specific supplements either recommended by your health practitioner or following the general guidelines in chapter 28. Most important, you need to increase your intake of pure water to 1³/₄ to 3¹/₂ pints (one to two liters) a day.

Let Food Be Your Medicine

Miso—pronounced MEE-so—is also known as fermented soybean paste. It is a savory paste made from soybeans and grain that has been cultured with *Aspergillus oryzae*—a microorganism highly beneficial to the human body due to its ability to help set up virtually ideal conditions in the colon so that intestinal flora support digestion in the best possible way. This, in turn, facilitates the body's manufacture of B vitamins important for energy and for protecting the body from excess stress, enabling a continuous effective elimination of toxic waste buildup.

For generations, Japanese folklore has insisted that miso broth is beneficial to health and longevity. As a result, it still forms the basis of breakfast for over 70 percent of the population of Japan. Recently, a number of scientific studies have been carried out to quantify the effects of taking miso regularly. Scientists have been able to identify some of the specific ways in which it benefits health. The daily use of miso has been shown to lower cholesterol, to alkalinize blood made acid by too much sugar, refined foods and meat, and to neutralize many of the negative effects of environmental pollution on our bodies, including cigarette smoke. In many ways, most fascinating of all is miso's apparent ability to neutralize many of the effects of radiation, helping to prevent the free radical damage that underlies early aging and the development of degenerative diseases from cancer to coronary heart disease.

The first inkling of miso's ability to do so came from the work of Dr. Shinchiro Akizuki. As director of Saint Francis Hospital in Nagasaki, Akizuki spent his life treating atomic bomb victims a few miles from ground zero and investigating the use of foods as preventative medicine. Although his team spent years close to the place in which the atomic bomb had been dropped, neither he nor his colleagues experienced the effects of radiation poisoning that devastated the lives of the patients whom they were treating. Akizuki wondered if this may have been because he and his staff drank miso soup regularly through each day. Then, in 1972, his hypothesis was confirmed when scientists discovered that miso is rich in an alkaloid called dipicolonic acid, which is able to link up with molecules of heavy metals in the body such as lead, mercury, aluminum, and radioactive strontium, and, by chelating them, carry them out of the body.

A few years later, at Japan's Cancer Research Center, other researchers discovered that people who regularly use miso soup have significantly lower levels of many forms of cancer and heart disease. And recently, scientists at Tohoku University in Hokkaido have been able to isolate compounds in miso that appear to wipe out the carcinogenic or cancer-causing effects of many chemicals on the body. Scientists at Hiroshima University's Atomic Radioactivity Medical Lab under the direction of Professor Akihiro Ito have confirmed with animal experiments the free radical protection against radiation that the regular use of miso can infer. The liver cancer rate of animals not fed miso and then exposed to radiation is 100 to 200 percent higher than those of animals that *are* fed miso.

Miso Detox and Rebuild

Miso comes in many flavors, and ranges in color from the sweet pale tan varieties to the dark rich brown and red misos. Some misos are made from barley, others from rice or chickpeas. In texture, they resemble a soft nut butter that can be spread on bread; added to soups, grain dishes, and casseroles; and used in salad dressings. The cornerstone of the miso diet for detoxification is the use of miso broth. The kind of miso that is best for this is organic *genmai* miso, made from soya and brown rice. It is dark, rich in flavor, and has a thick texture. Although the preparation of miso soup in Japan is an art in itself and makes use of their famous dashi broth and superbly cut vegetables, it is simple to put together an instant broth by placing a heaped teaspoon to a tablespoon of the miso in the bottom of a large cup or bowl and pouring boiling water over it. Then you can add sea vegetables such as flaked nori or other sea plants, spirulina flakes or other green powerhouses like green barley or wheatgrass to taste. I like to add a splash of good soya milk and sometimes a crushed clove of garlic or two. Once you break through old habit patterns that force us all to look upon breakfast as a time for packaged cereals and coffee, you find that such a breakfast is not only satisfying, it also helps keep your energy levels steady all through the morning and beyond. After a couple of weeks of miso broth taken once or twice a day, all of the body's elimination processes move into top gear, enabling it to cast off all kinds of stored wastes, gently yet inexorably.

The basic principles of the Miso Detox and Rebuild are simple. Remove all foods that can interfere with the body's natural abilities to cleanse itself. These include heavy proteins such as meat, dairy products, wheat, sugar, junk fats, and other highly processed items. Cut out stimulants such as coffee and tea, and depressants such as alcohol, which tend to distort body energies and build up toxicity. Then you take in foods with deep-cleansing abilities such as raw fruits and vegetables and miso to encourage the elimination of stored wastes from the cells. Finally, you supply a high level of easily available nutrients from power foods such as sea plants; sprouted seeds and grains; and the green foods; as well as low-fat easily absorbed protein foods rich in phytohormones, such as the soy products tofu, tempeh, soya milk, and miso itself. While carrying out a Miso Detox and Rebuild, the foods to use and those not to use are given below.

Choose from:	Avoid:
sprouted seeds and grains	coffee
organic miso	tea
fresh fruits	alcohol
fresh vegetables	sugar or anything containing sugar
seaweeds	artificial colorings and flavorings
green foods (spirulina, Chlorella, green barley, wheat grass)	convenience foods
buckwheat and buckwheat noodles	wheat and wheat products
organic brown rice	meat
fresh seeds	fish
fresh nuts	game
soya milk	cigarettes
fresh herbs	drugs
low-salt vegetable bouillon powder	chocolate
soya seasonings (elgl, organic tamari)	colas
raw honey	milk and milk products
tofu	
tempeh or soya cheese	
legumes	
extra virgin olive oil	
herb teas	

Here is what two weeks of the Miso Detox and Rebuild looks like. Breakfast is simple: a bowl of miso broth every day. It is important to experiment with miso broth in the beginning. You will probably find that some of the green foods I have suggested you add to it will appeal to you, while others will not. You will also discover by trial and error the amounts of these various foods your body needs and wants. This is likely to vary from time to time as well. You may find at the beginning that you want only the miso broth with a little soya milk by itself. It doesn't matter. But do try to add the green foods bit by bit as you get used to this new kind of breakfast.

The other two meals of the day are interchangeable and can be adjusted to fit what is available on the menu of a restaurant when you need to eat out.

SAMPLE WEEK'S MENU FOR MISO DETOX AND REBUILD

	Main Meal	Light Meal
Monday	Grilled tofu spread with tamari. A fresh salad of raw beetroot and apple dressed with fresh orange juice and curry powder. A fresh peach.	Vegetable soup made with root vegetables, green vegetables, garlic, onions, and low-salt vegetable bouillon. Melon.
Tuesday	Risotto of organic brown rice, vegetables. A salad of fresh sprouted seeds or grains topped with mixed three seeds: pumpkin, sesame, and sunflower. Half a grapefruit or tangerines.	Crudités with a dip made by blending organic tofu with garlic, lemon juice, seasoning and Worcester sauce. Miso broth with soba (100% buckwheat noodles).
Wednesday	Sweet potatoes or baked yams topped with grated	Fresh spinach, mushroom and garlic salad with dressing

fresh ginger and extra virgin olive oil. Salad of grated celeriac, carrots, red pepper, and black olives with olive oil and lemon dressing.

Baked apple with raisins and cinnamon.

made by blending tofu with brown rice vinegar, garlic, vegetable bouillon powder, and herbs.

Fresh fruit salad.

Thursday

Baked carrots and parsnips with almonds or cashews spread with miso. A cooked buckwheat and raw vegetable salad, including whatever fresh vegetables and sprouts are available.

Slices of orange topped with raisins that have been plumped by soaking in spring water overnight.

Dairy-free muesli (for recipe, see the end of chapter 27).

Bowl of miso broth if desired.

Friday

Leek, parsnip, and yellow split-pea soup made with garlic, seaweeds, and vegetable bouillon. Fresh cucumber slices topped with a dressing of olive oil, finely chopped onions, grated fresh ginger, slivered mushrooms, and miso.

Sliced tomato and sesame seed salad with fresh basil if available, cubes of organic tofu, and crushed cloves of garlic. Dress with cider vinegar, olive oil, miso, and honey.

Saturday

Tofu slices spread with miso then grilled served with wok-fried fresh vegetables.

A bunch of grapes.

Brown rice salad with chopped carrots, green onions, olives, tomatoes, parsley, celery, and garlic; dressed with olive oil, lemon, sesame seeds, and sprinkled with sea salad vegetables.

Sunday

Scrambled tofu with green salad made from Chinese leaves, herbs, celery, green pepper, spring onions, and rocket.

Half a melon filled with blueberries or strawberries.

Barley pilaf salad with miso sauce.

Cook and cool the barley and mix with finely chopped raw vegetables. For miso sauce: 1$\frac{1}{2}$ cups water, 2 tablespoons arrowroot, $\frac{1}{2}$ cup miso, juice of 1 lemon, 6 tablespoons apple concentrate. Mix half the water with the fruit concentrate and the miso in a food processor until thoroughly blended. Mix arrowroot into a small amount of the remaining water and blend, adding more and more water until all the water is used. Heat on medium heat, stirring briskly, until the starch gels. Remove from the heat and stir in the miso mixture. Squeeze in the lemon juice at the last minute. Mix thoroughly.

Almond milk made in a blender from $\frac{1}{2}$ cup of blanched almonds, raw honey, spring water, and pure vanilla essence.

Secrets of Water

Water is the principal constituent from which your blood, your cells, your muscles—even your bones—are mostly made. A healthy person who weighs just over 140 pounds carries about 15 gallons of water around—7 gallons inside the cells, 4 gallons outside, including 2 gallons in the blood. Let yourself become dehydrated, and the chemical reactions in the cells involved in fat burning become sluggish. Your cells cannot build new tissue, toxic products build up in your bloodstream, your blood volume decreases so that you have less oxygen and nutrients transported to your cells—all of which are essential to fat burning. Dehydration also results in your feeling weak and tired and can lead to overeating, as it disturbs appetite mechanisms so you think you are hungry even when you are not. The role of water in weight control and health in general is almost completely ignored. The brain, too, is 75 percent water. This is why the quantity and quality of water you drink also affects how you think and feel. If the water you drink is polluted by heavy metals or chemicals, then the biochemical reactions on which clear thought and emotional balance depend will become polluted as well.

Liquid Energy

Drinking enough brings dynamic energy. Yet few of us drink enough. When Sir Edmund Hillary set out to conquer Everest, he had a shrewd doctor named George Hunt on his ascent team. Hunt knew this precept well. He had studied the records of the recent failed attempt by the Swiss team and discovered that their climbers had drunk less than two glasses of water per day per man. So he ordered special battery-operated snow-melting equipment for the kit and urged the British climbers to take a minimum of 12 glasses of water each day of the climb to reduce their fatigue as they scaled the peaks.

Since then, research carried out with athletes at Harvard University and Loma Linda University explored the relationship between water drinking and energy. It was demonstrated that drinking extra water reduces fatigue and stress, and increases stamina and energy, to a remarkable degree. During one of the Harvard studies, researcher G. C. Pitts set athletes walking at three and a half miles an hour, allowing them to rest regularly but not allowing them to drink extra water. They reached exhaustion after three and a half hours with temperatures of 102 degrees Fahrenheit. Under the same conditions, he allowed them to drink as much as they wanted. The same athletes lasted six hours before collapsing. On the third occasion, the athletes were forced to drink more water than thirst dictated—in quantities calculated by researchers to replace what was being lost in perspiration. This time, they were able to continue indefinitely without fatigue or fever until finally, after running out of time, the researchers were forced to bring the experiment to a close. Few of us drink as much water as we need to remain in top form. Even if you pay attention to your thirst and quench it regularly, you are likely to replace only about a half to two-thirds of the water your body needs for optimal health.

Water Power

Water plays a major part in digesting your foods and absorbing nutrients, thanks to enzymes that are themselves mostly water. If you fail to drink enough water between meals, your mouth becomes low in saliva, and digestion suffers. Water is also the medium through which wastes are eliminated from your body. Each time you exhale, you release highly humidified air—about two big glasses' worth a day. Your kidneys and intestines eliminate another six or so glasses every 24 hours, while another two glasses' worth are released through the pores of your skin. That makes eight glasses a day—and this is on a *cool* day. When it gets hot, when you are exercising, or when you are working hard, the usual ten glasses lost in this way can triple. On average, in a temperate climate—not sweating from exertion or heat—we need about six pints a day for optimal health, although few of us consume as much as two pints. The important thing to remember is that how thirsty you are is *not* a reliable indication of how much water you need to drink. If you want to grow lean and stay that way, you need to do as French women have done for decades. Keep a large bottle or two of pure, fresh mineral water on your desk, and make sure you consume your quota of this clear, delicious, health-giving drink. Here's how to work it out.

Divide your *current* weight in pounds by 18. If you weigh 152 pounds, then 152 divided by 18 equals 8.4 big glasses. Then round the figure up or down to the next glass, and there you have it: 8 glasses a day. But remember that is only a base calculation for a cool day. *You will need a lot more during exercise or on a hot day.*

Provided you do not suffer from a kidney or liver disease, drinking eight big glasses or more of water a day not only helps you to lose weight and keep it off permanently, but also improves the functioning of your whole body.

There is another way in which drinking optimal quantities of water plays a central role in detoxifying the body. It has to do with your kidneys. The kidneys are responsible for recycling all the water in your body—some 800 glasses of it a day—and for filtering out any wastes present. The filtering mechanism responsible for all this in the kidneys is made up of millions of microscopic bodies known as glomeruli. They identify waste products such as urea, which need to be removed, as well as screening out other chemicals and unwanted metals and minerals. At the same time, they pour back into the bloodstream the minerals you do need and regulate your body's acid-alkaline balance.

When some part of you needs more water, your kidneys make sure it arrives. For instance, when you are hot and sweating, a message is sent to the pituitary gland in the head telling it to release the antidiuretic hormone, which, in turn, tells your kidneys to let more water be reabsorbed into the blood. Your urine at such times can become highly concentrated and a dark color. Provided you replenish the water you are losing in sweat by drinking more, your kidneys remain happy and well functioning, and the appetite/thirst messages from your brain do not become confused. When your body's water level gets too low, however, your kidneys cannot carry out their cleansing efficiently, and the liver's role in detoxification becomes overburdened. Water is also the world's best natural diuretic. If your body tends to retain water, this is often because you don't drink *enough,* so it tries its best to hold on to the water there is. Once you do begin to drink enough, this tendency to waterlogging decreases and usually disappears completely.

And, by the way, if you are worried about puckered thighs, the best way to help eliminate them easily is simply to *drink more water*. During a Miso Detox and Rebuild, you need to drink plenty of water. Keep a quart bottle on your desk or in your room, and see that you drain it every day, no matter what else you drink.

Only the Best

The quality of water you drink matters a lot, too. If you can afford the best spring waters, buy them. If not, at least get yourself a good water filter and use it, always changing it regularly. Bottled waters differ tremendously from one to another. Some are nothing more than tap water that has been run through conditioning filters to remove the taste, while doing nothing to improve the quality. Just because they say "spring" on the label doesn't mean a thing. The word may be nothing more than the brand name used to sell the product. Other bottled waters are excellent in taste and quality. Few countries do much to regulate standards for bottled water, and what regulations there are, are generally even poorer than those applied to tap water— except in France.

There are some 1,200 springs in France. Several dozen of them supply bottled waters, the quality of which has long been monitored and controlled by official government bodies. A few have been granted the title *eau minerale naturelle*. This means that they maintain a constant mineral content. It also means that they have a reputation for specific therapeutic properties.

These waters should be safe from bacterial or chemical contamination, and you can be sure they have not been mixed with any foreign substance when they are bottled. Two of the best mineral waters are Volvic, an exceptionally pure still water from the Auvergne mountains in central France, and the sparkling Perrier, which arrives in a carbonated form from a spring in Verg'ze in southern France. The Volvic spring is surrounded by 17 square miles of countryside free from industry, intensive farming, and other nearby sources of pollution. Volvic is lightly mineralized, with a lot of character and a vibrant quality. Vittel is also good, as is Evian.

At first it takes a bit of practice to make sure you get your water quota each day, but soon it will become second nature. Start by drinking two glasses of water first thing in the morning when you get up, either plain or with a twist of lemon or lime. You can heat the water if you like. This helps with elimination. Then, drink two or three glasses between breakfast and lunch, and another two or three between lunch and dinner. When you exercise or when it is hot, remember to drink more. Getting into the water habit will quench your appetite, improve your body's ability to eliminate wastes, heighten your energy levels, improve the look of your skin, and help your metabolic processes function at their peak. You will be amazed to discover just how potent its gifts are.

During a Miso Detox and Rebuild, it is also important to get plenty of rest—you will need more than usual, for much of the body's energy will be involved in deep cleansing itself. Take a nap in the middle of the day whenever you can, and spend more time in bed at night reading, listening to music, or doing anything else that brings you pleasure. It can be helpful to take long walks and get plenty of gentle exercise.

Brush your skin before a bath or shower using a natural bristle dry brush that encourages good lymphatic drainage and cleansing.

The Detox is also an excellent time to explore what meditation or a deep relaxation exercise practiced once or twice a day can do for you, or to begin recording your dreams or writing spontaneously in a journal—whatever happens to come into your mind without censoring any of it. The whole process of deep-cleansing the body—breaking out of living habits that do not support health and energy—is but one part of cleansing the whole being. It can open up new vistas and help you to see your whole life in new ways.

When you stop eating the foods you are accustomed to eating and substitute the cleansing and regenerating foods, your body begins to throw off its stored wastes at an incredible rate. This can sometimes lead to a coating of the tongue and teeth with a most unpleasant-tasting stuff, headaches, a feeling of being unwell for a few hours, or, in the case of those who have been heavy drinkers or who have long polluted their bodies through poor nutrition, even temporary nausea or diarrhea. Sometimes one will even run a bit of a fever in the first few days, which comes about as a result of the toxin-burning processes that have begun. These unpleasant symptoms (and they by no means occur in every case) are simply a sign that the detox is working; they need no special treatment, just patience and rest, and they usually pass quickly. Then, as stored wastes are eliminated from your body, your skin takes on a new glow and translucence. Lines on the face are softened, and your eyes become clear and bright. In addition, your mind becomes clearer so that thinking is easier.

Many writers and artists use detoxification regimes such as this or a high-raw diet before beginning a new project since it can heighten creativity. It is no accident that throughout history, saints and philosophers have turned to abstinence as a way of increasing spiritual awareness and improving mental clarity. Following this kind of regime for one to several weeks can actually help create a bridge between a woman's previous existence and a new way of living. It is a midlife ritual that can carry with it not just regeneration on a physical level, but in a very real sense, the resurrection of one's being.

CHAPTER TWENTY-SEVEN

SEEDS OF CHANGE

Foods and Fixings for New Vitality

he basic principles of balancing a woman's hormonal system are, by and large, the same nutritional principles that keep you vibrant and full of energy. Much of what follows I have already investigated in previous books, but it forms the core of using food to enhance health and life energy. Never were these more important to any woman than after she passes the age of 35.

Making changes in the way you eat means making changes in how you cook. Not only are the methods of food preparation and the equipment you need in preparing life-generating foods special, but so is the shopping. You may find your kitchen stocked with a whole new set of ingredients—particularly if until now you have been living on convenience foods or meat and two vegetables.

The foods that you will use for most of these recipes are not only good for you, they are delicious—grains and legumes, nuts and seeds, fruits, vegetables, and herbs. These can either be bought at great cost, or, if you shop around, purchased very cheaply. I buy many of my fruits in crates from a wholesaler at less than half the price I would pay at the grocery store. You can pay dearly for nuts and seeds and grains and legumes in some health-food stores where they come in tiny packages (and are often not very fresh). But beans and legumes and nuts and seeds can also be bought cheaply in good supermarkets or in bulk at reasonable cost from many of the new whole-food emporiums that are beginning to appear everywhere. Obviously, the more you buy at one time, the cheaper they are. Be sure to refrigerate your nuts after purchase to keep their oils from going rancid. And if you ever buy a package of anything that you find on returning home is not absolutely fresh, take it back and complain. That is the only way to protect yourself, while improving the quality of what is being sold. Here is a brief guide to stocking a larder with life-generating foods to give you some idea of just how much variety you have to choose from.

Fruit

Not only are fruits some of the most delicious natural foods available, they also have remarkable properties for spring-cleaning the body and are excellent biochemical antidotes to the stress that ages. Because fruits contain many natural acids such as citric and malic acid, they have an acid pH reaction in digestion. However, since they are also a rich source of alkaline-forming minerals, their reaction in the blood is always alkaline. This reaction helps neutralize the acid by-products of stress as well as the waste products of metabolism that are also acidic. That is why fruits are so highly prized as a means of internally cleansing the body.

Fruit contains very little protein, but it is very high in the mineral potassium that needs to be balanced with sodium for perfect health in the body. Because most people in the West eat far too much sodium in the form of table salt and an excess of protein as well (which leaches important minerals from the bones and tissues), eating good quantities of fruit can help rebalance a body, improve its functioning, and make you feel more energetic as well.

Finally, because fruits are naturally sweet and because we are born with an innate liking for sweet things, a dessert of fresh fruit after a meal can be tremendously satisfying to the palate. And there is such a variety of beautiful textures, colors, and tastes to choose from—from the sensuous softness of persimmons and the super-sweetness of fresh figs, to the exhilarating crunch of the finest apple.

Vegetables

The best vegetables are those you grow yourself organically. If you are lucky enough to have a garden—even a small one—save all the leftovers and turn them into compost for fertilizer. Even in winter, you can grow some delicious salads and root vegetables in a greenhouse. The quality of organic produce is far superior to chemically fertilized fruits and vegetables—not to mention all the vitamins that are lost in foods when they are picked, stored, shipped, and sit on shop shelves. During the summer, I go to the garden to pick my vegetables, and 15 minutes later they are gracing the dinner table. That is the best way to preserve their nutritional value, as well as to experience the fullness of their flavor. If you are an apartment dweller without a garden, you can sprout fresh seeds and grains in jars or trays on your windowsill.

How you treat your vegetables once you cut them or buy them determines how they will taste and how much of their energy-enhancing goodness you preserve. Scrub anything that will stand up to a good scrubbing, using a brush marked *veg only*. Scrubbing vegetables is better than peeling, since many of the valuable vitamins and minerals are stored directly beneath their skins. Never soak vegetables for long periods. They are better washed briefly under running water so you don't allow water-soluble vitamins to leach out of them. Always keep vegetables as cool as possible (even carrots and turnips are best kept in the fridge), and use them as soon as you can. When shopping for fresh things, be demanding—choose your own cauliflower, and make sure it is a good one. Don't be intimidated by pushy grocers who want to foist the leftovers on you before they bring in their new stock. Demand the best, and you will get it. Your palate and your health will be grateful that you do.

Grains

Thousands of years ago, Zarathustra, the Persian, sage, waxed ecstatic about grains. "When the light of the moon waxeth warmer," he said, "golden hued grains grow up from the earth during the spring." I have always thought that his words beautifully captured the richness and delight of the grain foods. When a good portion of what you eat comes from grain foods, because of the effect on the brain of the complex carbohydrates they contain, it tends to improve your disposition, make you feel calm, and bring you energy that lasts and lasts. Grains, like legumes, need special handling. They should not be eaten raw. This is why many of the packaged mueslis cause digestive upset in many people. It is only by cooking them (or by sprouting or soaking them) that you break the chemical bonds, turning hard-to-digest starches into more easily digested sugars. All grains can be toasted lightly. This process, which is called dextrinizing, not only helps turn starches into natural sugars, but also enhances the flavor of grains used as cereals or cooked in other recipes.

To dextrinize grains, spread them on a baking sheet and pop them into an oven at 300 degrees F (150 degrees C). Bake two sheets for about 20 minutes, stirring every now and then. This is not necessary if you are going to boil them, but it does enhance the flavor and is particularly good if you want to use grains to make oatmeal or other hot breakfast cereals. The other important thing to remember about grains is that it is best to get as wide a variety as possible, so if you have oatmeal at breakfast, at lunch you might choose whole rye bread or a bulgur wheat salad or brown rice. The more variety the better, since each grain boasts a different balance of essential minerals and micronutrients.

GUIDE TO COOKING GRAINS

Grain (1 cup)	Water (cups)	Cooking time	Yield (cups)
Barley (whole)	4–5	2–3 hours	$3^1/_2$
Barley (flakes)	3	45–60 minutes	3
Brown rice	2–$2^1/_2$	1 hour	3
Buckwheat	2	20 minutes	$2^1/_2$
Bulgur wheat	2	15–20 minutes	$2^1/_2$
Couscous	1	15 minutes	$2^3/_4$
Millet	$2^1/_2$–3	45–60 minutes	$3^1/_2$
Oats (whole groats)	5	2–3 hours	$2^1/_2$
Polenta	5	45–60 minutes	$3^1/_2$
Rye	5	2–3	2
Quinoa	2	20 minutes	$2^1/_2$
Wild rice	3	1–$1^1/_2$ hours	$3^1/_2$
Wheat (whole grain)	5	2–3	$2^3/_4$
Wheat flakes	2	45–60 minutes	3

Oils

It is wise not to use oils, except for soya oil and cold-pressed extra virgin olive oil. In heat-processed oils, usable "cis" fatty acids have been chemically changed into "trans" fatty acids—junk fats (see chapter 11). These can not only be actively harmful, but can actually block the use of any "cis" fatty acids in the rest of your diet. Olive oil adds a distinctive flavor to salad dressings. It is quite heavy, though, and some people prefer a lighter oil.

The oil found in flaxseed or linseed is an almost perfect balance of linoleic and linolenic acid—both the omega 6 and omega 3 fatty acids. Linoleic acid is prominent in many seeds. Linolenic acid belongs to the omega 3 family. These are the fatty acids that are generally most prevalent in fatty fishes. What makes flaxseed oil so exceptional is that it has such a high degree of the omega 3 fatty acids, which are, incidentally, particularly important in fat burning. The way to take flaxseed oil is by eating the seeds themselves—flaxseed oil that has been extracted is too easily made rancid. I grind flaxseed in a coffee grinder and then put it into a tightly covered jar and store it in the refrigerator. I use two to four teaspoons a day. It is important to go for the very best German vacuum-packed linseeds, however, in order to make sure that the precious fatty acids that they contain are protected from rancidity. It is as easy as that to make sure you get all the essential fatty acids, provided you steer clear of junk fats and processed oils. Your body will do the rest.

Nuts

Fresh nuts are a good source of essential fatty acids when used in small quantities. The rancid oils in old nuts are harmful to the stomach. They retard pancreatic enzymes and destroy vitamins. If nuts are fresh and whole (unbroken), you can buy a kilo or so at a time, and, provided they are kept airtight in a cool dry place (best in the fridge), they will keep for a few months. You can even freeze them and keep them longer. It is a good idea to buy a few different kinds, then if you mix them, you will get a good balance of essential amino acids. You will also have more variety in your recipes. Choose from: almonds, Brazils, cashews, coconut (fresh or desiccated), hazelnuts, macadamia nuts, pecans, pine kernels, pistachios, tiger nuts, and walnuts.

Seeds

Be sure you buy really fresh seeds with no signs of decay. The three seeds that provide a particularly valuable combination of protein and essential fatty acids are sunflower, pumpkin, and sesame. They can be ground fresh in a coffee grinder and sprinkled on salads or cereals. Other seeds worth trying, mainly for seasoning, are poppy, celery, caraway, dill, fennel, and anise.

Legumes

Nutritious, economical, and delicious when well prepared, beans and legumes are rich in complex carbohydrates, protein, and fiber, as well as minerals and essential fatty acids. It is important to know how to handle them and to cook them well in order to avoid digestive upset. All legumes should be washed and cleared of any small pieces of stone or spoiled food. Then everything except lentils, split peas, and mung beans should be soaked for at least six hours, preferably overnight, before cooking. The soak water should then be thrown away, and fresh water should be added. There are two ways to minimize digestive upset when cooking legumes. I use both of them. The first is, after soaking and rinsing, put the legume in the freezer overnight and cook the next day. The second is, after soaking, throw the soak water away, boil up the beans for 20 minutes, throw the boil water away, rinse the beans, then put them in more water, plus whatever vegetables, herbs, and seasonings you may be putting in with them. Then cook in a covered saucepan by bringing the beans to a boil, reducing the heat and simmering them until they grow tender.

BEANS AND LEGUMES

Legumes (1 cup)	Soak	Water (cups)	Cooking time (hours)	Yield (cups)
Adzuki	Yes	4	3	2
Baby lima	Yes	3	2	1³/₄
Black beans	Yes	5	2	2
Cassoulet	Yes	4	3¹/₂	2
Chickpeas	Yes	4	3¹/₂	2¹/₂
Kidney	Yes	3	1¹/₂	2
Lentils	No	4	1	2¹/₄
Lima	Yes	5	2	1¹/₄
Mung	No	2¹/₂	1¹/₂	2
Navy	Yes	3	2¹/₂	2
Pinto	Yes	3	2¹/₂	2
Red	Yes	3	3¹/₂	2
Split peas	No	3	1	2¹/₄

There are so many things that you can make with legumes that you could fill ten cookbooks with wonderful recipes. I like to make thick soups with them and casseroles. They are great cooked and used cold the next day as a base for a whole-meal salad. In either case, I add whatever vegetables I intend to cook with the beans, plus some low-salt vegetable broth powder, and whatever other seasoning I am going to use. I then bring the beans to a boil and allow them to simmer for the prescribed length of time. Alternatively, I will bring the beans to a boil and put them in a slow cooker or the bottom of the Aga oven and forget about them for six to eight hours. I sometimes cook beans overnight this way. I soak various kinds of beans, such as lima beans, black-eyed beans, kidney beans, or a mixture of them; I pour the soak water away and rinse them, then store them frozen in bags so that I can pull them out whenever I need them to make a casserole or a soup.

Many legumes sprout well, particularly lentils, mung, and adzuki beans. Legumes contain a trypsin inhibitor, a substance that blocks the action of some of the enzymes that break down protein in your body, and because of this they must never be eaten raw. Trypsin inhibitors are destroyed when legumes are well cooked. Sprouting also neutralizes them.

Sprouts

Seeds and grains are latent powerhouses of nutritional goodness and life energy. Add water to germinate them, let them grow for a few days in your kitchen, and you will harvest delicious, inexpensive fresh foods of quite phenomenal health-enhancing value. The vitamin content of seeds increases dramatically when they germinate. The vitamin C content in soybeans multiplies five times within three days of germination—a mere tablespoon of soybean sprouts contains half the recommended daily adult requirement of this vitamin. The vitamin B_2 in an oat grain rises by 1,300 percent almost as soon as the seed sprouts, and by the time tiny leaves have formed it has risen by 2,000 percent. Some sprouted seeds and grains are believed to have anti-cancer properties, which is why they form an important part of the natural methods to treat the disease.

When you sprout a seed, enzymes that have been dormant in it spring into action, breaking down stored starch and turning it into simple natural sugars and splitting long-chain proteins into amino acids. What this means is that the process of sprouting turns these seeds into foods that are very easily assimilated by your body when you eat them. Sprouts are, in effect, predigested. As such, they have many times the nutritional efficiency of the seeds from which they have grown. They provide more nutrients gram for gram than any natural food known.

Because of the massive enzyme release that occurs when a seed or grain is sprouted, the nutritional quality of a sprout is extremely good. These enzymes not only neutralize such factors as trypsin inhibitors, but also destroy other substances that can be harmful, such as phytic acid. Phytic acid, which occurs in considerable quantity in grains, particularly wheat, tends to bind minerals so that the digestive system cannot break them down for assimilation. When a grain is sprouted, this mineral-binding capacity is virtually eliminated.

Another attractive thing about sprouts is their price. The basic seeds and grains are cheap and readily available in supermarkets and health-food stores—chickpeas, brown lentils, mung beans, wheat grains, and so forth. And since you sprout them yourself with nothing but clean water, they become an easily accessible source of organically grown fresh vegetables, even for city dwellers. In an age when most vegetables and fruits are grown on artificially fertilized soils and treated with hormones, fungicides, insecticides, preservatives, and all manner of other chemicals, the homegrown-in-a-jar sprouts emerge as a pristine blessing—fresh, unpolluted, and ready to eat in a minute by popping them into salads or sandwiches. As such, they can be a wonderful health food to any family concerned about the rising cost of food and the falling nutritional value in the average diet. They are the cheapest form of natural food around. Different sprouts mixed together will indeed support life all on their own. While I would never suggest that anybody live on sprouts alone, I think they are an ideal addition to the table—particularly if the budget is tight.

Growing Sprouts

When you discover how economical and easy it is to grow sprouts you will want to have some on the go all the time. Once germinated, you can keep sprouts in polythene bags in the fridge for up to a week—just long enough to get a new batch ready for eating. Most people grow sprouts in glass jars covered with nylon mesh held in place with an elastic band around the neck, but I have discovered an even simpler method that allows you to grow many more and avoids the jar-method problem of seeds rotting due to insufficient drainage. You will need the following:

- Seeds (e.g., mung beans).
- Seed trays with drainage holes, available from gardening shops and nurseries.
- A jar or bowl to soak seeds in overnight.
- A plant atomizer—from gardening or hardware shops.
- A sieve.
- Nylon mesh—available from gardening shops.

1. Place two handfuls of seeds or beans in the bottom of a jar or bowl, and cover with plenty of water. Leave to soak overnight.

2. Pour the seeds into a sieve, and rinse well with water. Be sure to remove any dead or broken seeds or pieces of debris.

3. Line a seedling tray with nylon mesh (this helps the seeds drain better), and pour in the soaked seeds.

4. Place in a warm dark spot for fast growth.

5. Spray the seeds twice a day with fresh water in an atomizer, and stir them gently with your hand in order to aerate them.

6. After about three days, place the seeds in sunlight for several hours to develop the chlorophyll (green) in them.

7. Rinse in a sieve, drain well, and put in a polythene bag in the fridge to use in salads, wok-fries, etc.

There are many different seeds you can sprout—each with its own particular flavor and texture. Use the chart that follows as a guide to the variety of sprouts you can try.

SPROUTING

Seeds and soak time	To yield 1 quart	Ready to eat in	Length of shoot	Growing tips and notes
Alfalfa (6–8 hours)	3–4 tbsp	5–6 days	1½ inches (3.5 cm)	Rich in organic vitamins and minerals, and natural estrogens.
Fenugreek (6–8 hours)	½ cup	3–4 days	½ inch (1 cm)	Has quite a strong "curry" taste. Good for ridding the body of toxins.
Adzuki beans (10–15 hours)	1½ cups	3–5 days	1–1½ inch (2.5–3.5 cm)	Have a nutty flavor. Especially good for the kidneys.
Chickpeas (10–15 hours)	2 cups	3–4 days	1 inch (2.5 cm)	May need to soak for 18 hrs. to swell to their full size. Replace the water during this time.
Lentils (10–15 hours)	1 cup	3–5 days	¼–1 inch (0.5–2.5 cm)	Try all different kinds of lentils. They are good eaten young or up to 6 days old.
Mung beans (10–15 hours)	1 cup	3–5 days	½–2½ inches (1–5 cm)	Soak at least 15 hours. Keep in the dark for a sweet sprout.
Sunflower seeds (10–15 hours)	4 cups	1–2 days	same length as seed	Soak them and sprout for just a day. They bruise easily, so handle carefully.

Wheat (12–15 hours)	2 cups	2–3 days	same length as grain	An excellent source of the B vitamins. The soak water can be drunk straight or added to soups and vegetable juices.

SPECIAL FOODS

Carob (St. John's Bread)

Carob powder/flour is a superb chocolate substitute—and good for you, too. Unlike chocolate, it does not contain caffeine. Instead, it is full of minerals—calcium, phosphorus, iron, potassium, magnesium, and silicon—as well as vitamins B_1, B_2, niacin, and a little vitamin A plus some protein. Carob powder is often sold toasted, but the best kind is raw. It is lighter in color than the cooked kind. It can be bought from most health-food stores and used to make chocolate drinks, desserts, and treats.

Agar-Agar

This starch comes from seaweed. You can use it to make vegetarian gelatin-based sweets and salads, and to thicken sauces and toppings. It comes in flakes or granules and sometimes in sheets. Soak the agar-agar in a little water to soften it before adding hot liquid to dissolve it. Use about one teaspoon to each cup of water or liquid.

Arrowroot

Made from the pulp of the tuberous rootstocks of a tropical American plant, arrowroot is a nutritious, easily digested food high in calcium. When you heat it in water, it thickens (use $1\frac{1}{2}$ teaspoons per cup of liquid). It is better than cornstarch or corn flour to thicken gravy, fruit sauces, soups, and stews.

Sea Vegetables

If you have never used the sea vegetables for cooking, this is an ideal time to begin. Not only are they delicious—imparting a wonderful, spicy flavor to soups and salads—they are the richest source of organic mineral salts in nature, particularly of iodine. Iodine is the mineral needed by the thyroid gland. As your thyroid gland is largely responsible for the body's metabolic rate, iodine is very important to a woman's energy.

I like to use powdered kelp as a seasoning. It adds both flavor and minerals to salad dressings, salads, and soups. I am also very fond of nori seaweed, which comes in long thin sheets or tiny flakes. It is a delicious snack food that you can eat along with a salad or at the beginning of the meal; it has a beautiful, crisp flavor. I often toast it very, very quickly by putting it under a grill for no more than 10 or 15 seconds. It is also delicious raw.

Get to know some of the sea vegetables, and start to make use of them. Your nails and hair and the rest of your body will be strengthened by the full range of minerals and trace elements such as selenium, calcium, iodine, boron, potassium, magnesium, iron, and others, which are not always found in great quantities in our ordinary garden vegetables. You can use nori to wrap around everything from a sprout salad to cooked grains in order to make little pieces of vegetarian *sushi*. It's often a good idea to soak some of the other sea vegetables such as dulse, arame, and hiziki for a few minutes in enough tepid water to cover. This softens them so that they can be easily chopped to be put into salads or added to soups. Sea vegetables are available in health-food stores and in Asian food shops. Recommended ones are:

- arame
- hiziki
- mixed sea salad
- laver bread
- wakame
- dulse
- kelp
- combu
- nori

SEASONINGS

Mustard

Mustard can be bought in dry or paste form. The dry powder is sometimes useful in dressings. I think the most delicious mustards are French. They are milder and more aromatic than English mustard. Moutarde de Meaux is particularly delicious and is great in dressings for all sorts of salads. Dijon and Bordeaux are also nice.

Tahini (preferably unroasted)

A paste made from ground sesame seeds that is delicious and very nutritious. It has many uses, including tahini mayonnaise, and is delicious as an addition to many seed and nut dishes.

Low-Salt Vegetable Bouillon Powder

This is something I use a lot to season just about everything. Use it for soup stocks, to flavor pizzas, grains like brown rice and kasha, and even salad dressings, stews, and casseroles. It is my favorite of all seasonings. The very best is Marigold's Low-Salt Swiss Vegetable Bouillon. I even take it with me when I travel.

Yeast Extract

This can be used as a substitute for "vegetable bouillon." It is rich in B complex vitamins but very salty, so it should also be used in moderation.

Food Yeast

This is sometimes called primary yeast or nutritional yeast. It is not brewer's yeast, which is a by-product of beer making. Food yeast is grown specifically to be used as a flavoring. It is light yellow-beige and slightly spiky in its texture and is good to add to soups, sauces, cheeses, and dips. You can even sprinkle it on popcorn.

Vanilla Essence

Try to find real vanilla essence, rather than the more common vanilla flavoring, which is synthetic. It gives a delicious, warm flavor.

PLANT STEROLS HELPERS

So many fresh foods are rich in plant hormones. Include them often in your meals. The fresher they are, the better: yams, peas, papayas, bananas, cucumbers, raw nuts, bee pollen, sprouted seeds, and grains; and the herbs licorice root, alfalfa, red clover, sage, sarsaparilla, and sassafras. The green vegetable juices, particularly figs and garlic, dates, avocados, grapes, apples, Chlorella, seaweed, and wheat germ can all be helpful in countering menopausal and menstrual problems. Grapes, cherries, citrus fruits, and red clover are excellent sources of the bioflavonoids, which also have weak estrogenic activity and have shown themselves to be useful in countering hot flashes, mood swings, and in helping to prevent heavy irregular menstrual flow. Plant foods high in phytosterols are good insurance against cancer, too, since they help prevent estrogen dominance in the body. They also help prevent xenoestrogens in the environment from binding with hormone receptor sites and causing long-term damage.

The antioxidants in fresh plant foods also offer protective properties against cancer. These include vitamin C from fresh fruits and vegetables; vitamin E, which is rich in fresh whole grains; and vitamin A from fish liver and beta-carotene. The fiber found in plants is protective against estrogen dominance and cancer via another mechanism. Breast cancer is highly related to estrogen levels, as well as to the consumption of high levels of meat and fat. Women on a vegetarian diet high in fiber excrete a much higher level of estrogen than other women and have much lower blood levels of the hormones. In Britain and the United States, the use of milk products has been correlated with breast cancer. Sea plants, green vegetables, and Chlorella are far better sources of calcium than cheese and milk. Some of the best products of all are the soya-based foods from the Orient, together with naturally fermented foods—often of Japanese origin.

TOFU

Its other name is bean curd. This white, bland, soft food made from soybeans is easy to digest, high in protein, low in calories and fat, cheap, and you can use it for just about anything. It behaves a bit like a sponge, which will absorb whatever flavor you soak it in. When you cook it, it becomes firmer. You can mix it with herbs, make sauces or low-fat mayonnaise from it, dips for vegetables, pizza toppings, and stir-fries. You can even substitute it for cheese in some of your favorite recipes, except that it doesn't melt under the grill. Buy it in the supermarket, health-food store, or Asian food shop, and keep it sitting in water in the fridge so it doesn't dry out.

Miso

Miso is a fermented soybean paste that is rich in digestive enzymes and high in protein. It can be used for seasoning soups and sauces. It is also a delicious addition to dips for crudités and salad dressings (see chapter 26).

Tamari

This is a type of soya sauce made from fermented soybeans, but unlike soya sauce, it contains no wheat, although it does contain sea salt so should be used in moderation. It is good for giving a "Chinese" taste to dishes, as well as a rich flavor to bland dressings or sauces.

Soya Flour

Made from cooked, ground soy beans, soya flour is sometimes added to grain-based flours to increase their protein content. It can be used to make soya milk and soya cheese.

Soya Milk

Made from cooked, ground, and strained soybeans, this is often used for bottle-fed infants who are allergic to cow's milk. I use it as a substitute for milk on cereals and in recipes. You can make your own very cheaply. I prefer this since ready-made varieties are often packed in aluminum-lined cartons, and it is best to avoid aluminum (see Resources for the best soya milk).

HERBS

The magicians of life-generating cooking, fresh herbs can transform a humble recipe into a pasha's delight. I use them constantly, lavishly, and occasionally with utter abandon. I have been known to add as many as seven different leafy herbs to a simple green salad, which becomes more of an herb salad than a green salad by the time I have finished. I grow most of my herbs in the garden because there is something about freshness that you can't recapture from the dried varieties. With fresh herbs, you needn't worry much about choosing the wrong ones. Some of my favorites for salads include lovage (which I also use to season many salad dressings), basil, dill, the mints, winter savory, fennel, chives, and the parsleys. In the summer, I cull them from the garden. Some I dry by hanging from beams in the kitchen for a few days, and then store them in airtight jars for winter use. Others—the more succulent herbs such as parsley, basil, and chives—can be deep frozen in sprigs, then simply chopped and used when needed. If you live in an apartment or don't have a garden, you can grow herbs in pots in the kitchen window where they lend their own beauty to the room, as well as offering a constant supply of culinary delights. Thyme, marjoram, and winter savory will grow beautifully in pots indoors over the winter. So will parsley. Once you begin to play about with herb magic, you will probably find, as I have, that you never want to be without these lovely plants. Here are some of the most common herbs and what I find them useful for.

Herb Magic

Basil—I probably use this herb far too much because it is available only in the summer months and because it is simply so lovely. It has a distinctive flavor that is an ideal garnish for tomatoes, or in large amounts mixed in a green salad. Use the leaves whole for the best possible flavor.

Chervil—This herb is a cousin to parsley, with a delicate aniseed flavor. We use it lavishly in salads. It mixes particularly well with chives, tarragon, and parsley.

Chives—More beautiful in looks than in flavor, I think, chives are great for sprinkling onto sunflower wafers or in seed cheeses. I don't find them strong enough for most salads, preferring spring onions or a some chopped shallots instead.

Dill—It goes wonderfully with dressings, cucumbers, and beetroot and apple salads, and has a gentle delicate flavor that reminds me of quiet afternoons under sun-shaded willows.

Fennel—A lacy aniseed-flavored herb that grows quite large in the summer. It goes well with salads and with cucumbers, tomatoes, and in vegetable loaves. It is also a lovely decorative herb to place around the edge of a dish of salads.

Lovage—Perhaps the most underrated of the common herbs, lovage is wonderful mixed with the mints and yogurt as the base of an herbal salad dressing, which is as beautiful in color as it is in flavor. We use lots of it in our dish salads.

Marjoram—This herb comes in many varieties—sweet marjoram, pot marjoram, winter marjoram, and golden marjoram. Each is a little different. The sweet variety is lovely with plain green salads and goes well with tomatoes and Mediterranean vegetables. Oregano is a wild marjoram akin to our winter variety.

The mints—There are even more varieties than the marjorams—spearmint, peppermint, apple mint, pineapple mint, ginger mint, and eau de cologne mint. I use spearmint and apple mint in green salads and many dressings. Pineapple mint, with its splendid variegated leaves, makes a wonderful garnish for fruit salads, drinks, and also salad platters. Ginger mint is great in summer drinks, sorbets, and punches.

Parsley—This common herb comes in two main varieties—fine and broadleaf. For most raw dishes, we prefer the broadleaf parsley because it is more delicate and pleasant to munch. Both have a rich "green" flavor that works well with other herbs. It is great chopped in patties and loaves, in green salads and for dressings, as well as being a lovely garnish for almost any dish.

Sage—This herb has a strong individual flavor and a particular affinity for onions. It is good in savory nut dishes and adds flavor to seed and nut ferments.

Thyme—It comes in many varieties, some of which are much richer in flavor than others, but all have a wonderful warming sweet flavor that enhances peppers, courgettes, and nut dishes, as well as giving a unique flavor to sprout salads.

SEVEN DAYS OF SUPERMEALS

For energy that lasts, eat breakfast like a king, eat lunch like a prince, and supper like a pauper. For example, breakfast would be a bowl of miso broth with green foods or a grain dish—that is, porridge, raw muesli, or sugar-free granola. In addition, you might eat one or two pieces of fruit, wholegrain bread (best wheat-free), or toast with a fruit or nut spread. Lunch would become your main meal, consisting of a main course plus some vegetables—crudités, salads, or sprouted seeds and grains, plus a yellow and green vegetable if not already incorporated. You might want to add wholegrain bread (best wheat-free) with a fruit spread. Supper now becomes a light meal consisting of a fruit dish or fresh fruit salad or perhaps a light soup.

Monday

Main meal—100 percent corn pasta with garlic olive oil and steamed vegetables. Charismatic carrot salad made with shredded fresh raw carrots and tangerine sections dressed with orange juice, curry powder, and chopped parsley.

Baked bananas made using organic brown rice syrup, a dash of rum, and a squeeze of lemon juice.

Light meal—A dish salad where whatever raw vegetables are available have been arranged in segments—grated carrots, red or yellow bell peppers, half an avocado, radish slices, a handful of Chinese bean sprouts, a few slices of cucumber, a grated raw beetroot or white radish, and some mustard and cress dressed with tofu vinaigrette. For this, you will need ¾ cup of tofu, 3 tablespoons of rice wine vinegar or cider vinegar, the juice of two lemons, a tablespoon of Dijon mustard, one clove of crushed garlic, salt, and fresh herbs put into a blender and processed. (This dressing will keep for a few days in the fridge.)

Tuesday

Main meal—Carrot soup with orange and fresh ginger made with: $1/2$ cup chopped green onions, one cup orange juice, one cup water, 2 cups diced carrots, 2 teaspoons chopped fresh ginger, 2 tablespoons low-salt vegetable bouillon (to taste), freshly ground pepper, and a teaspoon of coriander. Boil the carrots until tender, then add the orange juice and bouillon powder, reheat, and serve.

Can be served with slices of organic tofu that have been spread with miso and grilled along with raw mushrooms.

Serve with a selection of steamed vegetables all cooked in the same pot—that is, cauliflower, broccoli, spinach, green beans, onions.

Raw pineapple slices dusted with shredded coconut.

Light meal—A jacket potato stuffed with sprouted seeds or grains and tofu dip made with: one cup tofu, juice of one lemon, one teaspoon wholegrain Meaux mustard, one tablespoon low-salt vegetable bouillon powder, a few leaves of fresh basil or some chopped parsley. Combine well in a food processor. This will keep for several days in the fridge.

Wednesday

Main meal—Grilled fresh mackerel with garlic and lemon juice served with a selection of steamed vegetables. Or split-pea soup made with: one cup dried split peas (soaked overnight), one onion, 2 medium carrots, 2 sticks celery, $1^3/4$ pints spring water, one tablespoon low-salt vegetable bouillon powder, 2 tablespoons chopped fresh herbs. Put the peas, vegetables, and water into a pot, boil and simmer for $1^1/2$ hours until the peas are tender. Add the vegetable bouillon and fresh herbs five minutes before serving. If you want a smooth soup, put into a food processor and blend.

Salad of fresh young spinach leaves and sliced white mushrooms dressed with lemon and olive oil and sprinkled with toasted sunflower seeds.

Orange sorbet made from eight oranges with skin and seeds removed and pulped in a processor. Add a tiny amount of honey to sweeten and some nutmeg, ginger, or fresh mint. Pour the mixture into ice-cube trays or a plastic container, and freeze. Remove from the freezer and leave to thaw slightly for about ten minutes. Blend the mixture again immediately before serving.

Light meal—100 percent buckwheat soba noodles in a bowl of miso broth. To cook soba noodles, bring a big pot of water to a firm boil and add the noodles slowly so the water continues to boil. When it begins to foam, pour a cup of cold water into the pot. When it comes to a boil the second time, add another cup of water, repeating this process three times. Once the noodles are *al dente*, drain them and rinse immediately under cold water to prevent their sticking together. Make the miso broth and place the cold noodles into it immediately and serve. You can cook more soba than you will eat at one meal and store them in the fridge for later. Doing this makes soba and miso broth an almost instant meal.

Thursday

Main meal—Fresh vegetables, either with tofu or chicken, wok-fried in a little olive oil or soy oil. Serve on a bed of steamed organic brown rice made from one cup brown rice, 2–3 cups spring water, 2 teaspoons vegetable bouillon powder, 3 tablespoons fresh parsley, one teaspoon marjoram, and 2 cloves garlic. Wash the rice three times under running water, and put into a saucepan. Boil the water in a kettle, and pour over the rice. Add seasonings except for parsley. Bring to a boil and cook gently for 45 minutes or until all the liquid has been absorbed. Garnish with parsley and serve.

Apple ginger salad made from 6 green apples, 1/4 cup fresh orange juice, 1 teaspoon grated fresh ginger, 2 teaspoons clear honey, and 3 tablespoons toasted sesame seeds. Baked apples made from 4 large apples, 1/2 cup date butter or raisins that have been soaked in water for 2 hours, 1/4 cup chopped almonds or pecans, 2 tablespoons vanilla essence, 2 tablespoons rum, 2 tablespoons fresh lime or lemon juice. Wash and core the apples. Mix other ingredients together in a small bowl, and stuff the core of each apple. Place in a nonstick oven dish, and pour remaining mixture over the apples, adding a tablespoon or two of water if necessary. Bake for 45 minutes at 350 degrees F (180 degrees C).

Light meal—Corn soup made from 2 fresh corn on the cob, $1/2$ pint warm spring water, 2 spring onions, one teaspoon low-salt vegetable bouillon powder, $1/4$ red bell pepper, $1/4$ green pepper, one tablespoon watercress, one tablespoon tahini. Wash the corn and cut off the kernels. Mix together with the water, spring onions, and vegetable bouillon powder; season with tahini and blend until creamy in a blender or food processor. Add the chopped peppers and watercress. Toast made from rye bread and spread with soya cottage cheese made from 2 cups tofu, $3/4$ cup mayonnaise, one teaspoon low-salt vegetable bouillon powder, one teaspoon caraway seeds, one teaspoon mild curry powder, one clove garlic, handful fresh herbs and 2 tablespoons chopped chives. Mash the tofu well, add all the other ingredients, and blend. This will keep for several days in the fridge.

Friday

Main meal—Dahl stew made from $3/4$ to one cup red lentils or split peas, one large cauliflower broken into florets, 3 large carrots, pinch of turmeric, 3 cloves garlic, 2 tablespoons low-salt vegetable bouillon powder, one large onion, one red pepper, one yellow pepper, 2 teaspoons ground cumin, 2 teaspoons coriander, 2 teaspoons fresh ginger, 1 to 2 teaspoons mild curry powder, 1 large parsnip, 1 cup broccoli florets, 2 large tomatoes or 3 tablespoons tomato paste with $1/2$ cup water. Put the lentils or peas into a large pot and cover with 3 cups water and one tablespoon low-salt vegetable bouillon powder. Cook for 45 minutes until tender. Pureé in a food processor and set them aside. While the peas are cooking, braise the onion in a little water with the garlic, turmeric, ginger, and one tablespoon vegetable bouillon. When they have softened, add the vegetables, except the broccoli, and other seasonings, and simmer until cooked. Pour the pureéd legume mixture into the vegetables, add the broccoli, and serve immediately.

Sunshine salad made from a few leaves of crisp lettuce, one medium-sized fresh pineapple, 2 coarsely grated carrots, 2 finely chopped sticks celery, 2 handfuls soaked sultanas, $1/2$ teaspoon celery seeds. Dress with an oil-free French dressing made from $3/4$ cup tomato juice, $1/4$ cup lemon juice or cider vinegar, one teaspoon wholegrain mustard, a little low-salt vegetable bouillon powder, one clove garlic and black pepper.

Carob and banana ice cream made from 4 cups soya milk, 4 ripe bananas, 3 tablespoons granular lecithin (optional), one cup unheated carob powder, $1/2$ cup pear concentrate, and one teaspoon vanilla essence. Freeze the milk in a low, flat plastic container. When frozen, remove from the freezer and let it sit for about half an hour until it is just soft enough to slice into pieces. Put the bananas into the food processor, add about a cup of the frozen milk, the lecithin, carob powder, pear concentrate and vanilla, and blend until it is just mixed. Add the remainder of the soya milk. Should it become too liquid, return to the freezer for a few minutes, then stir before serving.

Light meal— Nut milk shake made from: $1/3$ cup almonds (blanched), $2/3$ cup soya milk, 5 pitted dates, a few drops vanilla essence, and one teaspoon honey. Blend the almonds and the soya milk really well until the mixture is smooth. Add the other ingredients, and process well. Serve immediately.

An orange or apple.

Saturday

Main meal—Scrambled tofu made from $1/2$ cup diced onions, $1/2$ cup diced carrots, $1/2$ cup chopped celery, 2 cloves garlic, one teaspoon olive or soya oil, 2 cups mashed tofu, one tablespoon soy sauce, 2 teaspoons low-salt vegetable bouillon powder, and one teaspoon mild curry powder.

Sprout salad made from one cup lentil sprouts, one cup fenugreek sprouts, one cup alfalfa sprouts, one cup shredded Chinese leaves, 3 sliced carrots, and 4 diced tomatoes. Dress the salad with $1/2$ cup tofu or 3 medium-ripe tomatoes, $1/2$ cup fresh garden herbs, one tablespoon sesame seeds, 2 tablespoons lemon juice, one teaspoon onion powder, and one teaspoon celery salt.

Fresh fruit salad with cashew cream made from $1/2$ cup cashews, $3/4$ cup soya milk, and a dash of cinnamon or nutmeg. Put all the ingredients in a food processor, and blend well.

Light meal—Sprouted lentil salad made from $1 1/2$ cups fresh lentil sprouts, one large red pepper, 4 oz. (100 g) broccoli florets, 4 oz. cauliflower florets, 6 oz. (150 g) button mushrooms garnished with $1/4$ cup of splintered raw almonds and dressed with $1/4$ cup tomato juice, 2 tablespoons cider vinegar, 1 teaspoon freshly grated root ginger, 2 tablespoons fresh orange juice, 2 teaspoons vegetable bouillon powder or soy sauce, and one teaspoon mild curry powder.

Sunday

Main meal—Spicy shishkebab made from one large aubergine, chunks of tofu, 10 fresh tomatoes, 24 large mushrooms, one red pepper, one green pepper, 2 large onions, one large swede or 2 small turnips. Marinade: 1¼ cups olive oil, juice of 3 lemons, 2 tablespoons red wine, 3 cloves garlic, one teaspoon coriander, 2 tablespoons parsley, ½ teaspoon nutmeg, one tablespoon fresh basil, and one teaspoon dried oregano. Place all the marinade ingredients together in a large bowl and mix thoroughly. Grill the aubergine until just soft, and put with the rest of the vegetables into the marinade. Allow to sit for 2–4 hours. Skewer the vegetables and baste with the marinade as they are grilled.

Serve with brown rice or kasha made from 2 cups buckwheat, spring water to cover, 2 teaspoons vegetable bouillon powder, and 2 tablespoons chopped fresh parsley or other herbs. Place buckwheat in a heavy-bottomed pan and roast it dry over a medium heat while stirring with a wooden spoon. As it begins to darken, pour hot water over the buckwheat and add the vegetable bouillon powder and one tablespoon of the herbs. Cover and simmer very slowly for about 15 to 20 minutes until all the liquid has been absorbed. Serve with remaining herbs as a garnish.

Sliced tomato and fresh basil or parsley salad dressing with lemon, garlic, and olive oil.

Raspberry ice cream made from 4 tablespoons agar flakes, 2½ cups soya milk, ¼ cup apple juice concentrate, and one pound (450 g) frozen raspberries. Place the agar flakes and soya milk in the top of a *bain-marie*, and boil gently, stirring constantly until the agar is dissolved. Take off the heat and pour in the apple juice concentrate, while still stirring. Add the raspberries, stir, and chill. Stir the mixture from time to time until it has thickened, then freeze until firm.

Light meal—Dairy-free muesli made from 2 tablespoons oat flakes or a combination of oat, rye, and wheat soaked overnight in a little spring water or fruit juice. A handful of raisins also soaked overnight, one grated apple or pear, juice of ½ lemon, 3 tablespoons soya milk or yogurt, one tablespoon apple concentrate or pear or strawberry juice, and ½ teaspoon powdered cinnamon or ginger. Mix together the soaked oat flakes and raisins, and combine with the grated apple or pear, lemon juice, and the soya milk or yogurt. Drizzle with fruit juice, and sprinkle with cinnamon or ginger. You can also sprinkle with fresh ground pecans, hazelnuts, or three seeds (sesame, pumpkin, and sunflower). Serve immediately.

THE PROFESSIONALS

Advanced Nutritional Supplements for
Energy, Protection, and Good Looks

here is no substitute for healthy eating. Throughout evolution, your body has relied upon natural foods to supply it with the vitamins, minerals, trace elements, essential fatty acids, and all the other elements of nutrition it needs to maintain health and life. All nutrients are synergistic—they work together in highly complex ways. The body is genetically set up to receive these elements bound together in plant complexes, and a pill full of vitamins and minerals can never take the place of that. That being said, unless you have lived an exemplary life, eaten foods you have grown yourself organically, and not been exposed to high levels of pollutants in the environment, you may benefit by taking certain carefully chosen nutritional supplements. There are also some quite remarkable natural substances—L-pyroglutamic acid, DMAE, N-acetyl-carnitine, and melatonin—which used as nutritional supplements can revolutionize the way the brain functions. Some of these cognitive enhancers can heighten intelligence and improve memory. Others enhance immune functions or neuroendocrine regulation. Still others improve the body's ability to relax or regulate body rhythms or help protect against premature aging. All are life enhancers capable in one way or another of improving the quality of life and the energy levels of healthy people who use them. They are the next generation of professional supplements, and as such, can be very useful to women in midlife and beyond.

The Powerfoods

The first rank of nutritional supplements—the very best of all—are the powerfoods: dried green barley, wheat grass, alfalfa, spirulina, or blue-green algae, chlorella, flaxseed, seaweeds, and apple cider vinegar. Spirulina or blue-green algae is a fine source of easily assimilated protein, chlorophyll, beta-carotene, and vitamin B_{12}, plus many other important trace elements. Green barley is also full of vitamins, minerals, enzymes, and chlorophyll, as is wheat grass. Flaxseeds are the best single source of essential fatty acids. The green foods can be added to fresh vegetables, fruit juices, miso broth, or salads. Seaweeds go well in soups, casseroles, stir-fries, salads, and miso broth. They are just about the best source of minerals and trace elements you can find anywhere. A tablespoon a day of apple cider vinegar in a glass of spring water cures dietary indiscretions. Spirulina and green barley are the two most important green powerfoods.

Spirulina—A rich source of an amazing variety of essential nutrients, spirulina contains significant quantities of the essential fatty acid, linoleic; plus GLA, B_{12}, iron, RNA, DNA, chlorophyll, and a blue pigment called phycocyanin found only in blue-green algae, which has been shown to increase the survival rate of animals with liver cancer. It is also a rich source of essential amino acids, being 60 to 70 percent protein. Easy to digest, spirulina helps protect immunity and aids mineral absorption. It also helps to stabilize blood sugar and curb appetite. Spirulina is available in tablet form but is easiest to take either in powder stirred into broth or juice or (my favorite form) as flakes that I sprinkle over salads and soups. A teaspoon or two a day of this powerfood brings excellent nutritional support, but be careful about the kind that you buy. Some spirulina is not good quality, and it must be pure—preferably organic (see Resources).

Green barley—This is a dried form of the natural juice taken from young barley leaves. It needs to be organically grown and pesticide-free. Rich in proteins, flavonoids, minerals including iron, vitamins such as K and B_{15}, as well as chlorophyll and other nutrients, green barley is also rich in thousands of enzymes, not all of which are destroyed in the digestive process and many of which can play important roles in supporting metabolic processes. It also contains a high concentration of superoxide dismutase (SOD)—an antioxidant enzyme. Sprinkle from $1/2$ to one teaspoon of green barley onto salads or mix into juices, miso broth, or water.

Antioxidants

Free radicals are toxic species of atoms or molecules that are highly reactive simply because they are electrochemically unbalanced. They are common and necessary to all biological systems and are formed naturally during a wide variety of biological processes from respiration to the carrying out of enzyme activities that are a normal part of energy production and cell metabolism. The body has important antioxidant enzymes—superoxide dismutase, catalase, and glutathione peroxidase—designed to deactivate free radicals before they can cause damage to the body. The problem is, when we are subjected to physical, chemical, and electromagnetic stress, then our bodies create more free radicals than our antioxidant enzymes can handle. When free radicals get out of hand, they can precipitate a relentless process of destruction and degeneration in the body as a whole. Recent findings in the field of free radical pathology—the study of free radicals "gone wrong"—are nothing short of revolutionary. They make it possible for the first time in scientific terms to formulate a *unified* theory of disease.

Thanks to free radical biochemistry, doctors well versed in the subject are beginning to make sense of a lot of what until now appeared to be contradictory clinical and epidemiological observations and to create a scientific rationale for both the treatment and prevention of a number of the major causes of degeneration and death: arteriosclerosis, cancer, arthritis, dementia, and other age-related diseases. We know now that free radical damage underlies the pathology of *all* of these conditions despite the difference in their manifestations in the body. Free radical damage is the very foundation of premature aging. To counteract it, certain antioxidant nutrients can be enormously effective: vitamins C and E, beta-carotene or the mixed carotinoids, zinc, selenium, the flavonoids, co-enzyme Q10, and the sulphur-based amino acids such as methionine, cysteine, n-acetyl cysteine, glucose-cysteine, and taurine.

Troublesome though it may seem, with the exception of the B complex vitamins, which are often best taken together, antioxidants and other specific nutrients are best taken singly—each on its own. This is much better than using multivitamin and mineral supplements. It is also important to take only fresh supplements. Vitamins, minerals, and other supplements that are not fresh are toxic to the body and can do harm. Always buy the best-quality supplements you can find. Most will stay fresh for 12 weeks after you have opened the container. Never remove vitamins from bottles more than one day before you are going to take them, and keep all supplements away from sunlight and warmth. It is a good idea to smell the bottle whenever you remove supplements. If it has a strong odor, the vitamins may have gone bad and should be thrown away.

Vitamin C—A water-soluble antioxidant, vitamin C plays an important role in the formation of collagen and the building of connective tissue in skin, tendons, and cartilage. It is also important in supporting the action of the adrenal glands in their manufacture of essential hormones such as cortisone, adrenalin, and the estrogens—particularly in the case of menopausal and postmenopausal women when the adrenals take over this task from the ovaries. Vitamin C is also important for the health of other glands in the body, as well as for the strength of teeth, gums, bones, and organs. Also, vitamin C looks after immunity, helping to protect from the common cold, physical and mental stress, and the toxic effects of drugs, pollutants, and chemicals in food and water. Vitamin C is found in fresh fruits and vegetables, especially rose hips, blackcurrants, acerola cherries, green peppers, turnip greens, and watercress. Tables of recommended daily doses of vitamin C will tell you that you need no more than 30 to 70 mg of the vitamin a day. However, most nutritionists recommend 1,000 to 2,000 mg (1 to 2 g a day), and most women find that at such levels they look and feel better and have more energy. A good form of vitamin C as a supplement is so-called buffered vitamin C—calcium ascorbate or magnesium ascorbate—together with the bioflavonoids (see Resources).

Vitamin E—This vitamin might be said to be the fat-soluble counterpart of vitamin C. It protects the unsaturated fatty acids, sex hormones, and fat-soluble vitamins from free radical destruction. This is why it is often added to oils. It is also used as a base for the sublingual drops of progesterone—to protect against rancidity and degradation. Vitamin E supports good circulation, guards the lungs from free radical damage as a result of pollution, counters blood clots, and helps retard aging. It is also used to prevent and counter menstrual and menopausal problems, blood sugar problems, heart conditions, arthritis, varicose veins, and benign breast lumps. Vitamin E is found in whole grains, dark green leafy vegetables, nuts, seeds, brown rice, and wheat germ. The recommended daily allowance of vitamin E is a mere 15 to 30 IU. Most nutritionists, however, use 100–200 IU for a healthy person and between 200 and 2,000 IU a day for therapeutic purposes. People with high blood pressure need to be careful when taking vitamin E since the dosage has to be increased gradually under the watchful eye of a practitioner trained in nutrition, or it can exacerbate the condition.

Beta-carotene and the mixed carotinoids—The carotinoids, of which beta-carotene is the best known and most widely studied, are precursors to vitamin A. They occur naturally in vegetables and can be turned into this vitamin in the body. This makes them a safe source of vitamin A since the body will metabolize only as much as it needs. Vitamin A is another important antioxidant that helps make the body resistant to infection by enhancing immunity. It is also needed to enhance the repair of epithelial tissue and to make strong bones. It helps prevent premature aging (most so-called aging is premature), fights free radical damage, improves the permeability of capillaries, and protects against infection and cancer. Either vitamin A or the carotinoids are found in fish liver oils, animal livers, and green and yellow fruits and vegetables—especially alfalfa, apricots, dandelion greens, garlic, parsley, watercress, yams, and carrots. The recommended daily allowance for vitamin A (or vitamin A activity present in beta-carotene or the mixed carotinoids) is 5,000 IU per day. It is important not to take too much vitamin A itself—doses over 25,000 IU a day taken over a long time can cause toxicity. The same is not true of the carotinoids. Many nutritionists recommend a supplement of beta-carotene or mixed carotinoids, giving an activity of 15,000 IU of vitamin A per day or even more.

Zinc—Necessary for protein synthesis and the health of skin and bones, zinc is a co-factor in many of the body's enzymic processes involved in hormonal activities. It is also essential for the formation of DNA and RNA, and is needed for the production and health of the sex organs. Like all the antioxidant nutrients, this mineral helps rid the body of toxic levels of pollutants, including carbon dioxide, accelerates the healing of wounds, and supports the metabolism of vitamin A. Zinc is found in legumes, oysters, poultry, seafood, egg yolks, liver, food yeast, pecans, mushrooms, soybeans, sunflower seeds, pumpkin seeds, onions, and herring. The recommended daily allowance of zinc is 15 mg. Most Western diets are low in zinc, and supplements of 30 to 45 mg a day are commonly used. The best form of zinc to take as a supplement is either zinc citrate or zinc picolinate, since they are most readily absorbed.

Selenium—Another important antioxidant, selenium is at the center of the enzyme glutathione peroxidase, which inactivates the excessive free radicals that destroy tissue. Selenium also helps protect the immune system and acts synergistically with vitamin E in the production of antibodies and to support a healthy heart. This trace element is also important for tissue elasticity and pancreatic deficiency, while a deficiency in selenium has been consistently linked with the development of cancer and heart disease. Selenium is found in meats and grains—depending upon its presence in the soils on which they have been raised—in Brazil nuts, food yeast, brown rice, chicken, garlic, liver, molasses, onions, deep sea fish, wheat germ and whole grains, mushrooms, and sea plants. The recommended daily allowance of selenium is estimated to be 50 to 200 mcg. Very high doses of the mineral—above 3,000 mcg a day—are known to be toxic and can result in hair loss, nail loss, and impairment of the nervous system.

D-glucose–L-cysteine—This compound, which is taken as a nutritional supplement for its antioxidant properties, is one of two substances known to human beings that acts as a precursor to intracellular glutathione peroxidase—the most important antioxidant enzyme in the body. When you take glyco-cysteine, it increases intracellular glutathionine peroxidase and has powerful antioxidant properties. *Like most amino acids, this should be taken on an empty stomach.* Nutritionists recommend 500–1,000 mg a day.

Gamma Linolenic Acid (GLA) This fatty acid, which is found in blackcurrant seed oil, borage oil, starflower oil, and evening primrose oil is another regulator of T-lymphocyte functions in the immune system. Borage and starflower oil can be extracted without chemicals or refining. In a healthy body, GLA can be made from the essential fatty acid, linoleic acid. However, if a woman is deficient in magnesium, vitamins A, C, B3, B6, or zinc, her body may be unable to make the conversion. Junk fats in the diet can also block this conversion. GLA has been shown to have a positive effect on the production of steroid hormones, including progesterone and the stress hormones, estrogen and testosterone. GLA is also important in helping to prevent heart disease, arteriosclerosis, PMS, and high blood pressure. In addition to being found in the natural plant oils, GLA is produced by biotechnology in a pure form. Nutritionists generally recommend between 500 and 1,500 mg of GLA a day when it is used as a supplement.

Co-enzyme Q10—A vitaminlike substance related to vitamin E, CoQ10 is a powerful antioxidant found in human tissue. Its concentration diminishes with age. In Japan it is used in the treatment of heart disease. It has also shown itself to be useful in the treatment of allergies, asthma, and respiratory complaints, as well as anomalies of brain function. CoQ10 is believed by many to be a major step forward in the prevention of cancer and premature aging. It is also used by athletes. CoQ10 is found in mackerel, salmon, and sardines. In supplement form it must be protected from light and heat, as it readily deteriorates.

Women-Power Nutrients

In addition to the antioxidants and powerfood supplements, there are three more nutrients that are particularly important to menstruating and menopausal women and which you might consider taking as supplements: the B complex, B6, and magnesium.

B complex—This group of water-soluble vitamins work together in the body and can profitably be taken together in the form of a B complex to help keep the nervous system and circulation functioning well, help build red blood cells, and look after the health of the skin. B complex vitamins are co-enzymes involved in energy production and can be useful to counter depression and anxiety. Buy only a top-quality, well-balanced B complex with 50 mg of B_1, B_2, B_3, B_6, pantothenic acid, choline, PABA and inositol, with 400 mcg of folic acid, 50 mcg of B_{12}, and 50 mcg of biotin (see Resources).

Vitamin B6—B6 works together with magnesium as a co-factor in a great many enzyme reactions in the body. It is involved in the production of antibodies, is essential for the synthesis and actions of DNA and RNA in the cells; and aids in assimilation, fat metabolism (including essential fatty acids), and protein metabolism. It also facilitates the body's manufacture of progesterone and reduces inflammatory reactions, as well as preventing nervous disorders. B6 is needed for the production of hydrochloric acid in the stomach and for the absorption of vitamin B_{12} from foods. Antidepressant drugs, estrogen, and oral contraceptives all increase the need for B6, and carpal tunnel syndrome, where the hands and fingers grow numb, is linked to a B6 deficiency. B6 is found in food yeast, wheat germ, soybeans, blackstrap molasses, leafy vegetables, egg yolks, walnuts, and carrots. Raw food contains much higher quantities of this vitamin, since cooking and food processing destroys it. The recommended daily allowance for B6 is a mere 2 mg.

However, virtually every doctor who is nutritionally aware, and all nutritionists, insist that for optimal health we need a great deal more than this. As John Lee says, "Since this vitamin is inexpensive and remarkably safe at effective levels (50 mg once or twice a day), it is wise to supplement it along with magnesium." An intake above 200 mg of B6 a day taken over long periods of time—that is, two years—may cause neurological problems.

Magnesium—This mineral is also an important catalyst in a huge number of enzyme reactions, particularly those involved in energy production and the metabolism of sugars. It helps the body make use of B vitamins and vitamin E, as well as essential fatty acids, calcium, and other minerals. Magnesium is needed for a healthy heart, to regulate acid-alkaline balance, and as a natural tranquilizer. It also helps prevent the buildup of cholesterol in the arteries. Adequate magnesium in the body increases calcium absorption and helps its role in mineralizing bones. Deficiencies of this mineral are common, since nonorganic farming, where fields are spread with lots of potassium, which is an antagonist to magnesium, food processing, and long-term storage of food all deplete our diet of this mineral.

Sugar and alcohol rob the body of magnesium, too. A deficiency of magnesium causes loss of calcium and potassium from the body and can lead to premature aging of the skin, depression, irritability, epileptic seizures, arteriosclerosis, muscle cramps, impaired metabolism, and confusion. Good food sources of magnesium include alfalfa, apples, kale, seafood, seaweeds, tofu, green leafy vegetables, whole grains, sunflower seeds, brown rice, unsulphured black molasses, and sesame seeds. The recommended daily allowance of magnesium is generally considered to be 350 mg. Up to 750 mg of magnesium is used daily for therapeutic purposes, split into three 250 mg doses. As part of his osteoporosis treatment and prevention program, John Lee uses 300 mg supplements of magnesium a day. The best form of magnesium is chelated magnesium, since it is well absorbed, and many other forms are not.

Hydrochloric acid (HCL)—Under normal conditions, the stomach secretes adequate amounts of HCL and pepsin for the digestion of food and to prepare it for further enzymic actions. For all of this to happen, the pH needs to be around two, which is optimum for pepsin activity. In many women, as they get older, levels of hydrochloric acid in the stomach decrease so that they do not digest foods as efficiently, and neither are they able to assimilate important minerals into their bloodstream. A supplement of HCL and pepsin taken with each meal can provide optimal conditions for pepsin activity, as well as acidifying important minerals such as calcium, iron, and zinc for bonding to other compounds for use by the body.

Next-Generation Helpers

This is where the whole business of nutritional supplements gets exciting, since most of these supplements are capable of taking healthy people to even greater levels of energy, well-being, and clarity of mind. These are substances that in one way or another affect brain functioning. The brain's biochemistry is more complex than that of any other organ in the body. It functions in highly elaborate ways to regulate an enormous range of control mechanisms mostly by transmitting (together with the nervous system as a whole) electrical impulses.

Only recently have the biochemical mechanisms that underlie the transmission of these electrical impulses begun to be explained by science. The many billions of functional units in the brain—the neurones—are rarely close enough to each other to be able to communicate directly. Instead, they communicate by chemical means through specialized structures called *synapses*, which lie at the end of an axon or nerve branch. The chemicals that carry the electrical impulses from synapse to synapse are known as *neurotransmitters*. Each neurotransmitter has its own characteristic. Some are excitatory in character. They rapidly trigger electrical discharge. Others are inhibitory. Science has so far isolated scores of neurotransmitters, but there could turn out to be hundreds as yet undiscovered. They are made in the body out of nutrients from the foods you eat, and there is very good evidence that many of the most important neurotransmitters are diet dependent—the levels of them in your brain are directly related to how many of the specific nutrients such as amino acids, vitamins, and minerals needed for their manufacture are supplied through the diet.

There is also much evidence that there is no reason for brainpower to decline with age. Neither should anyone expect that feelings of depression or apathy or even long-standing fatigue are "normal." But when the nuts and bolts of neurotransmitter manufacture are not present in adequate quantities in the body or when they are unable to pass through the blood-brain barrier, any of this can occur. Most of the next-generation supplements are able with remarkable speed and efficiency to restore high-level energy, clarity of mind, and brain function by supplying these nuts and bolts. That is why you will sometimes find them referred to as "smart drugs," although they have nothing to do with drugs. With all of the next-generation supplements, experts insist that it is important to start small and go slow, gradually increasing the amounts you are taking for maximum effects.

Everyone is different. If you take more than your body considers optimal, then the benefits from them begin to decrease. The trick is to find just the right amount for you. When it comes to the brain stimulants, if you take more than one, they can be taken together first thing in the morning on an empty stomach. I use them often, for when the brain functions well, you feel so much more alive and positive, not to mention all the body's other organs and systems that can be affected for the good. Melatonin needs to be taken in the evening.

L-Pyroglutamic Acid—One of the major mood-enhancing and stimulating neurotransmitters for the brain is glutamic acid. Unfortunately, glutamic acid taken as a nutritional supplement does not easily cross the blood-brain barrier, so it is not useful as a cognitive enhancer. L-pyroglutamic acid, however, is. It is one of the best supplements for elevating mood and energizing mental functions. Alcoholics have less than normal amounts of glutamic acid in the brain. L-pyroglutamic acid is frequently given to alcoholics to help them break the addiction. Doses vary between 1,000 mg and 3,000 mg a day.

DMAE (dimethylaminoethanol)—This is a precursor to choline, which in turn becomes acetylcholine—an important brain neurotransmitter. DMAE when taken on an empty stomach is able to cross the blood-brain barrier and deliver choline to brain neurons, stimulating concentration and enhancing memory and alertness. It can improve the ability to learn, raise physical energy, and improve intelligence. It also has a wonderful effect on mood, helping people without confidence to feel more confident and outgoing. Doses vary between 130 mg and 500 mg a day.

Acetyl-L-carnitine—This helps the transfer of lipids and fats and also acts as a precursor to acetylcholine, improving concentration, memory, and alertness. It is often taken with DMAE. Doses vary between 120 mg and 240 mg a day.

N-acetyl–L-tyrosine—This is a precursor to the important brain chemical noradrenaline—the stimulating neurotransmitter that is a mood elevator. Athletes have a naturally high level of noradrenaline, while chronically depressed people are known to have low levels. N-acetyl–L-tyrosine is useful in breaking addictions and is widely used for withdrawal from drugs. Doses vary between 300 and 900 mg a day.

Melatonin—Melatonin is the most interesting and the most broadly useful of all the next-generation supplements. It is a key element in the maintenance of the body's hormonal balance, in the regulation of immune integrity, and in the control of the body's daily metabolic functions or circadian rhythms. Melatonin is secreted by the tiny pinecone-shaped pineal—what the mystics call the "third eye"—which sits deep within the brain. The pineal is a kind of neuroendocrine transducer. It converts incoming nerve impulses received as bioelectrical messages about the outside environment into outgoing hormones. Even the way in which electromagnetic fields affect the body is mediated through the pineal gland and melatonin. During the daylight hours, the pineal, which is highly responsive to the amount of light to which you are exposed, releases very little melatonin. However, with the coming of darkness, levels rise two- to three-fold to help regulate the circadian rhythms or bodily processes that depend upon our internal "clocks." As melatonin rises, you begin to experience a hypnotic state that helps bring sleep on. Then in the morning when the daylight returns, melatonin production decreases again.

When you are subjected to a lot of bright sunlight during the day, melatonin secretion is stimulated in the hours of darkness that follow. When, however, enough full-spectrum sunlight is not available during the day, melatonin production declines in the evenings. In some people, this can produce Seasonal Affective Disorder (SAD) or chronic depression. This can be counteracted either by the use of artificial full-spectrum light boxes during the day or by taking melatonin supplements in the evening, or both. In recent years, melatonin supplements have been used to counter jet lag, clear away SAD, and even to treat cancer.

One of the most effective treatments for insomnia in women over the age of 40 is to take between 3 and 20 mg of melatonin as a nutritional supplement in the evening. When you suffer from jet lag after crossing several time zones, this is largely because melatonin secretions become temporarily out of sync with the rhythms of day and night in the new time zone. Much jet lag can be eliminated by taking from 3 to 15 mg of melatonin at around 9 P.M. each evening, local time. Start this three days before you leave home, and continue for up to 10 days at your new destination—depending on how many time zones you have crossed.

Researchers such as Dr. Steve Levine and his colleague John Fontenot, who have looked closely at melatonin, have discovered both that its production tends to decline with age and also that a melatonin deficiency may be a critical starting point for degeneration. Studies have shown that the pineal gland inhibits the growth of tumors through the release of melatonin. As a result, melatonin is one of the compounds used in the natural treatment of cancer by some practitioners. There is also a strong indication that supplements of this important hormone can exert anti-aging effects on the body, enhance the immune system, help to normalize menstrual cycles, lift depression, and (most important of all for women who awaken regularly in the night), counteract insomnia. In numerous studies, it has been shown that when people with insomnia take melatonin in the evening, both their total sleep time and their daytime alertness is improved within a couple of weeks.

Like all next-generation supplements, melatonin demands that you experiment for a while to find the right dose and the right time to take it. Some people find within an hour of taking it that they are ready to go to sleep. Others need to take it early on in the evening, just after dusk, and a few respond best to it being taken just before going to bed. There is also a wide range of optimal doses, depending upon individual biology. Most of the studies of melatonin used 20 mg of the substance a day. However, as a nutritional supplement, it is usually sold in 3 mg doses. Most people find that five of these 3 mg capsules (that is, 15 mg) at night work well, although some do better on very low doses of 3 to 9 mg. Nutritionists advise that you monitor its effects and also how you feel the next day. You should feel bright and good. If you feel sluggish, try reducing the dose and see what happens.

SECOND COMING

Metamorphosis of Body and Spirit
Through Exercise at Any Age

*W*hat a woman can accomplish through exercise is impressive, not only in terms of protecting her body from the ravages of female troubles and even from time itself, but also in preventing her from illness and in rejuvenating her body in medically measurable ways. But exactly what kind of exercise *is* the right kind? It is an important question to answer, because so much of what has become fashionable—fancy clothing and tossing weights around in a gym—is mostly the *wrong* kind. Walking or running along roads filled with air pollution and subjecting your body to the stress this brings can also do more harm than good.

Aware of the benefits of exercise, most people who exercise regularly do aerobic movement—swimming, cycling, running, or walking. There is much to be said for this kind of exercise. It improves the functioning of the heart, lowers cholesterol, and shifts brain chemistry so that you produce natural opiates that make you feel good. It also increases noradrenaline—a brain chemical that improves your self-image and confidence. Aerobic exercise can also enhance your body's ability to burn fat, not only while you are working out, but for many hours afterwards as well. This makes aerobic exercise an important part of any good exercise program. So get out and walk briskly as often as you can. But aerobic exercise doesn't go far enough. It does not offer the body enough weight resistance to maintain muscle mass.

One interesting study compared the Lean Body Mass (LBM)-to-fat ratio in three groups of women—non-exercisers, aerobic exercisers, and weight trainers. Researchers found significant differences. In sedentary women, 21.8 percent of their body weight was fat. Among the aerobic exercisers, 16.2 percent was fat, while among resistance trainers, only 14.7 percent of their body weight was fat. This, and the kind of research looked at in chapter 12, is revolutionizing fitness advice. Exercise physiologists have come to realize that although aerobic exercise has a place as *part* of an exercise program, it does not maintain bones and muscle the way resistance exercise does. The bottom line is that we need both, although resistance exercise is the more important of the two. As a member of the advisory board of the American College for Sports Medicine (which has in the past promoted aerobic exercise as the best form for overall health and fitness) said: "Done correctly, weight training is the most efficient, effective, and safest form of exercise there is, and it won't be long before people realize it."

Let's Get Started

What does a confirmed lounge lizard do once she decides she wants to explore how exercise can change her life? First, she gets approval from her doctor to make sure that there is no reason she should not start on a simple graded program. Then go easy. If you start small and work up, you will win. If you start big, you can not only wear out your body, but also lose your taste for movement. The whole effort will then have become counterproductive, since you will end up hating exercise and getting nowhere. For exercise to work, it has to become an ordinary part of your daily life. It needs to be done regularly at least three times a week. Begin with only 15 minutes when you get up in the morning or at any other time of the day that is convenient. The great news is that right from that very first session, your body will begin to rejuvenate itself.

Exercise routines progress well when you work out at the same time each day. Try to do this if you can. Your body will get used to the routine and love it. When it comes to resistance training, you don't need to own a lot of fancy equipment either. Nor do you need to join a gym. A couple of dumbbells will do. Later on, if you catch the exercise bug, you might like to have a barbell as well. Dumbbells and barbells are what are known as *free weights*, as opposed to the kind of gym equipment you find in a multitude of sizes and shapes and glitzy finishes these days. They are also far simpler, since you can tuck them under the bed out of sight when they are not in use, and you can make use of them anytime you want without having to dress in special clothes and go to the gym.

Choose the kind of dumbbells—each of which fits into one hand—that have six removable weights on each so that you can add and then take off weights as needed for each exercise. Your body and their weight against gravity offer all the resistance you need to work muscles deeply. The machines you find in gyms are designed to mimic the effects of free-weight exercises, but with a couple of minor exceptions, no matter how flashy they look, they are not as good as simple free weights because the range of movement that you go through in each exercise is restricted by the machine. Free weights should form the basis of any good weight-training routine, whether you are a complete beginner or a professional weight lifter.

There are three things you want to accomplish in your exercise program. First, you want to maintain and improve your heart and lung fitness. For this you will use weights plus some form of aerobic activity for warming up and cooling down. Second, you want to maintain and increase your muscle mass. Finally, you want to maintain and improve your flexibility, and for this you need some kind of slow stretching afterwards.

Warm Up

It is important at the beginning of any exercise session that you spend a few minutes doing an aerobic activity. (You must never pick up a weight when your muscles are cold.) This can be running on the spot, slow and steady jumping jacks, using a rowing machine (my favorite), or bouncing on a rebounder (mini trampoline). In the beginning, your total exercise session may last only 15 to 20 minutes, in which case you will want to devote five minutes at the beginning to the aerobic warmup. Later on it can be longer. I generally row on a Concept II rowing machine for about 10 minutes at a slow, steady pace to get my heart and lungs moving and to warm up before beginning my weights. As the length of your exercise session grows week by week, until it is ideally 45 minutes to an hour at a time, so will the time you spend on your aerobic activities at the beginning and end of the session and perhaps in the middle, too.

Stretch Out

After this initial period, which should last long enough so that you feel fully warmed up, you should then spend 5 to 10 minutes stretching. Stretch slowly and smoothly toward the ceiling, toward your toes, and to the side. Never jerk when stretching, and breathe deeply. Stretching before a workout but after a warmup is done to allow major muscle groups along with associated tendons and ligaments to be gently stretched, ensuring that possible injuries are greatly reduced. Now you are ready for your muscle work.

Weights Workout

To work with weights properly, you need to split your sessions into different body parts and work one or two body parts per session, leaving at least 48 hours between that session and the next time you work that body part. The muscle and bone strengthening that comes with resistance training does not take place *while* you are using the weights. In fact, working out stresses the muscles and bones, causing tiny breakdowns in the cells to occur. It is during the *rest* that comes after a workout that new muscle and bone is built in direct response to the piezoelectric stimulation at a molecular level. If you come to the point of using quite heavy weights and training five times a week, then it is important to work out each body part only once a week, for it can take about 48 hours for the breakdown process to take place and between 48 and 72 hours to build new strong tissue to replace it. Ignorant of these facts, many gung-ho body builders and weight trainers overtrain their muscles and end up undermining their immune system, while getting nowhere near the benefits in terms of strengthening LBM that they should. Exercising a particular muscle group every five to eight days is ideal for optimum progress.

Stand in any gym, and watch weight trainers do their stuff. It can be highly instructive in showing you how *not* to work with weights. Ninety percent of the men and women who use weights let their bodies swing all over the place, and when they are doing an exercise such as a dumbbell curl, they let the weight just fall back after each movement instead of being in control. When you do your movements, be sure to keep your body absolutely centered with each movement, only using the particular muscle group that is supposed to be working, and emphasize the *eccentric* contraction or return movement, where you are returning the weight to its original position. Resist the movement all the way back. It is the stress placed on your muscles of lengthening again when they are under resistance load that brings about most of the gains in strength and LBM you are after. Be sure while you are working out that you drink lots of water between each set and eat plenty of alkaline-forming foods (see chapter 22), since any kind of exercise tends to make your system more acid.

The Cool Down

It is important to spend a few minutes at the end of a weights session again doing some kind of aerobic activity to cool down. How long depends on the length of your session. You can go through the same kind of activity you have used in the beginning of your session or even take a brisk walk; but make sure you stay warm by adding an extra sweater, for your body will cool down fast and you don't want to become chilled.

The Stretch Out

Then do some more stretching for a couple of minutes. You will find that your body stretches more easily now since your muscles are full of blood and energized. Go slow and enjoy the feeling. It can be wonderful.

Beginner's Program

All of the exercises here are classic weight-training movements. They are simple and straightforward. They require nothing more than a couple of dumbbells (the kind that have six weights on each). Start with the lightest weights. You will be able to tell for yourself if something feels right. Never strain. As your body becomes accustomed to the lighter weight, you can add a bit more. The object of the exercise is not to use heavy weights, but simply to provide your body with enough weight to create resistance against which your muscles do their work. You will find pictures of the movements given below in any standard book on weight training, or you can ask a fitness instructor to show them to you.

Each exercise is done smoothly and with complete control, both on the contraction of the muscle group and on the relaxation. While one muscle group is working, the rest of the body remains still and centered. Start off by doing only three training sessions a week with one set per exercise. A set is the same exercise repeated a certain number of times: so 2 x 10 would mean ten repetitions of the movement, rest for two to three minutes, then ten more repetitions of the movement; 3 x 10 means the ten repetitions are done three times with two minutes' rest between each set. Increase reps by adding more exercises for each muscle group you are working with and doing one warm-up set of easy repetitions (10–15) followed by a heavier set using a little more weight (5–10 repetitions). Begin with very light weights—just enough for you to feel that your muscles are being worked as you near the end of your repetitions. Then by the time you are ready to add your second set, put on a little more weight until at the end of your repetitions your muscles feel tired.

Session One: Shoulders and Arms

Dumbbell press: 2 x 10
Side lateral raise: 2 x 10
Single arm tricep extension: 2 x 10
Tricep kickback: 2 x 10
Dumbbell curl: 2 x 10
Concentration curl: 2 x 10

Session Two: Chest and Back

Dumbbell bench press: 2 x 10
Dumbbell flies: 2 x 10
Single-arm rowing: 2 x 10
Dumbbell shrug: 2 x 10
Floor hyperextensions: 2 x 10

Session Three: Legs and Abdominal Muscles

Dumbbell squat: 2 x 10
Dumbbell lunge: 2 x 10
Calf raise: 2 x 10
Abdominal crunch: 2 x 10–15
Reverse crunch: 2 x 10–15

The Result

Each woman is, in reality, two women: an outer woman and an inner counterpart that is an individual self, utterly unique. Each woman has a stable center of strength and growth. Each inner woman sees the world in her own way, has her own brand of creativity, her own needs and desires, and is a law unto herself. The inner self holds the power to create, change, build, nurture, and transform. The outer woman is the vehicle for what the self creates. When her self is allowed free expression, then a woman is truly beautiful, for she is fully alive. Her body is strong, her skin is clear and healthy; and her movements, speech, and actions radiate a kind of vitality that is unmistakably charismatic because it is *real*, an outward expression of who she truly is. Many of the secrets to calling forth this kind of aliveness are to be found within the body itself—secrets that are best learned by working with muscle. Once you get the hang of it, working with weights is like meditation—one of the most mind-stilling activities in the world. Meanwhile, as your LBM begins to develop, you will find that your muscles and whole body have come alive. Then, as you work out, your muscles will begin to glow, until after a few months your body often begins to feel the way it did when you were a child—radiant with life and spirit.

MAGNUM FORCE

Putting the Power of Natural Progesterone into Practice

s far back as the 1940s, natural progesterone—chemically the exact same molecule produced by the corpus luteum in a woman's body—was known to offer protection against the dangers of excess estrogen, including miscarriage. It was also considered to be a natural contraceptive believed to offer protection against pregnancy without harmful side effects via a completely different mechanism than that which would later be developed as drug-based contraceptives. So important is progesterone to a woman's health that the body produces it not in micrograms or picograms, as in the case of the estrogens and other hormones, but in milligrams.

Since 1948 in Britain and 1981 in the United States, natural progesterone has been used in the treatment of PMS. In 1953, Dr. Katherina Dalton and Dr. Raymond Green in Britain published the first paper on PMS in medical literature, "The Premenstrual Syndrome." Dalton, who describes premenstrual syndrome as the most common of endocrine disorders, was the first to test the use of progesterone on women as a treatment for the condition. She was soon to become the leading investigator on PMS and the use of progesterone for its treatment in the world. Dalton's work is always quoted by later investigators who have further explored the use of natural progesterone, not only in the treatment of PMS, but also menopausal problems and other conditions.

Progesterone is a natural hormone—that is, chemically identical to the hormone naturally found in a woman's body—not a chemically altered patentable drug as are the progestogens or progestins. Progesterone is available under prescription in oral form, by injection, and as a suppository or implant. It is also available without prescription in most countries (Britain is presently excluded, although it can be ordered for personal use from abroad by any woman wanting to buy it) in the form of a cream to rub on the surface of the body or in a vitamin E oil. In both cases, the progesterone has been derived from diosgenin found in the wild yam—usually either *Dioscorea villosa* or *Dioscorea Mexicana*. Some doctors who frequently use progesterone prefer tablets or the injectable form (this is what Dalton still does). Increasingly, however, for ease and economy, the cream and oil are preferred. There are a number of creams and oils available. The best (see Resources) have been on the market for a long time and have been well tested by doctors and the women who have used them. A 2-oz. (50 g) jar of the cream—technically marketed as a cosmetic in many countries—contains between 900 and 1,000 milligrams of progesterone. Natural progesterone oil in d-alpha tocopherol (vitamin E) is more potent than the cream; a 1-oz. (25 g) bottle of the oil, technically a food supplement, contains between 2,500 and 3,000 milligrams of progesterone.

On the next few pages, you will find some of the most frequently asked questions about natural progesterone, as well as a few general protocols following the practices of doctors who frequently use it: Dr. John Lee in California; Barry Durrant-Peatfield and Shamim Daya in Britain; Joel T. Hargrove, director of the PMS and Menopause Clinics at Vanderbilt University in Nashville; Neils Lauersen, professor of Obstetrics and Gynecology at New York Medical College and author of *PMS: Premenstrual Syndrome and You*; and others, including investigative biochemist Dr. Ray Peat. Many have much experience in the use of the natural hormone: orally, by injection or by topical application; and in the treatment of PMS, osteoporosis, menopausal disturbances, infertility, and for skin care.

In many ways, progesterone cream and oil have advantages over other forms of the hormone. A typical patient on injected progesterone therapy may need ten or more injections a month, which can mean trips to the doctor's office, expense, and inconvenience. Some of the solvents in which progesterone by injection is dissolved can have toxic side effects. The oil—which is placed under the tongue and allowed to absorb through the mucosa of the mouth for five minutes rather than swallowed—is able to bypass breakdown by the liver. Like the cream, it can enter the bloodstream directly so that far less is needed than when given orally.

Apart from its reported actions in countering so many female ailments, natural progesterone is directly related to the biosynthesis of all of the adrenal corticosteroids and all the other sex hormones such as testosterone and the estrogens. It is a precursor for them. This means the body can transform progesterone into all these other hormones when needed (see the diagram in chapter 5). In contrast, the synthetic progestogens are end-product molecules incapable of being converted to other hormones by the body. When you lack progesterone, by following the arrows in the diagram you will see which biosynthetic pathways are eliminated and which hormones will have to be produced via an alternative pathway (such as DHEA) for your body to have them at all.

When natural progesterone is adequately supplied, the body is able to make all of whatever else it needs. On the other hand, when there is not enough progesterone present, this can be a major reason why people wake up with morning stiffness or suffer arthritis, injury to a joint, carpal tunnel syndrome, or tendinitis—conditions that never seem to get better since the body is simply not making all the cortisone that is needed to suppress inflammation and arrest the deleterious action in the joints. Doctors working with the progesterone cream report that such conditions frequently clear up when the cream is used for other purposes.

How Does Natural Progesterone Differ from the Synthetic Progestogens?

Natural progesterone, which was first crystallized in 1934, is now derived from plant sources and is an exact molecular match of the progesterone produced in a woman's body. It is not known to have any side effects except for altering the menstrual cycle temporarily in some women and bringing about a state of relaxation. By contrast, pharmaceutical manufacturers' product information on the various synthetic progestogens or progestins commonly used as oral contraceptives and in HRT carry a long list of small print cautions, contraindications, and adverse reactions. These include life-threatening pulmonary embolism, cerebral hemorrhage, cerebral thrombosis, and cancers, as well as dozens of minor complaints such as depression, migraine, fibroid enlargement, loss of hair, nausea, and vomiting. To quote Dr. Neils Lauersen:

> Progestogens are chemically formulated from progesterone, but rather than duplicating the properties of progesterone, these synthetic hormones react differently. When a woman is treated with synthetic progestogens, her body becomes confused and produces less natural

progesterone, causing salt buildup, fluid retention and hypoglycemia...synthetic progestogens generally make PMS symptoms
worse, so if a woman is about to be treated with progesterone, she should
be sure that it is *natural* progesterone.

The synthetic progestogens can also cause breast cancer and hirsutism,
while natural progesterone counters both.

What Are the Side Effects of Synthetics?

Here are a few side effects of one of the most commonly prescribed
synthetic progestogens—Provera—medroxyprogesterone acetate, as
reported in the 1995 edition of *Physicians' Desk Reference.*

Warnings—Increased risk of birth defects. Beagle dogs given the drug
have been reported to develop malignant nodules in the mammary glands;
must be discontinued if sudden or partial loss of vision occurs; may contribute to thrombophlebitis. Usage in pregnancy is not recommended.

Contraindications—Thrombophlebitis, thromboembolic disorders, cerebral apoplexy, liver dysfunction or disease, known or suspected malignan-
cy of breast or genital organs, undiagnosed vaginal bleeding, missed abortion, or known sensitivity.

Precautions—May cause fluid retention, epilepsy, migraine, asthma, cardiac
or renal dysfunction, breakthrough bleeding or menstrual irregularities, and
may cause or contribute to depression. The effect of prolonged use of this
drug on pituitary, ovarian, adrenal, hepatic, or uterine function is unknown.
May decrease glucose tolerance—diabetic patients must be carefully monitored—and may increase thrombotic disorders associated with estrogens.

Adverse reactions—May cause breast tenderness, sensitivity reactions
such as urticaria, pruritus, edema, or rash; may cause acne, alopecia, and
hirsutism, edema, weight changes, cervical erosions, and changes in cervical secretions, cholestatic jaundice, mental depression, nausea, insomnia or
somnolence, anaphylactiod reactions and anaphylaxis (severe allergic reactions), thrombophlebitis and pulmonary embolism, breakthrough bleeding,
spotting, menorrhea, or changes in menses.

When taken with estrogens, the following have been observed—Rise in blood pressure, headaches, dizziness, nervousness, fatigue, changes in libido, hirsutism, and loss of scalp hair, decrease in T-3 uptake values, premenstrual-like syndrome, changes in appetite, cystitis-like syndrome, erythema multiform, erythema, hemorrhagic eruption, and itching.

Besides Its Use in the Treatment of Female Complaints, Is Natural Progesterone Good for Other Things, Too?

Apart from its well-known reproductive functions, progesterone—unlike the progestogens, which are end-molecules—is a precursor to a whole family of other molecules (of steroid hormones) that are not easily made without it: the cortisone that your adrenal gland makes, for instance. In men, who make progesterone in their testes, it is also a precursor to testosterone. So progesterone is needed for the production of other hormones such as the estrogens, as well as cortisol, which is often called the "fight or flight" hormone since it comes into play when you are under stress. At such times, your body diverts progesterone away from being converted into the estrogens needed for female functions, changing it instead into cortisol. This can result in a deficiency in female hormones, including progesterone itself if the stress is prolonged enough, and produces symptoms such as hot flashes at or near menopause, and PMS earlier on. That is the down side. The up side is that when enough natural progesterone is available to the body, it can be turned into other steroids (including the estrogens), which help balance emotions, increase your ability to handle stress, and counter hot flashes and vaginal dryness.

It can also do so many other things for some women that when you attempt to list them, it makes progesterone look like a panacea, while in reality it is only part of a total approach to natural health care for women. As a result of its providing the raw materials for the production of other steroid hormones, progesterone has a remarkable ability to counter the dangers implicit in estrogen dominance in the body, through its interaction with other glands, organs, and systems of the body. Doctors and women using it claim that many symptoms, such as those listed below, respond to progesterone therapy.

- anxiety
- blurred vision
- cold hands and feet

- black circles under the eyes
- breast pain and problems
- constipation

- cyclic acne
- disturbances in appetite
- exhaustion
- infertility
- irritability
- lethargy
- migraines
- muscle and joint pains
- poor concentration
- sciatica
- spontaneous bruising
- thinning hair

- depression
- dry skin
- fibroids
- insomnia
- lack of sex drive
- low blood sugar
- mood swings
- panic attacks
- poor digestion
- spontaneous abortion
- stiffness
- water retention

How Do You Use a Cream?

That partly depends on what it is being used for (see below for specific protocols). All gonadal hormones, being small, fat-soluble molecules, are easily absorbed through the skin—in fact better than when given orally. Natural progesterone dissolved in a moisturizing emulsion is readily absorbed through the skin and taken into the bloodstream. It can be applied to the face, belly, breasts, back, thighs—almost anywhere on the body. Go for the largest possible areas of relatively thin skin. It is rapidly taken up, and after a few minutes leaves no trace on the skin surface. At the beginning in progesterone-deficient women, a lot of the progesterone is absorbed into body fat. After a while, as the receptors in the fatty tissues become saturated, successive doses of progesterone bring about an increase in blood levels and physiological effects. This is why it can take three months of use for some women to begin to experience the benefits of progesterone cream. Others, however, seem to experience results much more quickly.

Transdermal progesterone bypasses the liver (where breakdown of oral progesterone occurs) and travels to specific receptor sites where it is needed. Only small quantities of progesterone are needed to make big changes in the body and mind. Where doctors who prescribe oral progesterone or injectable progesterone are working with doses of from 200 mg to as much as 500 mg or even 800 mg a day, the dose you need to have the same effect absorbed from a cream is likely to be at least ten times less than that—more on the order of 20–25 mg a day.

When applying the cream—which you can do once or twice a day—it is a good idea to rotate its application around different areas of the body. When the cream is taken through the skin, it is absorbed into the fat cells, and if the receptors there become saturated, they can't absorb any more. So it is advisable to apply it to the abdomen one day, on the thighs the next, on the breasts the next, and so forth, returning to the original site every four or five days. Many women discover that the progesterone cream is just about the best thing you can use as a skin moisturizer. It has such a good effect on the face that they want to use it every day. It is probably not necessary to use it every day but only a couple of times a week. Also, there is always the danger that you could develop an allergic reaction to some ingredient any cream contains if you use it every day in the same place.

How Much of a Cream Should I Use?

Most doctors suggest you start with $1/4$ to $1/2$ teaspoon a day, then monitor how rapidly it is absorbed. Every woman's requirement for natural progesterone is unique to her. In a menstruating woman, natural progesterone is usually used for 14 days a month starting on about day 13 or 14 of her menstrual cycle (counting the first day of a period as day one), then stopping on day 27 or 28 and increasing the amounts used in the last week or so before a period begins. A woman who is anovulatory would use the cream in a cyclical way each month from day 12 to day 26 for three months. An ovulation can result from lack of synchronous timing between the hypothalamus, the pituitary, and the ovaries so the chemical messages are not arriving at the right time. If a woman cycles this way, using progesterone cream for three months and then withdrawing it sometimes allows the normal ovulation to return. (This is the way it is used in treating infertility.)

After using the cream for a few months, many women no longer need to use as much, and the amount can be decreased, all the while monitoring the effect on symptoms. If symptoms increase, you use more. When they decrease, you need less. As biochemist Ray Peat says:

> Since progesterone is not known to have any side effects except for alteration of the menstrual cycle and production of euphoria...the basic procedure should be to use it in sufficient quantity to make the symptoms disappear, and to time its use so that menstrual cycles are not disrupted. This

normally means using it only between ovulation and menstruation unless
symptoms are sufficiently serious that a missed period is not important.

In menopausal women, doctors usually recommend using the cream 21 days
a month and leaving it off for 7 before beginning again. Although there is no
reason why a woman cannot use it continuously, if you do, the progesterone
receptor sites may become accustomed to a continual supply of progesterone
so they lose some of their receptivity to it. This is no more than a variation
on the principle of natural medicine that says that the body thrives on change
and that it is best—even with herbal supplements or brain stimulants or vitamins and minerals—to have periodic short breaks away from using them.

John Lee recommends that, instead of trying to measure $1/4$ to $1/2$ teaspoon each time you open the jar, simply begin by using a 2-oz. (50 g) jar
each month—whether or not you are using the cream for 14 days a month
or 21 days—for the first three or four months of use. Once it has been established—either by a doctor taking blood levels of progesterone or by an
improvement in symptoms—that the problems being treated are responding, you can gradually decrease amounts down to half a jar a month. Some
women absorb progesterone more easily through the skin than others. And
because estrogen and progesterone have so very many mutually antagonistic effects, how much estrogen there is in a woman's body will also to some
extent determine the quantity of progesterone needed to balance it. In PMS,
the dose usually needs to be high initially in order to counter the effects of
previously unopposed estrogen. After menopause, when estrogen levels are
low and a woman is using the progesterone for protection against osteoporosis, the effective doses are usually far lower. Blood progesterone levels
can be taken by a doctor, but Lee insists—and the many women I have spoken to confirm this—that women themselves are the best judge of how
much they need. Thanks to the great safety of natural progesterone, considerable latitude is allowed.

What Is the Difference Between the Natural Progesterone Creams and the Sublingual Granules and Oil?

The sublingual granules and oil have at least three times the concentration of progesterone found in the creams. They are taken sublingually by
putting a few drops of the oil or several of the pellets in the mouth and holding them there under the tongue—usually for five to eight minutes—until

they have been absorbed by the mucosa in the mouth. I personally believe that the sublingual pellets or granules are preferable to the oil; they are easier and more pleasant to use, and you have a greater control over how you are taking them, particularly since the oil can be hard to squeeze from the bottle. The oil can also be applied intravaginally by putting a few drops of it on the finger and introducing the finger into the vagina. The creams are effective for long-term use and maintenance; the granules and the oil are more immediate in their actions. Sometimes—in the case of severe PMS or hot flashes—it can be helpful to use both cream and sublingual applications together. Some suppliers make two varieties of the oil, one of which has the addition of essential oil of peppermint in an attempt to improve the flavor (in my opinion it doesn't!). Use only the oil *without* the peppermint for vaginal application. Some companies produce a cream without alcohol, which can also be applied directly to the vagina and vulva.

Should Application of a Cream Be Cycled?

Yes. When the body is continually exposed to signals from a hormone such as progesterone or any other compound, there is always the chance that this can lead to reduced receptor sensitivity as receptors, in effect, turn down the volume. During regular monthly menstruation, there occurs a week or so each month during which hormone levels are low. Doctors recommend that progesterone be cycled monthly. In postmenopausal women, it can be used for two to three weeks a month and then discontinued for a week before beginning again so that at least five to seven days a month remain hormone free. In menstruating or perimenopausal women, the timing of progesterone use is made to coincide with the normal luteal phase of menstruation—from about day 12 or 13 of the cycle to day 26 or 27. Sometimes this can be difficult to do if a woman's periods are irregular. Occasionally, too, some spotting occurs mid-month when progesterone is started. Should this happen, John Lee recommends that the progesterone be halted for 12 days and then started anew.

How Long Do I Have to Use Natural Progesterone to See Results?

This varies enormously. In the case of hot flashes or PMS, some women notice relief immediately. In general, menopausal and menstrual difficulties will be relieved within three months. The action of the progesterone oil taken sublingually is much faster than the cream in its actions since it gets into the bloodstream right away. This is why it can be so helpful to use the oil every 15 minutes or so when a woman is experiencing hot flashes. The oil can also be useful in this way for migraine. In the case of osteoporosis, bone scans taken six months after beginning progesterone treatment and following a good nutritional regime generally show an increase of at least 5 percent in bone density—often much greater depending upon the state of the bones at the beginning of treatment.

How Will I Know When to Use Progesterone Cream More or Less Frequently?

You'll know by keeping an eye on the symptoms for which you have been using the cream and by seeing how quickly the cream is absorbed into the skin from day to day. If you find it is absorbed in less than a minute— which often happens five to seven days before a period—then increase the number of applications a day to two, three, or four times. Similarly, if symptoms are present, use more until they abate, increasing the quantity slightly until menstruation. As for how long to use the cream, this depends on your own body and on what you are using it for. Some women find that after three or four months, they can cut down on the cream and gradually stop it altogether. Others—particularly menopausal and postmenopausal women—choose to use it permanently in whatever dose they themselves find appropriate to protect against osteoporosis, care for skin, and improve the body's ability to handle stress. Each woman's biochemistry is unique. It is a question of listening to your own body and feelings.

Can Progesterone Be Used to Enhance Fertility?

Infertility now affects one in six women in the West. Many women who have difficulty conceiving or who have had several unexplained miscarriages in the first trimester of pregnancy are low progesterone producers— a condition known as *luteal phase deficiency*—where the corpus luteum in the second half of the menstrual cycle produces so little progesterone that the endometrium (the womb lining) is not properly prepared for secured implantation of a fertilized egg. Others, because of estrogen dominance, are not ovulating normally. It is worth trying progesterone for three months as a means of conceiving. John Lee recommends that such a woman use a progesterone cream starting with day 10 or 12 of her menstrual cycle—just before ovulation should take place—through day 28 of the cycle. Then she should stop using the cream and begin counting again from day one when her period begins. This is done for three months. Cycling in this way suppresses ovulation and ensures that hormonal cycles become regular.

In the fourth month, he tells the woman to stop using the cream, anticipating that the follicles and ovulation will proceed with the right timing and that the woman will now have a better chance of becoming pregnant. Lee has had this happen so successfully with so many women that he knows it works. They call him to say, "Hey, I'm pregnant. We're going to name it after you!" Lee believes that estrogen dominance and the inability to get pregnant probably have a common cause—that a woman may not be completing ovulation, and this may be putting her ovaries at risk. The progesterone that such a woman is given helps bring about full follicle development and ovulation, which makes becoming pregnant less difficult.

Is It Okay to Use a Progesterone Cream When I Am Pregnant?

There is generally no reason for a woman to take progesterone when she is pregnant since the production of progesterone rises dramatically during pregnancy anyway. However, unlike the synthetic progestogens, natural progesterone is completely safe in pregnancy. It is even used by doctors to help protect against threatened miscarriage. During pregnancy, the body's own production of progesterone rises from 15, 20, or 25 mg a day during luteal peak periods to 350–400 mg a day. Progesterone plays an important role in the development of the baby. Studies carried out in the 1940s show that the subsequent IQ of a child as it grows can be related to whether the mother was making sufficient progesterone. Human milk from healthy mothers contains significant quantities of progesterone. This appears to be important for the development of the child's nervous system. John Lee often recommends progesterone to women just after birth—especially to those with postnatal depression. Progesterone is at its highest level in a woman's body just before birth, then it falls close to zero. It appears that the rapid fall of progesterone that occurs with birth and the elimination of the placenta, which produces progesterone during pregnancy, tends to precipitate depression in some women.

Does Natural Progesterone Cream Help Vaginal Dryness?

Vaginitis and a tendency to recurrent urinary tract infections can occur in women of all ages, but especially after menopause when the production of estrogen and progesterone decreases. Natural progesterone cream used on the perineum and intravaginally is generally successful in treating both vaginal dryness and vulvar dystrophy, both of which tend to return to normal after three or four months of using the cream. In a very few women for whom progesterone itself does not completely solve the problem, a small quantity of estrogen cream applied topically (on the skin) is useful.

Is There a Relationship Between Progesterone and Good Thyroid Function?

Yes. Optimal levels of progesterone help thyroid hormones work. Many women who are told by their doctors that they have symptoms of hypothyroidism get to a point where their body is still making estrogen but not progesterone. Then they can have trouble with weight gain. They tend to be tired and to be easily affected by the cold. Often the doctor believes this to be hypothyroidism and will prescribe thyroid hormones. Doctors who regularly use progesterone with their patients have found that many of these women are simply not making enough progesterone. Adding progesterone improves thyroid function so that many women who would otherwise need thyroid hormones do not require them, while others on thyroid hormones generally need to reduce the dose once progesterone levels are improved. It is important to monitor the TSH (thyroid-stimulating hormone) levels of any woman on thyroid hormones who uses a progesterone cream, since the continued use of thyroid medication once the progesterone level in the body has improved cellular utilization of thyroid hormone could lead to a woman becoming hyper thyroid.

Are There Any Side Effects to Using Natural Progesterone?

To quote biochemist Ray Peat: "Progesterone is not known to have any side effects except for alteration of the menstrual cycle and production of euphoria...The basic procedure should be to use it in sufficient quantity to make symptoms disappear, and to time its use so that menstrual cycles are not disrupted."

Joel Hargrove, M.D., director of the PMS and Menopause Clinics at Vanderbilt University in Nashville, has been using 300, 400, 500—even 1,000 mg—of oral progesterone a day and has found no undesirable side effects. "I've been prescribing progesterone for 12 years, and I haven't seen any long-term effects....It doesn't affect cholesterol levels, it doesn't affect Mother Nature—basically it is a wonderful thing."

The levels of progesterone that enter the body through the cream are far lower (usually in the realm of 10 to 15 mg a day) than are produced by a woman's body. When progesterone is being used for PMS by menstruating women too much over a few months, it can occasionally delay a period a day or so. Stopping its use for a week and then resuming it at a lower dose clears this up. Sometimes women with irregular periods get some spotting at ovulation when they start progesterone use. Doctors say that the period is attempting to regulate to a 28-day cycle. In time, periods become regular, and spotting is alleviated. Women who are starting menopause sometimes see some spotting when they start using progesterone, which also clears. Very occasionally a postmenopausal woman using progesterone will get a small period for the first month or two, then this stops permanently. Should this happen, it is a sign that the progesterone is causing the body to eliminate excess stored estrogen, which can trigger a shedding of the endometrium, or breakthrough bleeding.

It can be a big help to work with a doctor who is familiar with natural progesterone use if you feel you need reassurance about anything (the vast majority are not at all well versed, unfortunately). If any kind of breakthrough bleeding continues past three months or so, it is important to consult a doctor. Unlike the synthetic hormones, no human cancer has ever been reported as a result of natural progesterone treatment. There are, however, reports in the scientific literature that natural progesterone has been used to protect from and even to treat uterine cancer. In using the cream, you are getting very small amounts of progesterone. As John Lee says:

> During pregnancy the placenta makes as much as 300 to 400 mg of progesterone a day. You will be lucky using the cream or the oil to even get to the level of the corpus luteum production in a menstruating woman, which is about 20 to 25 milligrams a day. This is why I maintain without exception that there is no way that progesterone supplementation can cause anyone any harm. If that were to happen, it would mean that a woman's own menstrual monthly production of progesterone would also be harmful. I don't believe that there is a supplement that has the safety record that progesterone does.

Is There a Test to Determine If a Woman is Anovulatory?

The only way to know for sure is to have a laboratory test done for low-serum progesterone—that is, low levels of progesterone in the blood—between day 18 and 26 of your menstrual cycle. A normal serum progesterone level after ovulation is in the range of 7–28 picograms. If a woman does not ovulate that month, then the level tends to be around 0.3 picograms. However, many experts in the use of natural progesterone, such as John Lee, claim that the only real test comes not from laboratory results but from how a woman feels.

Is There a Test to Determine Optimal Progesterone Levels in a Postmenopausal Woman?

Again, serum levels of progesterone can be taken. Generally, a progesterone level of about nine is optimal for most women. It is far more important, however, that a woman judge for herself how much she needs by being aware of her symptoms or lack of them.

Can Natural Progesterone Supplementation Help Protect Me from Heart Disease and Cancer?

The latest study on hormone therapy for older women—the results of which have been called "dramatic" by the president of the American Heart Association—shows that natural progesterone used with estrogen is better than estrogen and Provera in relation to protection from the risks of heart disease. The nationwide study of 875 women, including 147 at Stanford University, has produced a gold mine of information about what combinations work best. However, experts on the use of natural progesterone have commented that it is a shame that the study did not look at the use of *progesterone alone*. In the mid-1940s, an interesting study was begun by Johns Hopkins University in a clinic established for women with possible hormone problems. Among the many things measured were progesterone levels. Almost 30 years later, in 1978, researchers looked up the cancer incidence of women who'd had normal progesterone levels and compared it with women who'd had low levels. They discovered that the cancer rate was ten times higher in the women who had been low in progesterone.

Their findings were reported in the prestigious *American Journal of Epidemiology* in 1981, but, like so many important findings, they disappeared without a trace. The cancer-protective capacities of progesterone were not restricted to breast cancer or uterine cancer either—they applied to all cancer. Mounting levels of xenoestrogens in the environment, and the estrogen dominance that is much more widespread now than it was 30 years ago, make it important for women in the industrialized world to be aware of the protective actions they can take. At least now we have a chance.

How Does a Woman in Perimenopause Begin Using the Cream?

In the years just preceding menopause, when women are experiencing changing patterns of menstruation such as irregular flows or missed periods, using a progesterone cream can bring menstruation back to normal and keep it that way until the moment at which menopause arrives and periods cease altogether. When you first add progesterone in this case, sometimes *estrogen rebound* can take place. This is a temporary phenomenon where the sensitivity of the estrogen receptors is heightened by the presence of progesterone. A woman can get a temporary worsening of her symptoms, such as tender breasts or PMS symptoms. She may also get an irregular or unexpected period where the endometrial proliferation that has built up because of the estrogen in her body is now able to be shed, thanks to sufficient progesterone being present. This is normal and will soon clear away once the extra sensitivity of estrogen receptors settles down. The progesterone cream is used between day 12 or 13 and day 26 or 27 of the menstrual cycle, beginning with half a jar a month during this period. However, be careful to adjust the dose according to the relief from symptoms that you get. Some women need to use a whole jar of the cream each month during this period. Stopping the use of the cream at day 26 or 27 usually brings on a normal period within the next 48 hours.

If Someone Is on HRT Already and Wants to Stop, How Does She Go About It?

HRT means that some sort of estrogen is being given to a woman, generally with a progestogen of some kind. Since estrogens contribute to estrogen dominance, with all that implies, and the progestogens are known to have many negative side effects and natural progesterone none, if a woman is taking both synthetic estrogen and a progestogen, the first step is generally to substitute natural progesterone for the progestogen, then gradually decrease the synthetic estrogen, allowing the progesterone to take effect while monitoring symptoms.

When a woman on HRT wishes to get off it, there are a few things that need to be kept in mind. The first is that the progestogens and progesterone compete for receptor sites in the body so that the full benefits of progesterone will be reduced until the progestogens have been cleared from the body. Second, blood levels of progesterone will not rise to optimal levels until two or three months after you begin to use the cream. Third, the use of a progesterone cream may temporarily sensitize estrogen receptors, leading to an experience of high-estrogen effects—fluid retention, tenderness, and swelling in the breasts, or even the appearance of scant vaginal bleeding. These are only temporary and will soon clear.

John Lee tells his patients that when they start progesterone, he wants them to use a 2-oz. (50 g) jar a month for two or three months, stopping for seven days a month, then beginning again the next month. He reduces the estrogen they are taking by 50 percent the moment they start on the progesterone and also the progestogen they have been taking by 50 percent. Then the next month they can reduce each of those again by 50 percent, and the same the next month, then they stop. It is important to allow time for the progesterone to reach physiological equilibrium as the synthetic hormones are reduced, because if they are stopped abruptly, women will tend to be flooded with hot flashes and think, *Oh, I can't stop.* By the end of the third month, the HRT can safely be discontinued completely. If natural progesterone does not completely clear up any symptoms within three or four months, then Lee considers adding a small amount of estrogen. However, with most women, natural progesterone is enough to handle everything.

How Does a Woman Who Has Had a Hysterectomy Use the Cream?

She can go by the calendar month, using the cream for 21 days and leaving off for the last week. In three months, the hypothalamus will have linked into the monthly cycles since the business of the ovaries following the cycle, intricate though it is, is remarkably *plastic*. This should enable her body to handle any hot flashes and bring protection against osteoporosis.

Why Not Use a Progesterone Cream Continually After Menopause?

Progesterone is best used in a cyclic fashion over the course of a month, and postmenopausal women should leave a minimum of four or five days when they are not using the cream. The reason for this is that hormones work by combining with a receptor that is already in the cell, which then migrates to the nucleus and to a DNA gene to create the response. It is like a key in a lock activating some response. If you occupy or stimulate a receptor continually, it will eventually tune down the response. It is as if you were working on a noisy street—at first the noise bothers you until you get used to it and you shut it out. Then if you go on vacation and come back again, the noise will be noticed again. Similarly, if you go out in bright sunlight, then come into a darkened room, it takes a few minutes for your eyes to see, since the bright sun has tuned down your receptor response for light. Then if you go back out into the bright sun, it will be so bright you cannot stand it. Using progesterone cream and then stopping it for a few days helps keep the receptor sites sensitive to it. If you used it continually, you would end up with reduced benefit from it.

Do You Get a Buildup of Progesterone, Or Do You Have to Use a Progesterone Cream Forever?

How long you use a progesterone cream depends upon your response to it. Using it for three or four months, you can monitor the improvement in the condition for which you have taken it. Often, menstruating women can then greatly reduce the amount they are using, always monitoring symptoms to see that they do not return. Similar advice applies to postmenopausal women. However, because of the protection natural progesterone offers a woman from osteoporosis, hirsutism, and so many other things, you might like to use a progesterone cream on an ongoing basis. It is likely that once any symptoms have been cleared up, you will need very little of the cream to maintain the benefits. When John Lee's patients ask him, "How long should I go on using this?" he says, "Do it until you are 96, and then we will reconsider." For, sadly, in the world we live in, the causes for women's estrogen dominance and progesterone deficiency are not likely to go away.

APPENDIX

Highly Recommended Books on the Science of Menopause

Brown, Ellen and Lynne Walker, *Breezing Through the Change,* Frog Ltd., Berkeley, CA, 1994.

Coney, Sandra, *The Menopause Industry,* Penguin Books, London, 1991.

Dalton, Dr. K., "The Premenstrual Syndrome," *British Medical Journal,* 1, 1007, 1953.

Dumble, Lynette, and Renate Klein, "Hormone Replacement Therapy: Hazards, Risks and Tricks," Proceedings of *Menopause: The Alternative Way: Facts and Fallacies of the Menopause Industry,* Australian Women's Research Center, Deakin University, Australia, 1993.

Lee, John R., M.D., *Natural Progesterone,* BLL Publishing, Sebastopol, California, 1993.

———, *Optimal Health Guidelines,* BLL Publishing, California, 1994.

Northrup, Christiane, M.D., *Women's Bodies, Women's Wisdom,* Bantam Books, New York, 1994.

Pearl, W., *Keys to the Inner Universe. The Encyclopedia on Weight Training,* Bill Pearl Enterprises, Phoenix, Oregon, 1982.

Reitz, Rosetta, *Menopause, a Positive Approach,* Unwin Paperbacks, London, 1985.

Vines, Gail, *Raging Hormones,* Virago, London, 1993.

Weed, Susun S., *Menopausal Years, The Wise Woman Way,* Ash Tree Publishing, New York, 1992.

Highly Recommended Books on the Mythology of Menopause

Achterberg, Jeanne, *Woman as Healer,* Shambhala, Massachusetts, 1990.

Baring, Anne, and Jules Cashford, *The Myth of the Goddess,* Viking Arkana, London, 1991.

Becker, Ernest, *The Denial of Death,* The Free Press, New York, 1973.

Campbell, Joseph, *The Hero With a Thousand Faces,* Bollingen Foundation, New York, 1972.

———, *Transformations of Myth Through Time,* Harper and Row, New York, 1990.

———, *Primitive Mythology, The Masks of God,* Arkana, Penguin, New York, 1991.

Downing, Christine, *Psyche's Sister,* Continuum Publishing Company, New York, 1988.

———, *Women's Mysteries,* The Crossroad Publishing Company, New York, 1992.

———, *The Goddess,* The Crossroad Publishing Company, New York, 1992.

Ereira, Alan, *The Heart of the World,* Jonathan Cape, London, 1990.

Foley, Helene P., *The Homeric Hymn to Demeter,* Princeton University Press, New Jersey, 1994.

Franz, Marie-Louise von, *Patterns of Creativity Mirrored in Creation Myths,* Spring Publications, Zurich, Switzerland, 1972.

———, *Shadow and Evil in Fairytales,* Spring Publications, New York, 1974.

George, Demetra, *Asteroid Goddesses,* ACS Publications Inc., CA, 1986.

———, *Mysteries of the Dark Moon,* HarperSanFrancisco, San Francisco, CA, 1992.

Gimbutas, Marija, *The Civilization of the Goddess,* HarperSanFrancisco, 1991.

Gleason, Judith, *Oya, In Praise of the Goddess,* Shambhala Publications Inc., Massachusetts, 1987.

Graves, Robert, *The White Goddess,* Faber and Faber, London, 1961.

Grof, Stanislav, and Christina Grof (eds), *Spiritual Emergency,* Jeremy Tarcher Inc., Los Angeles, CA, 1989.

Grof, Stanislav, and Christina Grof, *The Stormy Search for the Self,* Jeremy Tarcher Inc., Los Angeles, CA, 1990.

Hall, Nor, *The Moon and the Virgin,* The Women's Press, London, 1980.

Harding, Esther M., *A Woman's Mysteries Ancient and Modern,* Rider and Company, London, 1971.

Ingerman, Sandra, *Soul Retrieval,* HarperSanFrancisco, 1991.

———, *Welcome Home,* HarperSanFrancisco, 1993.

Lovelock, J.E., *Gaia,* Oxford University Press, Oxford, 1979.

Manheim, Ralph, *Grimm's Tales for Young and Old,* Victor Gollancz Ltd., London, 1977.

Mookerjee, Ajit, *Kali, The Feminine Force,* Thames and Hudson, London, 1988.

Morgan, Elaine, *The Descent of Woman,* Souvenir Press, London, 1972.

Murdock, Maureen, *The Heroine's Journey,* Shambhala Publications Inc., Massachusetts, 1990.

Owen, Lara, *Her Blood is Gold,* HarperSanFrancisco, 1993.

Pinkola Estés, Clarissa, *Women Who Run With the Wolves,* Rider, London, 1992.

Redgrave, Peter, *The Black Goddess and the Sixth Sense,* Bloomsbury, London, 1987.

Shuttle, Penelope, and Peter Redgrave, *The Wise Wound,* Victor Gollancz Ltd., London, 1978.

Walker, Barbara G., *The Crone, Woman of Age, Wisdom and Power,* HarperSanFrancisco, 1988.

Wolkstein, Diane, and Samuel Noah Kramer, *Inanna, Queen of Heaven and Earth,* Rider and Company, London, 1983.

———⊷———

Chapter One: Bloodless Revolution

Campbell, Joseph, *The Hero With a Thousand Faces,* Bollingen Foundation, New York, 1972.

———, *Transformations of Myth Through Time,* Harper and Row, New York, 1990.

———, *Primitive Mythology, The Masks of God,* Arkana, Penguin, New York, 1991.

Coney, Sandra, *The Menopause Industry,* Penguin Books, London, 1991.

Dumble, Lynette, and Renate Klein, "Hormone Replacement Therapy: Hazards, Risks and Tricks," Proceedings of *Menopause: The Alternative Way: Facts and Fallacies of the Menopause Industry,* Australian Women's Research Center, Deakin University, Australia, 1993.

Durrant-Peatfield, Barry, "The Premenstrual Syndrome," Monograph. Received December 1994.

George, Demetra, *Asteroid Goddesses,* ACS Publications Inc., CA, 1986.

———, *Mysteries of the Dark Moon,* HarperSanFrancisco, 1992.

Ingerman, Sandra, *Soul Retrieval*, HarperSanFrancisco, 1991.

———, *Welcome Home,* HarperSanFrancisco, 1993.

Khaw, K.T., "The Menopause and Hormone Replacement Therapy," *Postgraduate Medical Journal,* 68, 615-623, 1992.

——— (ed.), *Hormone Replacement Therapy,* Churchill Livingstein, London, 1992.

Lee, J. R., M.D., "Understanding Osteoporosis." Summary.

———, "Osteoporosis reversal; the role of progesterone," *International Clinical Nutritional Review,* Sydney, Australia, June 1990.

———, "Osteoporosis reversal with transdermal progesterone," *The Lancet,* 336, Letter, November 1990.

———, "Is natural progesterone the missing link in osteoporosis prevention and treatment?" *Medical Hypotheses,* 35, 314, 318, 1991.

———, "Hormonal and nutritional aspects of osteoporosis," *Health and Nutrition,* Vol. 6, Issue 4, Winter 1991.

———, *Natural Progesterone,* BLL Publishing, California, 1993.

———, "The Theory of Estrogen Dominance," Seminar given at St. Thomas's Hospital, London, June 4, 1994.

———, "Clinical Uses of Natural Progesterone," Seminar given at St. Thomas's Hospital, London, June 4, 1994.

———, "Dr. John Lee speaking at the Chelsea Hotel, London, June 5, 1994," Video.

———, "Effects of Progesterone on Osteoporosis and Menopausal Symptoms," Seminar given at St. Thomas's Hospital, London, June 4, 1994.

———, "Successful Menopausal Osteoporosis Treatment Restoring Osteoclast/Osteoblast Equilibrium," *The Townsend Letter for Doctors,* 900, August/September 1994.

Peat, R., "Progesterone: Safe Antidote for PMS," *McCall's,* 152-156, October 1990.

———, "The Progesterone Deception," *Ray Peat's Newsletter,* 44, May 4, 1986.

———, "Blocking Tissue Destruction," Unpublished Paper.

———, "Progesterone in Orthomolecular Medicine," Blake College Booklet, Eugene, Oregon. Available from Foundation for Hormonal and Nutrition Research, 8150 SW, Barnes Road, Portland, OR 97225.

———, "Progesterone Can Be Taken Orally," Letter to the Editor, *Townsend Letter for Doctors,* November 1994.

———, *Nutrition for Women,* Kenogen, Eugene, Oregon, 1981.

Pinkola Estés, Clarissa, *Women Who Run With the Wolves,* Rider, London, 1992.

Prior, J. C., "Progesterone as a bone-trophic hormone," *Endocrine Review:* 11:386-398, 1990.

———, "Spinal bone loss and ovulatory disturbances," *New England Journal of Medicine,* 323, 18, 1990.

Prior, J. C., Y. Vigna, and R.N. Alojado, "Progesterone and the prevention of osteoporosis," *Canadian Journal of Obstetric/Gynecology & Women's Health Care,* 3, 4, 1991.

———, "Progesterone and its relevance for osteoporosis," *Bulletin for Physicians,* vol. 2, no. 2, March 1993.

Prior, J. C., Y. Vigna, and R. Burgess, "Medroxyprogesterone increases trabecular bone density in women with menstrual disorders," University of British Columbia, Vancouver. Paper presented at annual meeting of the Endocrine Society, Indianapolis, IN, June 11, 1987.

Prior, J. C., Y. M. Vigna, and D. W. McKay, "Reproduction for the athletic woman: new understandings of physiology and management," *Sports Medicine,* 14, 190-199, 1992.

Shaffer, Willa, *Wild Yam, Birth Control Without Fear,* Woodland Health Books, Utah, 1986.

———, *Midwifery and Herbs,* Woodland Books, Utah, 1986.

Weed, Susun S., *Menopausal Years, The Wise Woman Way,* Ash Tree Publishing, New York, 1992.

Chapter Two: Cry Freedom

Aitken, M., D.M. Hart, and R. Lindsay, "Estrogen replacement therapy for prevention of osteoporosis after oophorectomy," *British Medical Journal,* 3, 515-518, 1973.

Barrett-Connor, E., "Postmenopausal estrogen replacement and breast cancer," *New England Journal of Medicine,* 5, 321, 1989.

Barzel, U.S., "Estrogens in the prevention and treatment of postmenopausal osteoporosis: a review," *American Journal of Medicine,* 85: 847-850, 1988.

Begley, S., and D. Glick, "The Estrogen Complex," *Newsweek,* March 21, 1994.

Berkgvist, L., H. O. Adami, I. Persson, R. Hoover, and C. Schairer, "The risk of breast cancer after estrogen and estrogen-progestin replacement," *New England Journal of Medicine,* 5, 321, 1989.

Biller, B.M., J.F. Coughlin, V. Saxe, et al., "Osteopenia in women with hypothalmic amenorrhea: a prospective study," *Obstetrics and Gynecology,* 78, 996-1001, 1991.

Bonnar, J., et al., "Coagulation system changes in postmenopausal women receiving estrogen preparations," *Post Graduate Medical Journal,* 52, 30, 1976.

Boston Collaborative Drug Surveillance Program, "Surgically confirmed gallbladder disease, venous thromboembolism, and breast tumors in relation to menopausal estrogen therapy," *New England Journal of Medicine,* 15, 290, 1974.

Bullen, B.A., G.S. Skriniar, I.Z. Beitins, et al., "Introduction of menstrual disorders by strenuous exercise in untrained women," *New England Journal of Medicine,* 312, 1349-1353, 1985.

Coney, Sandra, *The Menopause Industry,* Penguin Books, London, 1991.

Durrant-Peatfield, Barry, "The Premenstrual Syndrome," Monograph. Received December 1994.

Felson, D.T., Y. Zhang, M.T. Hannan, D.P. Kiel, P .W.F. Wilson, and J. J. Anderson, "The effect of postmenopausal estrogen therapy on bone density in elderly women," *New England Journal of Medicine,* 329:1141-1146, 1993.

Gambrel, R.D., "The menopause: benefits and risks of estrogen-progestogen replacement therapy," *Fertility Sterility,* 37, 457-474, 1982.

Grant, Dr. Ellen, *Sexual Chemistry, Understanding Our Hormones, The Pill and HRT,* Cedar Original, Mandarin Paperbacks, London, 1994.

Guyton, Arthur C., *Textbook of Medical Physiology,* Sixth Edition, W.B. Saunders Company, Philadelphia, 1981.

Hargrove, Joel T., et al., "Menopausal hormone replacement therapy with continuous daily oral micronized estradiol and progesterone," *Obstetrics and Gynecology,* 73, 606-612, 1989.

———, "Progesterone: Safe Antidote for PMS," *McCall's,* October 1990.

Henderson, B.E., R.K. Ross, M.C. Pike, and J.T. Casagrande, "Endogenous hormones as a major factor in human cancer," *Cancer Research,* 42, 3232-3239, 1982.

Hileman, Bette, "Environmental estrogens linked to reproductive abnormalities, cancer," *C&EN Washington.*

Hoover, R., L.A. Gray Sr., P. Cole, B. MacMahon, "Menopausal estrogens and breast cancer," *New England Journal of Medicine,* 295, 401-405, 1976.

Inman, W. H. W., et al., "Thromboembolic disease and the steroidal content of oral contraceptives. A report to the committee on Safety of Drugs," *British Medical Journal,* 203, 1970.

Kamen, Betty, *Startling New Facts About Osteoporosis,* Nutrition Encounter Inc., California, 1989.

———, *Hormone Replacement Therapy, Yes or No?* Nutrition Encounter Inc, California, 1993.

Lee, J. R., M.D., "Understanding Osteoporosis." Summary.

———, "The Theory of Estrogen Dominance," Seminar given at St Thomas's Hospital, London, June 4, 1994.

———, "Osteoporosis reversal with transdermal progesterone," *The Lancet,* Letter, 336, November 1990.

———, "Is natural progesterone the missing link in osteoporosis prevention and treatment? *Medical Hypotheses,* 35, 314, 318, 1991.

———, "Hormonal and nutritional aspects of osteoporosis," *Health and Nutrition,* Vol. 6, Issue 4, Winter 1991.

———, *Natural Progesterone,* BLL Publishing, California, 1993.

———, *Optimal Health Guidelines,* Second Edition, BLL Publishing, California, 1993.

———, Endocrinology Notes: Progesterone and Estrogen. February 6, 1993.

———, "The Theory of Estrogen Dominance," Seminar given at St. Thomas's Hospital, London, June 4, 1994.

———, "Clinical Uses of Natural Progesterone," Seminar given at St. Thomas's Hospital, London, June 4, 1994.

———, "Dr. John Lee speaking at the Chelsea Hotel, London, June 5th 1994," Video.

———, "Effects of Progesterone on Osteoporosis and Menopausal Symptoms," Seminar given at St. Thomas's Hospital, London, June 4, 1994.

———, "The Multiple Effects of Progesterone," Seminar given at St. Thomas's Hospital, London, June 4, 1994.

———, "The Theory of Estrogen Dominance," Seminar given at St. Thomas's Hospital, London, June 4, 1994.

Lees, B., et al., "Differences in proximal femur bone density over two centuries," *The Lancet,* 341:673-675, 1993.

McKinlay, John, Sonja McKinlay and Donald Brambilla, "Health status and utilization behavior associated with menopause," *American Journal of Epidemiology,* 125, 1, 110-121, 1987.

———, "The relative contributions of endocrine changes and social circumstances to depression in mid-aged women," *Journal of Health and Social Behavior,* 28, 4, 345-363.

McKinlay, Sonja, and John McKinlay, "Selected studies of the menopause: a methodological critique," *Journal of Biosocial Science,* 5, 533-555, 1973.

Metcalf, M.G., "Incidence of ovulatory cycles in women approaching the menopause," *Biosocial Science,* 11, 39-48, 1979.

Nabulsi, A.A., A.R. Folsom, A. White, et al., "Association of hormone replacement therapy with various cardiovascular risk factors in postmenopausal women," *New England Journal of Medicine,"* 328, 1069-1075, 1993.

Peat, R. Ph.D., "Estrogen in 1990," *Blake College Newsletter,* Eugene, Oregon, 1990.
———, "Progesterone in Orthomecular Medicine," Booklet.
Prior, J. C., Y. Vigna, and R. Burgess, "Medroxyprogesterone increases trabecular bone density in women with menstrual disorders," University of British Columbia, Vancouver. Paper presented at annual meeting of the Endrocine Society, Indianapolis, IN, June 11, 1987.
Prior, J. C., "Progesterone as a bone-trophic hormone," *Endocrine Review:* 11:386-398, 1990.
———, "Spinal bone loss and ovulatory disturbances," *New England Journal of Medicine,* 323, 18, 1990.
———, "Progesterone and its relevance for osteoporosis," *Bulletin for Physicians,* vol. 2, no. 2, March 1993.
Prior, J.C., Y. Vigna, and R.N. Alojado, "Progestone and the prevention of osteoporosis," *Canadian Journal of Obstetric/Gynecology & Women's Health Care,* 3, 4, 1991.
Prior, J.C ., Y.M. Vigna, and D.W. McKay, "Reproduction for the athletic woman: new understandings of physiology and management," *Sports Medicine,* 14, 190-199, 1992.
Shapiro, S., "Oral contraceptives—a time to take stock," *New England Journal of Medicine,* 315, 450, 1986.
Stadel, B.V., "Oral contraceptives and cardiovascular disease," *New England Journal of Medicine,* 305, 612, 1981.
Stevenson, J.C., P.C. Michael, F.G. Gangar, T.C. Hillard, B. Lees, and M.J. Whitehead, "Effects of transdermal versus oral hormone replacement therapy on bone density in spine and proximal femur in postmenopausal women," *The Lancet,* vol. 336, 2265-2269.
Stryer, Lubert, *Biochemistry,* W.H. Freeman and Company, San Francisco, CA, 1975.
Studd, John, and Rod Barber, "Mastering the Menopause," Leaflet presented with the compliments of Organon Laboratories Ltd., Cambridge, 1994.
Swenerton, K.D., P. Fugere, A.B. Miller, et al., "Menopausal progestins and breast cancer," *JSOCG,* 13, 7-9, 1991.
Tietz, Norbert W., Ph.D., *Textbook of Clinical Chemistry,* W.B. Saunders Company, Philadelphia, 1986.
Vollman, R.F., "The Menstrual Cycle," in *Major Problems in Obstetrics and Gynecology,* vol. 7, (ed.) E. A. Friedman, W.B. Saunders Company, Toronto, Canada, 1977.
Wise, P.W., "Influence of estrogen on aging of the central nervous system: its role in declining female reproductive function," *Menopause: Evaluation, Treatment and Health Concerns,* 53-70, 1989.

Chapter Three: Sleeping with the Enemy

The work of the following researchers is referred to in J. Raloff's "The Gender Benders": Michael Fry, Devra Lee-Davis, Louis J. Guillette, Neils Skakkebaek, Ana Soto, John P. Sumpter and Mary S. Wolff. Raloff's "Eco-Cancers" refers to the work of David E. Blask and Steven M. Hill, and Robert Liburdy. R. Weiss's "Estrogen in the environment" refers to the work of David Crews and Herman Aldercreutz.
Begley, S., and D. Glick, "The Estrogen Complex," *Newsweek,* March 21, 1994.
Berkgvist, L., H.O. Adami, I. Persson, R. Hoover, and C. Schairer, "The risk of breast cancer after estrogen and estrogen-progestin replacement," *New England Journal of Medicine,* 5, 321, 1989.
Colborn, T., vom Saal F. S., Soto A.M., "Developmental Effects of Endocrine-disrupting chemicals in wildlife and humans," in *Environmental Health Perspectives,* 101:378-384, 1993.
"Environmental Estrogens: Pathway to Extinction," xenoestrogen conference held May 13, 1995 in Santa Rosa, California. Speakers: Howard A. Bern, Ph.D., tumor and comparative endocrinologist at UC Berkeley in the Department of Integrative Biology and Cancer Research Laboratory; Theo Colborn, Ph.D., Senior Scientist and Manager of

Wildlife & Contaminants Project at World Wildlife Fund and editor of *Chemically Induced Alterations in Sexual & Functional Development: Wildlife/Human Connection*; Donald Michael Fry, Ph.D., Professor at UC Davis in Department of Avian Sciences—researches toxic effects of airborne and waterborne organochlorine pesticides on development and reproduction in birds; Louis Guillette Jr., Ph.D., Professor of Zoology, University of Florida, and expert adviser for US Environmental Protection Agency and US Fish and Wildlife Department—focuses on endocrine disrupting contamination in endangered species, reptiles, and other wildlife; John McLachlan, Ph.D., Chief of National Institute of Environmental Health Sciences (NIEHS), 1972-1994, in laboratory of reproductive and developmental toxicology—now director of Tulane/Xavier Center for Bioenvironmental Research; Marion Moses, M.D., President of San Francisco's Pesticide Education Center, who is both board certified in occupational medicine and an expert on the impact of chemical exposures, especially pesticides, on human health.

Gambrell, R.D., "The menopause: benefits and risks of estrogen-progestogen replacement therapy," *Fertility Sterility,* 37, 457-474, 1982.

Guillette, L.J. Jr., "Endocrine-disrupting environmental contaminants and reproduction: lessons from the study of wildlife, published in Woman's Health Today: Perspectives on Current Research and Clinical Practice, 201-207, 1994.

Guyton, Arthur C., *Textbook of Medical Physiology,* Sixth Edition, W.B. Saunders Company, Philadelphia, 1981.

Hiatt, R.A., R. Bawol, G.D. Friedman, and R. Hoover, "Exogenous estrogen and breast cancer after bilateral oophorectomy," *Cancer,* 54, 139-144, 1984.

Hileman, Bette, "Environmental estrogens linked to reproductive abnormalities, Cancer," *C&EN, Washington,* 19-23, January 31, 1994.

La Vecchia, C., A. Decarli, F. Parazzini, A. Gentile, C. Liberati, and S. Franceschi, "Non-contraceptive estrogens and the risk of breast cancer in women," *International Journal of Cancer,* 1886, 38, 853-858.

Lee, J. R., M.D., "Osteoporosis reversal; the role of progesterone," *International Clinical Nutritional Review,* Sydney, Australia, June 1990.

———, "Is natural progesterone the missing link in osteoporosis prevention and treatment?" *Medical Hypotheses* 35, 316-318, 1991.

———, *Natural Progesterone,* BLL Publishing, California, 1993.

———, Endocrinology Notes: Progesterone and Estrogen. February 6, 1993.

———, "The Theory of Estrogen Dominance," Seminar given at St. Thomas's Hospital, London, June 4, 1994.

———, "Dr. John Lee speaking at the Chelsea Hotel, London, June 5, 1994," Video. *Medical Tribune,* "Sperm-count drop tied to pollution rise," March 26, 1992.

McLachlan, I.A., "Functional Toxicology: a new approach to detect biologically active xenobiotics," in *Environmental Health Perspectives,* 10: 386-387, 1993.

Moses, Marion, M.D., "Pesticides and Human Health—An Interview with Dr. Marion Moses by Cincy Deuhring," in *Informed Consent,* 21-24, May/June 1994; also Moses, M., "Pesticides and Breast Cancer" in *Pesticide News,* 23: 3-5 Dec 1994.

Peat, R., Ph.D., "Estrogen in 1990," *Blake College Newsletter,* Eugene, Oregon, 1990.

———, "Progesterone in Orthomolecular Medicine," Booklet.

Raloff, J., "Eco-Cancers, do environmental factors underlie a breast cancer epidemic?," *Science News,* July 3, 1993.

Raloff, J., "The Gender Benders," Part Two, "That Feminine Touch," *Science News,* January 8, 1994, and February 22, 1994.

Skakkebaek, Neils E., et al., *British Medical Journal,* January 1992.

Soto, Ana, et al., *Science News,* 12, July 3, 1993.

———, *Science News,* 24, January 8, 1994.

Stadel, B.V., "Oral contraceptives and cardiovascular disease," *New England Journal of Medicine,* 305, 612, 1981.

Stevens, Richard G., *American Journal of Epidemiology,* April 1987.

Stone, Richard, "Environmental Toxicants Under Scrutiny at Baltimore Meeting—meeting brief review" in *Science*, 267: 1770-1771, March 24, 1995. And "Dioxins Dominate Denver Gathering of Toxicologists—meeting brief review" in *Science*, 266: 1162-1163, November 18, 1994.

Stryer, Lubert, *Biochemistry*, W.H. Freeman and Company, San Francisco, CA, 1975.

Tietz, Norbert, W., Ph.D., *Textbook of Clinical Chemistry*, W.B. Saunders Company, Philadelphia, 1986.

von Kaulla, F., et al., "Conjugated estrogens and hypercoagulability," *American Journal of Obstetrics and Gynecology*, 122, 688, 1975.

Weiss, R., "Estrogen in the environment," *Washington Post*, p. 10-13, January 25, 1994.

Wolff, Mary S., Devra Lee-Davis, et al., *Science News*, 262, April 24, 1993.

Chapter Four: Search for the Grail

Austin, Phylis, Agatha Thrash, and Calvin Thrash, *Natural Remedies, A Manual*, Yuchi Pines Institute, Seale, AL, 1983.

Barrett-Connor, E., "Postmenopausal estrogen replacement and breast cancer," *New England Journal of Medicine*, 5, 321, 1989.

Begley, S., and D. Glick, "The Estrogen Complex," *Newsweek*, March 21, 1994.

Berkgvist, L., H.O. Adami, I. Persson, R. Hoover, C. Schairer, "The risk of breast cancer after estrogen and estrogen-progestin replacement," *New England Journal of Medicine*, 5, 321, 1989.

Brown, Ellen and Lynne Walker, *Breezing Through The Change*, Frog Ltd., Berkeley, CA, 1994.

Christiansen, C., B.J. Riis, L. Nilas, P. Rodbro, and L. Deftos, "Uncoupling of bone formation and resorption by combined estrogen and progestogen therapy in post-menopausal osteoporosis," *Lancet*, October 1985.

Coney, Sandra, *The Menopause Industry*, Penguin Books, London, 1991.

Felson, D.T., Y. Zhang, M.T. Hannan, D.P. Kiel, P.W.F. Wilson, and J.J. Anderson, "The effect of postmenopausal estrogen therapy on bone density in elderly women," *New England Journal of Medicine*, 329:1141-1146, 1993.

Guyton, Arthur C., *Textbook of Medical Physiology*, Sixth Edition, W.B. Saunders Company, Philadelphia, PA, 1981.

Hudson, Tori, *Gynecology and Naturopathic Medicine*, TK Publications, Oregon, 1992.

Kamen, Betty, *Hormone Replacement Therapy, Yes or No?*, Nutrition Encounter Inc., California, 1993.

Lee, J.R., M.D., "Understanding Osteoporosis." Summary.

———, "Osteoporosis reversal; the role of progesterone," *International Clinical Nutritional Review*, Sydney, Australia, June 1990.

———, "Osteoporosis reversal with transdermal progesterone," *The Lancet*, Letter, 336, November 1990.

———, "Is natural progesterone the missing link in osteoporosis prevention and treatment?" *Medical Hypotheses* 35, 314, 318, 1991.

———, "Hormonal and nutritional aspects of osteoporosis," *Health and Nutrition*, Vol. 6, Issue 4, Winter 1991.

———, *Natural Progesterone*, BLL Publishing, California, 1993.

———, "The Theory of Estrogen Dominance," Seminar given at St. Thomas's Hospital, London, June 4, 1994.

———, "Clinical Uses of Natural Progesterone," Seminar given at St. Thomas's Hospital, London, June 4, 1994.

———, "Dr. John Lee speaking at the Chelsea Hotel, London, June 5th 1994," Video.

———, "Effects of Progesterone on Osteoporosis and Menopausal Symptoms," Seminar given at St. Thomas's Hospital London, June 4, 1994.

———, "Successful Menopausal Osteoporosis Treatment Restoring Osteoclast/Osteoblast Equilibrium," *The Townsend Letter for Doctors*, 900, August/September 1994.

Medical Research Publishers, *Amazing Medicines The Drug Companies Don't Want You To Discover!* Tempe, AZ 85281, 1993.

Peat, R., Ph.D., "Progesterone in Orthomolecular Medicine," Blake College Booklet, Eugene, Oregon. Available from Foundation for Hormonal and Nutrition Research, 8150 SW, Barnes Road, Portland, Oregon, 97225.

———, "Origins of Progesterone Therapy," *Townsend Letter for Doctors,* 112, 1016, November 1992.

Shaffer, Willa, *Wild Yam, Birth Control Without Fear,* Woodland Health Books, Utah, 1986.

Stevenson, J.C., P.C. Michael, F.G. Gangar, T.C. Hillard, B. Lees, M.J. Whitehead, "Effects of transdermal versus oral hormone replacement therapy on bone density in spine and proximal femur in postmenopausal women," *The Lancet,* Vol. 336, 2265-2269.

Studd, John and Rod Barber, "Mastering the Menopause," Leaflet presented with the compliments of Organon Laboratories Ltd., Cambridge, 1994.

Williams, David G., "The forgotten hormones," *Alternatives for the Health Conscious Individual,* Vol. 4, No. 6, 41-46, 1991.

Whitehead, M.I., D. Fraser, L. Schenkel, D. Crook, J.C. Stevenson, "Transdermal administration of estrogen/progestogen hormone replacement therapy," *The Lancet,* Vol. 335, 310-311, 1990.

Chapter Five: Cycles of the Moon

Coney, Sandra, *The Menopause Industry,* Penguin Books, London, 1991.

Guyton, Arthur C., *Textbook of Medical Physiology,* Sixth Edition, W.B. Saunders Company, Philadelphia, 1981.

Lee, J.R., M.D., "The Theory of Estrogen Dominance," Seminar given at St. Thomas's Hospital, London, June 4, 1994.

———, "Is natural progesterone the missing link in osteoporosis prevention and treatment?" *Medical Hypotheses,* 35, 314, 318, 1991.

———, *Natural Progesterone,* BLL Publishing, California, 1993.

———, Endocrinology Notes: Progesterone and Estrogen. February 6, 1993.

———, "Clinical Uses of Natural Progesterone," Seminar given at St. Thomas's Hospital, London, June 4, 1994.

Peat, R., Ph.D., "Estrogen in 1990," *Blake College Newsletter,* Eugene, Oregon, 1990.

———, "Progesterone in Orthomolecular Medicine," Blake College Booklet, Eugene, Oregon.

Stryer, Lubert, *Biochemistry,* W.H. Freeman and Company, San Francisco, CA, 1975.

Thomas, J. Hywel, and Brian Gillham, *Wills' Biochemical Basis of Medicine,* Butterworth Heinemann Ltd., Oxford, 1989.

Tietz, Norbert W., Ph.D., *Textbook of Clinical Chemistry,* W.B. Saunders Company, Philadelphia, 1986.

Vollman, R.F., "The Menstrual Cycle," in *Major Problems in Obstetrics and Gynecology,* vol. 7, (ed.) E. A. Friedman, W.B. Saunders Company, Toronto, Canada, 1977.

Williams, David G., "The Forgotten Hormone," *Alternatives for the Health Conscious Individual,* Vol. 4, No. 6, 41-46, 1991.

Chapter Six: Crazed Woman

The Amarant Trust Newsletter, "Feeling Good," The Amarant Center, London, Spring 1993.

Bewley, S., and T.H. Bewley, "Drug Dependence with Estrogen Replacement Therapy," *The Lancet,* 339, 290-291, 1992.

Boston Collaborative Drug Surveillance Program (A Report), "Surgically confirmed gall bladder disease, venous thromboembolism and breast tumors in relation to post-menopausal estrogen therapy," *New England Journal of Medicine,* 290(1), 15-19.

Brown, Ellen and Lynne Walker, *Breezing Through The Change,* Frog Ltd., Berkeley, CA, 1994.

Cabot, Sandra, *Don't Let Your Hormones Ruin Your Life,* Women's Health Advisory Service, NSW, Australia, 1991.

Colditz, Graham A., Kathleen Egan, and Meir J. Stampfer, "Hormone replacement therapy and risk of breast cancer: Results from epidemiologic studies," *American Journal of Obstetrics and Gynecology,* 186(5), 1473-1479.

Collings, Jill, "Suffering in Silence," *The Guardian,* November 24, 1988.

Coney, Sandra, *The Menopause Industry,* Penguin Books, New Zealand, 1991.

Cunningham, Gary, and Marshall D. Lindheimer, "Hypertension in pregnancy," *New England Journal of Medicine,* 326, 927-932, 1992.

Davis, Peter, *For Health or Profit? Medicine, the Pharmaceutical Industry, and the State in New Zealand,* Oxford University Press, Auckland, New Zealand, 1992.

Dumble, Lynette J., "Hormone Replacement Therapy: The Big Myth of Modern Medicine," *Healthsharing Women Research Issues Forum II: Hormone Replacement Therapy,* Melbourne, Australia, April 1992.

Dumble, Lynette, and Renate Klein, "Hormone Replacement Therapy: Hazards, Risks and Tricks," Proceedings of *Menopause: The Alternative Way: Facts and Fallacies of the Menopause Industry,* Australian Women's Research Center, Deakin University, Australia, 1993.

Dyerassi, C., "The Making of the Pill," *Science,* 84, 127-129, 1984.

Ehrenreich, Barbara, and Deirdre English, *For Her Own Good: 150 Years of the Expert's Advice to Women,* Anchor Books, New York, 1979.

Gaby, Alan R., "Premarin and Animal Cruelty," *Townsend Letter for Doctors,* November 1994.

———, *Preventing and Reversing Osteoporosis,* Prima, 1994.

Gangar, Kevin, and Elizabeth Key, "Individualising HRT," *The Practitioner,* 237, 358-360, April 1993.

Garnett, Timothy J., John Studd, A.F. Henderson, N.R. Watson, M. Savvas, and A. Leather, "Hormone Implants and Tachyphylaxis," *British Journal of Obstetrics and Gynaecology,* 97, 917-921, 1990.

Gorman, Theresa and Malcolm Whitehead, *The Amarant Book of Hormone Replacement Therapy,* Pan Books, London, 1989.

Greer, Germaine, *The Change,* Penguin Books, London, 1991.

Hall, C., "Caution Urged on Hormone Therapy," *The Independent,* June 3, 1993.

Hoover, Robert, et al., "Menopausal estrogens and breast cancer," *New England Journal of Medicine,* 295(8), 401-405, 1976.

Kaufert, R., "Myth and Menopause," *Sociology of Health and Illness,* 4, 141-166, 1982.

Khaw, K.T., "The Menopause and Hormone Replacement Therapy," *Postgraduate Medical Journal,* 68, 615-623, 1992.

———(ed.), *Hormone Replacement Therapy,* Churchill Livingstein, London, 1992.

Klein, Renate, and Lynette J. Dumble, "Disempowering Midlife Women: The Science and Politics of Hormone Replacement Therapy," Women's Studies International Forum, Australia, 1994.

The Lancet, Editorial: "Dangers in Eternal Youth," 2, 1135, 1975.

Lee, J.R., M.D., "Understanding Osteoporosis." Summary.

———, "Osteoporosis reversal; the role of progesterone," *International Clinical Nutritional Review,* Sydney, Australia, June 1990.

———, "Osteoporosis reversal with transdermal progesterone," *The Lancet,* Letter, 336, November 1990.

———, "Is natural progesterone the missing link in osteoporosis prevention and treatment?, *Medical Hypotheses,* 35, 314, 318, 1991.

———, "Hormonal and nutritional aspects of osteoporosis," *Health and Nutrition,* Vol. 6, Issue 4, Winter 1991.

———, *Natural Progesterone,* BLL Publishing, California, 1993.

——, *Optimal Health Guidelines,* Second Edition, BLL Publishing, California, 1993.

——, Endocrinology Notes: Progesterone and Estrogen. February 6, 1993.

——, "The Theory of Estrogen Dominance," Seminar given at St. Thomas's Hospital, London, June 4, 1994.

——, "Clinical Uses of Natural Progesterone," Seminar given at St. Thomas's Hospital, London, June 4, 1994.

——, "Dr. John Lee speaking at the Chelsea Hotel, London, June 5th 1994," Video.

——, "Effects of Progesterone on Osteoporosis and Menopausal Symptoms," Seminar given at St. Thomas's Hospital London, June 4, 1994.

——, "The Multiple Effects of Progesterone," Seminar given at St. Thomas's Hospital, London, June 4, 1994.

——, "Successful Menopausal Osteoporosis Treatment Restoring Osteoclast/Osteoblast Equilibrium," *The Townsend Letter for Doctors,* 900, August/September 1994.

Lewis, Jane, "Feminism, the Menopause and Hormone Replacement," *Feminist Review,* 43, 38-56, 1993.

Lindgren, R., G. Berg, M. Hammer, and E. Zuccon, "Hormone Replacement Therapy and Sexuality in a Population of Swedish Postmenopausal Women," *Acta Obstet. Gynecol. Scand.,* 72, 292-297 1993.

McCrea, F., "The Politics of Menopause: The Discovery of a Deficiency Disease," *Social Problems,* 31, 111-123, 1983.

McCrea, F., and G. Markle, "The Estrogen Replacement Controversy in the USA and the UK: Different Answers to the Same Question?" *Social Studies of Science,* 14, 1-26, 1984.

Mack, Thomas, et al., "Estrogens and endometrial cancer in a retirement community," *New England Journal of Medicine,* 294(23), 1262-1267, 1976.

Mannen, E.F., "Oral contraceptives and blood coagulation: a critical review," *American Journal of Obstetrics and Gynecology,* 142, 781-790, 1982.

National Advisory Committee on Core Health and Disability Support Services, "Hormone Replacement Therapy," Consensus Development Conference Report, Wellington, New Zealand, December 1993.

Northrup, Christiane, M.D., *Women's Bodies, Women's Wisdom,* Bantam Books, New York, 1994.

Peat, Ray, "The Progesterone Deception," *Ray Peat's Newsletter,* May 1986.

Psaty, Bruce M., et al., "A review of the association of estrogens and progestins with cardiovascular disease in postmenopausal women," *Archives of Internal Medicine,* 153, 1421-1427.

Reitz, Rosetta, *Menopause, A Positive Approach,* Unwin Paperbacks, London, 1985.

Rinzler, Carol Ann, *Estrogen and Breast Cancer: A Warning to Women.....,* Macmillan Publishing Company, New York, 1993.

Rochon Ford, Anne, "Hormones: Getting Out of Hand," in *Adverse Effects: Women and the Pharmaceutical Industry,* (ed.) Kathleen McDonnell, IOCU, Penang, Malaysia, 1986.

Rowland, Robyn, *Living Laboratories. Women and Reproductive Technology,* Pan Macmillan, Sydney, Australia, 1992.

Sadgrove, Judy, "HRT: older women's friend or foe?" *The Guardian,* February 20, 1990.

Saul, Helen, "The bad news about 'good' cholesterol," *New Scientist,* August 14, 1993.

Seaman, Barbara, and Gideon Seaman, *Women and the Crisis in Sex Hormones,* Bantam Books, New York, 1977.

Silberstein, Stephen D., and George R. Merriam, "Estrogens, progestins and headaches," *Neurology,* 41, 786-793, 1991.

Smith, Donald C., et al., "Association of exogenous estrogen and endometrial carcinoma," *New England Journal of Medicine,* 293(23), 1164-1167, 1975.

Sporrong, T., L.A. Mattsson, E. Stradbert, and M. Uvebrant, "Continuous combined HRT: long-term effects on the endometrium," Abstract 337. 7th International Congress on the Menopause, Stockholm, Sweden, June 20-24, 1993.

Stampfer, Meir, et al., "Postmenopausal estrogen therapy and cardiovascular disease," *New England Journal of Medicine,* 1991, 325, 756-762.

Studd, J., and M. Thom, "Letter to the Editor," *New England Journal of Medicine,* 300, 922-923, 1979.

Vines, Gail, "The Challenge to HRT," *New Scientist,* October 23, 1993.

———, *Raging Hormones,* Virago Press, London, 1993.

Whitecroft, S. I. J., M. C. Ellerington and M. I. Whitehead, "Routes of estrogen administration," *Annual Progress in Reproductive Medicine,* (eds) R.H. Asch and J. Studd, The Parthenon Publishing Group, Carnforth, UK, 1993.

Whitehead, M.I., T.C. Hillard, and D. Crook, "The role and use of progestogens," *Obstetrics and Gynecology,* 1990, 75(4), 59S-76S.

Wilson, R., *Feminine Forever,* M. Evans, New York, 1966.

Wilson, R.A., and T.A. Wilson, "The Fate of the Non-Treated Postmenopausal Woman: A Plea for Maintenance of Adequate Estrogen from Puberty to the Grave," *Journal of the American Geriatrics Society,* 11, 346-362, 1963.

Ziel, H.K., and Finkle, W.D., "Increased risk of endometrial carcinoma among users of conjugated estrogens," *New England Journal of Medicine,* 293(23), 1167-1170, 1975.

Chapter Seven: Dark Gods

Abraham, G.E., and J.T. Hargrove, "Effect of Vitamin B on Premenstrual Tension Syndrome: A double-blind crossover study," *Infertility,* vol. 3, 155, 1980.

Abraham, G.E., "Nutritional factors in the etiology of the Premenstrual Tension Syndromes," *Journal of Reproductive Medicine,* 1983, vol. 28, 446.

Aldercreutz, H., "Diet and Plasma Androgens in Postmenopausal Vegetarian and Omnivorous Women and Postmenopausal Women with Breast Cancer," *American Journal of Clinical Nutrition,* 1989, vol. 49, 433.

Aldercreutz, H., et al., "Determination of urinary lignans and phytoestrogen metabolites, potential antiestrogens and anticarcinogens in urine of women on various habitual diets," *J. Steroid, Biochem,* 1986, 25, 791-797.

———, "Dietary phytoestrogens and the menopause in Japan," *The Lancet,* 1992, vol. 339, 1233.

Balch, James F., and Phyllis A. Balch, *Prescription for Nutritional Healing,* Avery Publishing Group Ltd., New York, 1990.

Barrett-Connor, E., "Postmenopausal estrogen replacement and breast cancer," *New England Journal of Medicine,* 1989, 5, 321.

Barzel, U., "Estrogens in the prevention and treatment of postmenopausal osteoporosis: A review," *American Journal of Medicine,* 1988, 85, 847-850.

Begley, S., and D. Glick, "The Estrogen Complex," *Newsweek,* March 21, 1994.

Berkgvist, L., H.O. Adami, I. Persson, R. Hoover, C. Schairer, "The risk of breast cancer after estrogen and estrogen-progestin replacement," *New England Journal of Medicine,* 1989, 5, 321, 293-297.

Biskind, M.S., "The Effect of Vitamin B Complex Deficiency on the Inactivation of Estrone in the Liver," *Endocrinology,* 1942, vol. 31, 109-114.

Bloom, H., "The influence of delay on the natural history and prognosis of breast cancer," *British Journal of Cancer,* 1965, 19, 228-262.

Borysenko, Joan, *Guilt is the Teacher: Love is the Lesson,* Warner Books, New York, 1991.

Botez, M.I., "Neurologic Disorders Response to Folic Acid Therapy," *Canadian Medical Association Journal,* 1976, vol. 15, 217.

Boyd, N., "Effect of a Low-Fat, High-Carbohydrate Diet on Symptoms of Clinical Mastopathy," *Lancet,* 1988, vol. 2, 128.

Brown, Ellen, and Lynne Walker, *Breezing Through The Change,* Frog Ltd., Berkeley, CA, 1994.

Brown, R.R., et al., "Correlation of serum retinol levels with response to chemotherapy in breast cancer," *American Journal of Obstetrics and Gynecology,* vol. 148, no. 3, 309-312.

Buell, P., "Changing incidence of breast cancer in Japanese-American women," *Journal of the National Cancer Institute,* 1973, vol. 51, 1479-1483.

Bulbrook, P.D., M.C. Swain, and D.Y. Wang, et al., "Breast Cancer in Britain and Japan: Plasma OEstradiol-17B Oestrone, and Progesterone, and their Urinary Metabolites in Normal British and Japanese Women," *European Journal of Cancer,* 1976, vol 12, 725-735.

Carol, K. K., "Dietary factors in immune-dependent cancers," in M. Winick, ed., *Current Concepts in Nutrition,* vol 6, *Nutrition and Cancer,* John Wiley and Sons, New York, 1977.

Colditz, G.A., et al., "Prospective Study of Estrogen Replacement Therapy and Risk of Breast Cancer in Postmenopausal Women," *Journal of the American Medical Association,* 1990, vol. 264, 2648-252.

Colditz, G.A., et al., "Type of postmenopausal hormone use and risk of breast cancer: 12 year follow-up from the Nurse's Health Study," *Cancer Causes and Control,* 1992, 3, 433-439.

Cowan, L.D., L. Gordis, et al., "Breast cancer incidence in women with a history of progesterone deficiency," *American Journal of Epidemiology,* 1981, 114:209-217.

Cowley, G., et al., "In pursuit of a terrible killer," *Newsweek,* December 10, 1990, 66-68.

Cramer, D.W., et al., "Dietary Animal Fat and Relationship to Ovarian Cancer Risk," *Obstetrics and Gynecology,* 1984, Vol. 63, No. 6, 833-838.

DHHS publication no. (PHS) 90-1101, "Mortality," Part A, Washington D.C., U.S. Government Printing Office, 1990.

Dickinson, L.E., et al., "Estrogen Profiles of Oriental and Caucasian Women in Hawaii," *New England Journal of Medicine,* 1974, vol 291, 1211-1213.

Documenta Geigy, Scientific Tables, sixth edition, 493.

Facchinetti, F., et al., "Oral magnesium successfully relieves premenstrual mood changes," *Obstetrics and Gynecology,* 1991, Vol. 78, No. 2, 177-181.

Follingstad, Alvin, "Estriol, The Forgotten Estrogen?," *Journal of the American Medical Association,* January 2, 1978, Vol. 239, No. 1, 29-30.

Gambrell, R.D., "The menopause: benefits and risks of estrogen-progestogen replacement therapy," *Fertility Sterility,* 1982, 37, 457-474.

Gambrell, R.D., "Complications of Estrogen Replacement Therapy" in *Hormone Replacement Therapy,* D.P. Swartz, ed., Williams and Watkins, Baltimore, MD, 1992.

Goci, G.S., and G.E. Abraham, "Effect of Nutritional Supplement . . . on Symptoms of Premenstrual Tension," *Journal of Reproductive Medicine,* 1982, Vol. 83, 527-531.

Goldin, B., and J. Gorsback, "The effect of milk and lactobacillus feeding on human intestinal bacterial enzyme activity," *American Journal of Clinical Nutrition,* 1984, Vol. 39, 756-761.

Goodman, L., et al., *Pharmacological Basis of Therapeutics,* Macmillan Publishing Co., New York, 1975.

Guyton, Arthur C., *Textbook of Medical Physiology,* Sixth Edition, W.B. Saunders Company, Philadelphia, 1981.

Heimer, G.M., D.E. Englund, "Effects of Vaginally-Administered Oestriol on Post menopausal Urogenital Disorders: a Cytohormonal Study," *Maturitas,* March 14, 1992, Vol. 3, 171-179.

Henderson, B.E., R.K. Ross, M.C. Pike, and J.T. Casagrande, "Endogenous hormones as a major factor in human cancer," *Cancer Research,* 1982, 42, 3232-3239.

Hiatt, R.A., R. Bawol, G.D. Friedman, and R. Hoover, "Exogenous estrogen and breast cancer after bilateral oophorectomy," *Cancer,* 1984, 54, 139-144.

Hileman, Bette, "Environmental estrogens linked to reproductive abnormalities, cancer," *C&EN Washington.*

Hill, P., "Diet, Lifestyle and Menstrual Activity," *American Journal of Clinical Nutrition,* 1980, Vol. 33, 1192.

Hoeh, S.K., and K.K. Carroll, "Effects of dietary carbohydrate in the incidence of mammary tumors induced in rats by 7, 12-dimethylbenzanthracene," *Nutrition and Cancer*, 1979, Vol. 1, No. 3, 27-30.

Holl, M.H., et al., "Gut bacteria and aetology of cancer of the breast," *The Lancet,* 1971, Vol. 2, 172-173.

Hoover, R., L.A. Gray Sr, P. Cole, and B. MacMahon, "Menopausal estrogens and breast cancer" *New England Journal of Medicine,* 1976, 295, 401-405.

Hughes, R.E., "Hypothesis: a new look at dietary fiber in human nutrition," *Clinical Nutrition,* 1986, Vol. 406, 81-86.

Hunter, D.J., et al., "A prospective study of the intake of vitamins C, E, and A, and the risk of breast cancer," *New England Journal of Medicine,* July 22, 1993, Vol. 324, No. 4, 234-240.

Huppert, L., "Hormonal replacement therapy: Benefits, risks, doses," *Medical Clinics of North America,* 1987, 71, 23-39.

Ingram, D., "Effect of Low-Fat Diet on Female Sex Hormone Levels," *Journal of National Cancer Institute,* 1987, Vol. 79, 1225.

Iosif, C.S., "Effects of Protracted Administration of Estriol on the Lower Urinary Tract in Postmenopausal Women," *Archives of Gynecology and Obstetrics*, 1992, Vol. 3, No. 251, 115-120.

IpC, "Dietary Vitamin E Intake and Mammary Carcinogenesis in Rats," *Carcinogenesis,* 1982, Vol. 3, 1453-1456.

Journal of the National Cancer Institute, "Author of Canadian breast cancer study retracts warnings," June 3, 1992, 84, 832-834.

Kato, I., et al., "Alcohol consumption in cancers of hormone related organs in females," *Japan Journal of Clinical Oncology,* 1989, Vol. 19, No. 3, 202-207.

Kellis, T.T., and L.E. Vickery, "Inhibition of Human Estrogen Synthetase (Aromatase) by Flavonoids," *Science,* 1984, Vol. 255, 1032-1034.

Kelly, M., "Hypercholesterolemia: The cost of treatment in perspective," *Southern Medical Journal,* 1990, 83, 1421-1425.

Kinlen, L., "Meat and fat consumption and cancer mortality: a study of strict religious orders in Britain," *The Lancet,* 1982, 946-949.

Kirkengen, A.L., P. Anderson, E. Gjersoe, G. Johannessen, N. Johnsen, and E. Bodd, "Oestriol in the Prophylactic Treatment of Recurrent Urinary Tract Infection in Postmenopausal Women," *Scandinavian Journal Primary Health Care,* June 10, 1992, 139-142.

Kolata, G., "Studies say Mammograms fail to help many women," *New York Times,* February 26, 1993.

Kolata, Gina, "Breast cancer screening under 50: experts disagree if benefit exists," *New York Times,* December 14, 1993.

Kushi, M., *The Cancer Prevention Diet,* St. Martin's Press, New York, 1983.

Landau, R.S., et al., "The effect of alpha tocopherol in premenstrual symptomatology: a double-blind trial," *Journal of the American College of Nutrition,* 1983, Vol. 2, 115-123.

La Vecchia, C., A. Decarli, F. Parazzini, A. Gentile, C. Liberati, S. Franceschi, "Non-contraceptive estrogens and the risk of breast cancer in women" *Int J Cancer,* 1986, 38, 853-858.

Lee, H.P., et al., "Dietary effects on breast cancer risk in Singapore," *The Lancet,* May 18, 1991, Vol. 337, 1197-1200.

Lee, J.R., M.D., "Osteoporosis reversal; the role of progesterone," *International Clinical Nutritional Review,* Sydney, Australia, June 1990.

——, "Is natural progesterone the missing link in osteoporosis prevention and treatment?" *Medical Hypotheses* 1991, 35, 316-318.

——, *Natural Progesterone,* BLL Publishing, California, 1993.

——, Endocrinology Notes: Progesterone and Estrogen. February 6, 1993.

——, "The Theory of Estrogen Dominance," Seminar given at St. Thomas's Hospital, London, June 4, 1994.

———, "Dr. John Lee speaking at the Chelsea Hotel, London, June 5, 1994," Video.

———, *Optimal Health Guidelines,* Second Edition, BLL Publishing, California, 1993.

Lemon, H. M., "Oestiol and Prevention of Breast Cancer," *The Lancet,* March 10, 1973, Vol. 1, No. 802, 546-547.

———, "Estriol Prevention of Mammary Carcinoma Induced by 7, 12-Dimethylbenzanthracene and Procarbazine," *Cancer Research,* 1975, Vol. 35, 1341-1353.

———, "Clinical and Experimental Aspects of Anti-Mammary Carcinogenic Activity of Estriol," *Frontiers of Hormonal Research,* 1977, Vol. 5, No. 1, 155-173.

———, "Pathophysiologic Considerations in the Treatment of Menopausal Patients with Estrogens; The Role of Oestriol in the Prevention of Mammary Carcinoma," *Acta Endocrinologica,* 1980, Vol. 233, 17-27

Lemon, H.M., H.H. Wotiz, L. Parsons, and P.J. Mozden, "Reduced estriol excretion in patients with breast cancer prior to endocrine therapy," *Journal of the American Medical Association,* 1966, 196, 112-120.

Levy, J. A., et al., *Basic and Clinical Immunology,* 4th ed., Lange Medical Books, Los Angeles, CA, 1982.

London, R.S., et al., "Endocrine Parameters and Alpha-Tocopherol Therapy of Patients with Mammary Dysplasia," *Cancer Research,* 1981, Vol. 41, 3811-3813.

Lubran, M., and G. Abraham, "Serum and red cell magnesium levels in patients with Premenstrual Tension," *American Journal of Clinical Nutrition,* 1982, Vol. 34, 2364.

McConnell, K.P., et al., "The relationship between dietary selenium and breast cancer," *Journal of Surgical Oncology,* 1980, Vol. 5, No. 1, 67-70.

McCormick, J., "Cervical smears: A questionable practice?" *The Lancet,* July 22, 1989, 207-209.

McDougall, J., *McDougall's Medicine, A Challenging Second Opinion,* New Century Publishers, Piscataway, NJ, 1985.

McKenna, T., "Pathogenesis and Treatment of Polycystic Ovary Syndrome," *New England Journal of Medicine,* 1988, Vol. 318, 558.

MacMahon, B., et al., "Urine Estrogen Profiles in Asian and North American Women," *International Journal of Cancer,* 1974, Vol. 14, 161-167.

Medical Tribune, "Sperm-count drop tied to pollution rise," March 26, 1992.

———, "Late-cycle mastectomies may reduce recurrences," May 1992.

Michnovicz, J., and H. Bradlow, "Altered estrogen metabolism and excretion in humans following consumption of Indole-3-Carbinol," *Nutrition and Cancer,* 1991, Vol. 16, 59-66.

Miller, A., et al., "Canadian National Breast Screening Study: 1. Breast cancer detection and death rates among women aged 40-49 years," *Canadian Medical Association Journal,* 1992, 147, 1459-1476.

Moss, R., *The Cancer Industry: Unravelling the Politics,* Paragon House, New York, 1989.

National Center for Health Statistics, "Vital statistics of the United States," 1987, Vol. 2.

Nielson, M., et al., "Breast cancer and atypia among young middle-aged women: a study of 110 medical-legal autopsies," *British Journal of Cancer,* 1987, Vol. 56, 814-819.

Norris, Ronald, "Progesterone for Premenstrual Tension," *Journal of Reproductive Medicine,* August 1983, Vol. 28, No. 8, 509-515.

Peat, R., Ph.D., "Estrogen in 1990," *Blake College Newsletter,* Eugene, Oregon, 1990.

———, "Progesterone in Orthomolecular Medicine," Booklet.

Physicians Desk Reference, Medical Economics Co., Oradell, New Jersey, 1989.

Polson, D., "Polycystic Ovaries—A Common Finding in Normal Women," *The Lancet,* 1988, Vol. 1, 870.

Poyduck, M.E., "Inhibiting Effect of Vitamin C and B12 on the Mitotic Activity of Acites Tumors," *Experimental Cell Biology,* 1979, Vol. 47, No. 3, 210-217.

Price, F., "Theoretical Involvement of Vitamin B6 in Tumor Initiation," *Medical Hypothesis,* 1985, Vol. 15, 421-428.

Punnonen, R., S. Vilsak, and L. Rauramo, "Skinfold Thickness and Long-Term Post menopausal Hormone Therapy," *Maturitas,* April 5, 1984, Vol. 4, 259-262.

Raloff, J., "Eco-Cancers, do environmental factors underlie a breast cancer epidemic?" *Science News,* July 3, 1993, 144, 10-13.

Raloff, J., "The Gender-Benders," Part Two, "That Feminine Touch," *Science News,* January 8, 1994, and February 22, 1994.

Robin, E., M.D., *Matters of Life and Death: Risks vs. Benefits of Medical Care,* W.H. Freeman & Co, New York, 1984.

Rose, D., "Effect of a Low-Fat Diet on Hormone Levels in Women with Cystic Breast Disease, I: Serum Steroids and Gonadotropins," *Journal of the National Cancer Institute,* 1987, Vol. 78, 623.

Rose, D., "Effect of a Low-Fat Diet on Hormone Levels in Women with Cystic Breast Disease, II: Serum Radioimmunoassayable Prolactin and Growth Hormone and Bioactive Lactogenic Hormones," *Journal of the National Cancer Institute,* 1987, Vol. 78, 627.

Rosenberg, L., et al., "Breast cancer and alcoholic beverage consumption," *The Lancet,* 1982, Vol. 1, 267.

Rosenthal, Elisabeth, "Cancer Surgeons Debate Timing of Breast Operations," *Health,* Wednesday February 5, 1992.

Rossignol, A.M., "Caffeine-Containing Beverages and Premenstrual Syndrome in Young Women," *American Journal of Public Health,* 1985, Vol. 75, No. 11, 1335-1337.

Sanchez, A., "A Hypothesis on the Etiologic Role of Diet on the Age of Menarche," *Medical Hypotheses,* 1981, Vol. 7, 1339.

Sattilaro, Anthony, and Tom Monte, *Living Well Naturally,* Houghton Mifflin, Boston, 1984.

Schwartz, S., "Dietary Influences on the Growth and Sexual Maturation in Premenarchal Rhesus Monkeys," *Hormones and Behavior,* 1988, Vol. 22, 231.

Scott, J., "Hormones may increase cancer risk, study says," *Los Angeles Times,* August 2, 1989, 1-15.

Seely, S., and D.F. Horrobin, "Diet and breast cancer: the possible connection with sugar consumption," *Medical Hypotheses,* 1983, Vol. 3, 319-327.

Sillero-Arenas, M., et al., "Menopausal Hormone Replacement Therapy and Breast Cancer: A Meta-Analysis," *Obstetrics and Gynecology,* February 1992, Vol. 79, No. 2, 286-293.

Skrabanek, P., "False premises and false promises of breast cancer screening," *The Lancet,* August 10, 1985, 316-320.

Snowden, D.A., Letter to the Editor, *Journal of the American Medical Association,* 1985, Vol. 3, No. 254.

Speroff, L., "The Breast as an Endocrine Target Organ," *Contemporary Obstetrics and Gynecology,* 1977, Vol. 9, 69-72.

Stadel, B.V., "Oral contraceptives and cardiovascular disease," *New England Journal of Medicine,* 1981, 305, 612.

Stampfer, M., et al., "A prospective study of postmenopausal estrogen therapy and coronary heart disease," *New England Journal of Medicine,* 313, 1044-1049.

Stryer, Lubert, *Biochemistry,* W.H. Freeman and Company, San Francisco, 1975.

Thomas, J. Hywel, and Brian Gillham, *Will's Biochemical Basis of Medicine,* Second Edition, Butterworth Heinemann Ltd., Oxford, 1992.

Tietz, Norbert, W. Ph.D., *Textbook of Clinical Chemistry,* W.B. Saunders Company, Philadelphia, 1986.

Tzingounis, V.A., M.F. Aksu and R.B. Greenblatt, "Estriol in the Management of the Menopause," *Journal of the American Medical Association,* 1978, Vol. 239, 1638-1641.

van Haaften, M., G.H. Donker, A.A. Haspeis, and J.H. Thijssen, "Estrogen Concentrations in Plasma, Endometrium, Myometrium, and Vagina of Postmenopausal Women, and Effects of Vaginal Oestriol (E3) and Estradiol (E2) Applications," *Journal of Steroid Biochemistry,* 1989, Vol. 4A, 647-653.

von Kaulla, F., et al., "Conjugated estrogens and hypercoagulability," *American Journal of Obstetrics and Gynecology,* 1975, 122, 688.

Wattenberg, L.W., "Inhibition of neoplasia by minor dietary constituents," *Cancer Research* (supp), May 1983, 43, 2448-2453.

Weiss, R., "Estrogen in the environment," *Washington Post,* January 25, 1994, p. 10-13.

Welch, H. Gilbert, and William Black, "Advances in Diagnostic Imaging," *New England Journal of Medicine,* April 1993, Vol. 328, 1237-1243.

Werbach, Melvyn R., *Nutritional Influences on Illness,* Second Edition, Third Line Press, California, 1987.

Willet, W., et al., "Dietary fat and risk of breast cancer," *New England Journal of Medicine,* 1987, Vol. 316, No. 22.

Williams, D.G., "The Forgotten Hormone," *Alternatives,* 1991, Vol. 4, No. 6, 11.

Woods, M., "Low-Fat, High-Fiber Diet and Serum Estrone Sulfate in Premenopausal Women," *American Journal of Clinical Nutrition,* 1989, Vol. 49, p. 1179.

Wotiz, H.H., D.R. Beebe, and E. Muller, "Effect of Estrogens on DMBA-Induced Breast Tumors," *Journal of Steroid Biochemistry,* 1984, Vol. 20, 1067-1075.

Wynder, E.L., et al., "Diet and Breast Cancer. Causation and Therapy," *Gynecology and Obstetrics,* 1986, Springer-Verlag, 558-561.

Yang, C., et al., "Noncontraceptive hormone use and risk of breast cancer," *Cancer Causes and Control,* 1992, 3, 475-479.

Yuesheng, Z., et al., "A major inducer of anticarcinogenic protective enzymes from broccoli: isolation and elucidation of structure," *Proc. Natl. Acad. Sci.,* 1992, 89, 2399-2403.

Zussman, L., et al., "Sexual response after hysterectomy-oophorectomy: Recent studies and reconsideration of psychogenesis," *American Journal of Obstetrics and Gynecology,* 1981, 140, 725-729.

Chapter Eight: Gremlins in the Architecture (and Chapter Twenty-Two: Angels in the Architecture)

Abraham, G.E., "The Importance of Magnesium in the Management of Primary Post menopausal Osteoporosis," *The Journal of Nutritional Medicine,* 1991, 2, 165-178.

Abraham, G.E., and Harinder Grewal, "A Total Dietary Program Emphasizing Magnesium Instead of Calcium," *Journal of Reproductive Medicine,"* May 1990, Vol. 35, No. 5, 503-507.

Aihara, Herman, *Acid and Alkaline,* George Ohsawa Macrobiotic Foundation, Oroville, CA, 1980.

Aitken, M., D.M. Hart, and R. Lindsay, "Estrogen replacement therapy for prevention of osteoporosis after oophorectomy," *British Medical Journal,* 1973, 3, 515-518.

Albanes, A.A., et al., *Nutr Rep Internat,* 1985, 1093-1115.

Albright, F., et al., "Postmenopausal osteoporosis: its clinical features," *JAMA,* 1941, 116, 2465-2474.

Allen, L.H., "Protein-induced hypercalcuria: A longer term study," *American Journal of Clinical Nutrition,* 1974, 32, 741.

American Journal of Medicine, 1969, 46, 197.

Anand, C., and H.M. Linkswiler, "Effect of protein intake on calcium balance of young men given 500 mg calcium daily," *J. Nutr,* 1974, 104, 695.

Avioli, L.V., "Rationale for the use of cacitonin in postmenopausal osteoporosis," *Annale Chirugiae et Gynaecologiae,* 1988, 77, 224.

Bain, C., W. Willet, C.H. Hennekens, et al., "Use of Postmenopausal Hormones and Risk of Myocardial Infarction," *Circulation,* 1981, 64, 42-46.

Barzel, U.S., "Estrogens in the prevention and treatment of postmenopausal osteoporosis: a review," *American Journal of Medicine,* 1988, 85, 847-850.

Berkgvist, L., II.O. Adami, I. Persson, R. Hoover, and C. Schairer, "The risk of breast cancer after estrogen and estrogen-progestin replacement," *New England Journal of Medicine,* 1989, 5, 321.

Block, G.D., et al., *American Journal of Clinical Nutrition,* 1980, 33, 2128-2136.

Briscoe, A.M., and C. Ragan, *American Journal of Clinical Nutrition,* 1966, 19, 296. *British Medical Journal,* 1984, 289, 1103.

Brockis, J. G., A. S. Levitt, and S.M. Cruthers, "The effects of vegetable and animal protein diets on calcium, urate and oxalate excretion," *British Journal of Urology,* 1982, 54, 590.

Bryce-Smith, Professor D., "Boron: A Candidate for Essentiality," *Green Library Offprint,* Green Library Ltd., Surrey, No. 46.

Carlisle, E.M., "Silicon as an Essential Trace Element in Animal Nutrition," *Ciba Foundation Symposium,* 1986, 121, 123.

Cecil's Textbook of Medicine, 18th Edition, 1988, p. 1514.

Cohen, L., A. Laor, and R. Kitzes, "Bone Magnesium Crystallinity Index and State of Body Magnesium in Subjects with Senile Osteoporosis, Maturity-onset Diabetes and Women Treated with Contraceptive Preparations," *Magnesium,* 1983, 2, 70-75.

Christiansen, C., M.S. Christiansen, and I. Transbol, "Bone mass in postmenopausal women after withdrawal of oestrogen/progestogen replacement therapy," *The Lancet,* February 28, 1981, 459-461.

Christiansen, C., B. J. Riis, L. Nilas, P. Rodbro, and L. Deftos, "Uncoupling of bone formation and resorption by combined estrogen and progestogen therapy in post-menopausal osteoporosis," *The Lancet,* October 1985, 800-801.

Coats, C., "Negative effects of a high-protein diet," Family Practice Recertification, 1990, 12, 80-88.

Coney, Sandra, *The Menopause Industry,"* Penguin Books, London, 1991.

Cooper, C., C.A.C. Wickham, D.J.R. Barker, and S.J. Jacobsen, "Water fluoridation and hip fracture," *JAMA* 1991, 266, 513-514.

Cowan, L.D., L. Gordis, et al., "Breast cancer incidence in women with a history of progesterone deficiency," *American Journal of Epidemiology,* 1981, 114:209-217.

Cramer, D.W., et al., *American Journal of Epidemiology,* 1994, 139, 282-289.

Crane, Milton G., "The Use of Progesterone and/or an Estrogen in Osteoporosis," Unpublished, available from Weimar Institute, Weimar, CA 95736.

Cummings, S.R., "Are Patients with Hip Fractures More Osteoporotic?," *American Journal of Medicine,* 1985, 78, 487.

Cummings, S.R., et al., "Epidemiology of Osteoporosis and Osteoporotic Fractures," *Epidemiology Reviews,* 1985, 7, 178.

Cundy, T., M. Evans, H. Roberts, et al., "Bone density in women receiving depomedro-syprogesterone acetate for contraception," *British Medical Journal,* 1991, 303, 13-16.

Danielson, C., J.L. Lyon, M. Eger, and G.K. Goodenough, "Hip fractures and fluoridation in Utah's elderly population," *JAMA,* 1992, 268, 746-747.

DeLuca, H.F., *Vitamin D: Metabolism and Function,* Springer-Verlag, New York, 1979.

DeLuca, H.F., "The Latest Information on Vitamin D and Bone Status," *Complementary Medicine,* May/June 1986, 14.

Donaldson, C.L., et al., *Metabolism,* 1970, 19, 1071-1084.

Doppelt, S., *Harvard Medical School Newsletter,* November 1981, 3-4.

Dudl, R.J., et al., "Evaluation of Intravenous Calcium as Therapy for Osteoporosis," *American Journal of Medicine,* 1973, 55, 631.

Dyckner, T., and P.O. Wester, "Effect of Magnesium on Blood Pressure," *British Medical Journal,* 1983, 286, 1847.

Edgren, R.A., "Progestogens," reprinted from *Clinical Use of Sex Steroids,* Year Book Medical Publishers, Inc., 1980.

Ellis, F.R., S. Holesh, and J.W. Ellis, "Incidence of osteoporosis in vegetarians and omnivores," *Am Clin Nutr,* 1972, 25, 555.

Ettinger, B., H.K. Genant, and C.E. Cann, "Long-term estrogen replacement therapy prevents bone loss and fractures," *Ann Intern Med,* 1985, 102, 319-324.

Francis, R.M., and D.M. Beaumont, letters to the editor, "Involutional Osteoporosis," *New England Journal of Medicine,* 1987, 316, 216.

Fisken, R.A., "Osteoporosis: A Clinical Guide. Review of Books," *The Lancet,* 1988, 2, 996.

Friedman, G.L., "Diet in the Treatment of Diabetes," in *Modern Nutrition in Health and Disease,* (eds) R.S. Goodhart and M.E. Shils, 6th edition, Lea and Febiger, Philadelphia, 1980.

Gaby, A.R., *Preventing and Reversing Osteoporosis,* Prima Publications, Rocklin, CA, 1994.

Gaby, A.R., and J.V. Wright, "Nutrients and bone health," *JAMA,* 1988, 4, 2-6.

Gambrell, R.D., "The Menopause: Benefits and Risks of Estrogen-progestogen Replacement Therapy," *Fertility Sterility,* 1982, 37, 457-474.

Gambrell, R.D., C.A. Bagnell, and R.B. Greenblatt, "Role of estrogens and progesterone in the etiology and prevention of endometrial cancer. Review," *American Journal of Obstetrics and Gynecology,* 1983, 146, 696-707.

Gambrell, R.D., R.C., and Maier, S.L., "Decreased Incidence of Breast Cancer in Post-menopausal Estrogen-progestogen Users," *Obstetrics & Gynecology,* 1983, 62, 435-443.

Genant, H.K., G.S. Gordon, and P.G. Hoffman Jr, "Osteoporosis: Part II, Prevention of bone loss and fracture in women and risks of menopausal estrogen therapy," Medical Staff Conference, U. of Cal. SF. *West J Med,* 1983, 139, 204-211.

Gonzalez, E.R., *Journal of the American Medical Association,* 1980, 243, 309-316.

Goulding, A., *New Zealand Medical Journal,* 1990, 103, 120.

Gordon, G.S., J. Picchi, and B.S. Roots, "Antifracture efficacy of long-term estrogens for osteoporosis," *Trans Assoc Am Physicians,* 1973, 86, 326-332.

Guyton, Arthur C., *Textbook of Medical Physiology,* Sixth Edition, W.B. Saunders Company, Philadelphia, 1981.

Halioua, L., and J.J.B. Anderson, "Lifetime Calcium Intake and Physical Activity Habits: Independent and Combined Effects on the Radial Bone of Healthy Premenopausal Caucasian Women," *American Journal of Clinical Nutrition,* 1989, 49, 534.

Hall, F.M., M.A. Davis, and D.T. Baran, "Sounding Board: Bone Mineral Screening for Osteoporosis," *New England Journal of Medicine,* 1987, 316, 212.

Hammond, C.B., F.R. Jelvsek, K.L. Lee, W.T. Creasman, and R.T. Parker, "Effects of long-term estrogen replacement therapy. I Metabolic effects," *American Journal of Obstetrics and Gynecology,* 1979, 133, 525-536.

Hargrove, Joel T., et al., "Menopausal hormone replacement therapy with continuous daily oral micronized estradiol and progesterone," *Obstetrics and Gynaecology,* 1989, 73, 606-612.

——, "Progesterone: Safe Antidote for PMS," *McCall's,* October 1990.

Harrison's Principles of Internal Medicine, 12th Edition, 1991, p. 1925.

Harvard Medical School Health Letter, March 1976.

Heaney, R., et al., *American Journal of Clinical Nutrition,* 1986, 43, 299.

Hedlund, L.R., and J.C. Gallagher, "Increased incidence of hip fracture in osteoporotic women treated with sodium fluoride," *J Bone Miner Res,* 1989, 4, 223-225.

Hegsted, M., S.A. Schuette, M.B. Zemel, et al., "Urinary calcium and calcium balance in young men as affected by level of protein and phosphorus intake," *J Nutr,* 1981, 111, 553.

Holl, M.G., and L.H. Allen, "Comparative Effects of Meals High in Protein, Sucrose, or Starch on Human Mineral Metabolism and Insulin Secretion," *American Journal of Clinical Nutrition,* 1988, 48, 1219.

Holst, J., S. Cajander, and B. von Shoultz, "Endometrial effects of a continuous percutaneous estrogen/low dose progestogen regimen for climacteric complaints," *Maturitas,* 1987, 9, 63-67.

Hudleston, A.L., et al., *Journal of the American Medical Association,* 1980, 244, 1107-1109.

Human Nutrition Information Service, C.S.F. II, "Nationwide Food Consumption Survey Continuing Survey of Food Intakes by Individuals," 85-81, US Department of Agriculture, Washington DC, 1985.

Hutchinson, T.A., S.M. Polansky, and A.R. Feinstein, "Postmenopausal estrogens protect against fractures of hip and distal radius: a case control study," *The Lancet*, 1979, II, 705-709.

Jacobsen, S.L., et al., *JAMA*, 1990, 264, 500-502.

Johansen, J.S., S.B. Jensen, B.J. Riis, et al., "Bone formation is stimulated by combined estrogen, progestogen," *Metabolism*, 1990, 39, 1122-1126.

Johnston, F.A., et al., *Journal of American Dietary Association*, 1952, 28, 933-938.

Journal of the American Medical Association "National Institutes of Health, Consensus Conference: Osteoporosis," 1984, 252, 799.

Kabayashi, A., et al., *American Journal of Clinical Nutrition,* 1975, 28, 681-683.

Kamen, Betty, *Startling New Facts About Osteoporosis,* Nutrition Encounter Inc., California, 1989.

Kleerekoper, M.E., E. Petersen,E. Phillips, D. Nelson, et al., "Continuous sodium fluoride therapy does not reduce vertebral fracture rate in postmenopausal osteoporosis," *J Bone Miner Res*, 1989, Res. 4 (Suppl. 1), S376.

Kilner, B., and Pors Nielsen, S. *Clinical Science*, 1982, 62, 329-336.

Lane, N., et al., *Med Sci Sport Exer*, 1988, 20, suppl. 51.

Lee, J. R., M.D., "Understanding Osteoporosis." Summary.

———, "Osteoporosis reversal; the role of progesterone," *International Clinical Nutritional Review,* Sydney, Australia, June 1990.

———, "Osteoporosis reversal with transdermal progesterone," *The Lancet,* Letter, 336, November 1990.

———, "Is natural progesterone the missing link in osteoporosis prevention and treatment?" *Medical Hypotheses,* 1991, 35, 314, 318.

———, "Hormonal and nutritional aspects of osteoporosis," *Health and Nutrition,* Vol. 6, Issue 4, Winter 1991.

———, *Natural Progesterone,* BLL Publishing, California, 1993.

———, *Optimal Health Guidelines,* Second Edition, BLL Publishing, California, 1993.

———, "Dr. John Lee speaking at the Chelsea Hotel, London, June 5th 1994," Video.

———, "Effects of Progesterone on Osteoporosis and Menopausal Symptoms," Seminar given at St Thomas's Hospital, London, June 4, 1994.

———, "The Multiple Effects of Progesterone," Seminar given at St Thomas's Hospital, London, June 4, 1994.

———, "Successful Menopausal Osteoporosis Treatment Restoring Osteoclast/Osteoblast Equilibrium," *The Townsend Letter for Doctors,* August/September 1994, 900.

Lees, B., and J. C. Stevenson, "An evaluation of dual-energy X-ray absorptiometry," *Osteoporosis Int*, 1992, 2, 146-52.

Lees, B., T. Molleson, T.R. Arnett, and J.C. Stevenson, "Differences in proximal femur bone density over two centuries," *The Lancet*, 1993, 341:673-675.

Leichsenring, J. M., et al., *Journal of Nutrition*, 1957, 63, 425-435.

Lindsay, R., D. M. Hart, C. Forrest, and C. Baird, "Prevention of spinal osteoporosis in oopherectomized women," *The Lancet*, 1980, II, 1151-1154.

Lindsay, R., D. M. Hart, D. Purdie, M.M. Ferguson, A.S. Clark, and A. Karaszewski, "Comparative effects of estrogen and a progestogen on bone loss in postmenopausal women," *Clin Sc & Mol Med*, 1978, 54, 193-195.

Linksilver, H.M., et al., *Trans NY Acad Sci*, 1974, 36, 333.

Lufkin, E.G., et al., "Treatment of postmenopausal osteoporosis with transdermal estrogen," *Annals of Int Med,* July 1992, 117, 1-9.

McDougall, *McDougall's Medicine, A Challenging Second Opinion,* New Century Publishers, Piscataway, NJ, 1985.

MacIntyre, I., M.I. Whitehead, L.M. Banks, et al., "Calcitonin for prevention of post-menopausal bone loss," *The Lancet*, 1988, 1, 900.

Margen, S., et al., *American Journal of Clinical Nutrition*, 1974, 27, 584.

Marsh, A.G., et al., "Vegetarian Lifestyle and Bone Mineral Density," *American Journal of Medicine*, 1987, 82, 73.

Mazess, R.B., "On aging bone loss," *Clin Orthop*, 1982, 165, 239-252.

Mazess, R.B., H.S. Barden, M. Ettinger, and E. Schultz, "Bone Density of the radius, spine and proximal femur in osteoporosis," *J Bone Min Res*, 1988, 3, 13-18.

Monte, T., *New Age Journal,* September/October 1991, 25.

Munk-Jensen, N., S.P. Nielsen, E.B. Obel, and P.B. Eriksen, "Reversal of postmenopausal vertebral bone loss by estrogen and progestogen: a double-blind placebo-controlled study," *British Medical Journal,* 1988, 296, 1150-1152.

National Osteoporosis Foundation, *Medications and Bone Loss,* Washington DC, 1994.

National Osteoporosis Society, *Osteoporosis, A Decision-Making Document for Diagnosis and Prevention,* PO Box 10, Radstock, Bath, BA3 3YB.

National Osteoporosis Society, *Osteoporosis, A Guide to its Causes, Treatment and Prevention,* Number 1 in a series of Information Booklets, PO Box 10, Radstock, Bath, BA3 3YB, January 1993.

National Research Council, *Recommended Dietary Allowances,* 10th edition, National Academy Press, Washington DC, 1989.

Nielsen, F.H., et al., *Trace Element Research,* 1990, 9, 61.

Nilas, L., et al., *British Medical Journal,* 1984, 289, 1103-1106.

O'Mally, B.W., "Progesterone: Mechanism of Action," in *Metabolic effects of gonadal hormones and contraceptive steroids,* H.A. Salhanick, D.M. Kipnis, R.L. Vande Wiele, Plenum Press, New York, 1969.

Oski, Frank A., *Don't Drink Your Milk!* 9th edition, Teach Services, Brushton, New York, 1989.

Osteoporosis, *Yoga Journal,* March/April 1988, 44.

Ott, P., "Should Women Get Screening Bone Mass Measurements?," *Annals of Internal Medicine,* 1986, 104, 874.

Pak, C.Y.C., "Nutrition and Metabolic Bone Disease" in *Nutritional Diseases: Research Directions in Comparative Pathobiology,* Alan R. Liss, New York, 1986.

Peat, R., Ph.D., "Progesterone in Orthomolecular Medicine," Blake College Booklet, Eugene, Oregon. Available from Foundation for Hormonal and Nutrition Research, 8150, SW Barnes Road, Portland, OR 97225.

Peat, R.F., *Nutrition for Women,* Blake College Publishers, Eugene, Oregon, 1978.

Pfeiffer, C.C., *Mental and Elemental Nutrients: A Physician's Guide to Nutrition and Health Care,* Keats Publishing, New Canaan, 1975.

Pizzorno, Joseph E., and Michael T. Murray, *A Textbook of Natural Medicine,* John Bastyr College Publications, Seattle, Washington, 1985.

Prior, J.C., "Progesterone as a bone-trophic hormone," *Endocrine Review,* 1990, 11:386-398.

——, "Spinal bone loss and ovulatory disturbances," *New England Journal of Medicine,* 1990, 323, 18.

——, "Progesterone and its relevance for osteoporosis," *Bulletin for Physicians,* March 1993, Vol. 2, No. 2.

Prior, J. C., Y. Vigna, and R.N. Alojado, "Progesterone and the prevention of osteoporosis," *Canadian Journal of Obstetrics/Gynecology & Women's Health Care,* 1991, 3, 4.

Prior, J. C., Y. Vigna, and R. Burgess, "Medroxyprogesterone increases trabecular bone density in women with menstrual disorders," University of British Columbia, Vancouver. Paper presented at annual meeting of the Endocrine Society, June 11, 1987, Indianapolis, IN.

Rambaut, P.C., A.W. Goode, *The Lancet,* 1985, 2, 1050-1052.

Recker, R.R., *New England Journal of Medicine,* 1985, 313, 70.

Riggs, B.L., H.W. Wahner, L.J. Melton, L.S. Richelson, H.L. Judd, and W.M. O'Fallon, "Dietary calcium intake and rate of bone loss in women," *Journal of Clinical Investigation,* 1987, 80, 979-982.

Riggs, B.L., et al., "Effect of Fluoride Treatment on the Fracture Rate in Postmenopausal Women with Osteoporosis," *New England Journal of Medicine,* 1990, 322, 802-809.

Riis, B.R., et al., "Does calcium supplementation prevent postmenopausal bone loss?" *New England Journal of Medicine,* 1987, 316, 173-177.

Rowe, J. W., and R. D. Kahn, *Science,* 1987, 237, 143.

Rudy, D. R., "Hormone replacement therapy," *Postgraduate Medicine,* Dec 1990, 157-164. *Scientific American Medicine,* updated, chapter 15, section X, p. 9.

Saltman, P., et al., *Journal of Nutrition,* 1986, 116, 134.

Shapiro, J. R., et al., *Aren Intern Med,* 1975, 135, 563-567.

Sheikh, M.S., et al., "Gastrointestinal Absorption of Calcium from Milk and Calcium Salts," *New England Journal of Medicine,* 1987, 317, 532.

Smith, D.C., R. Prentice, D.J. Thompson, and W.L. Hermann, "Association of exogenous estrogen and endometrial carcinoma," *New England Journal of Medicine,* 1975, 293, 1164-1167.

Smith, E. L., et al., *Calcified Tissue International,* 1984, 36, Suppl. 129.

Smith, E. L., and C. Gilligan, *Physician Sportsmed,* 1987, 15, 91-100.

Sowers, M.F.R., M.K. Clark, M.L. Jannausch, and R.B. Wallace, "A prospective study of bone mineral content and fracture in communities with differential fluoride exposure," *Am J Epidemiol,* 1991, 134, 649-660.

Spencer, H., et al., *American Journal of Clinical Nutrition,* 1978, 31, 2167.

———, *American Journal of Clinical Nutrition,* 1982, 36, 32.

———, *Arch Intern Med,* 1983, 143, 657.

———, *Clinical Orthopaedics,* 1984, 184, 270.

Stepan, J. J., et al., "Castrated men exhibit bone loss: effect of calcitonin treatment on biochemical indices of bone remodeling," *J Clin Endocrinal Metab,* 1989, 69, 523-527.

Stevenson, J.C., B. Lees, M. Davenport, M.P. Cust, and K.F. Gangar, "Determinants of bone density in normal women: risk factors for future osteoporosis," *British Medical Journal,* 1989, 298, 924-928.

———, "Dietary Calcium and Hip Fracture," *The Lancet,* 1988, 1318.

Stevenson, J.C., P.C. Michael, F.G. Gangar, T.C. Hillard, B. Lees, and M.I. Whitehead, "Effects of transdermal versus oral hormone replacement therapy on bone density in spine and proximal femur in postmenopausal women," *The Lancet,* Vol. 336, 2265-2269.

Stevenson, J.C., M.I. Whitehead, M. Padwick, et al., "Dietary intake of calcium and post-menopausal bone loss," *British Medical Journal,* 1988, 297, 15-17.

Stryer, Lubert, *Biochemistry,* W.H. Freeman and Company, San Francisco, CA, 1975.

Thorne Research Inc, "Osteoporosis: Calcium and Beyond," *Capsulations*, 1990.

Tietz, Norbert W., PhD., *Textbook of Clinical Chemistry,* W.B. Saunders Company, Philadelphia, PA, 1986.

Underwood, E., *Trace Elements in Human and Animal Nutrition,* 4th edition, Academic Press, New York, 1977.

Vikkanski, L., "Magnesium May Slow Bone Loss," *Medical Tribune,* July 22, 1993, 9.

Virvidakis, K., et al., *International Journal of Sports Medicine,* 1990, 11, 244-246.

Watts, N.B., T.H. Steven, H.K. Genant, et al., "Intermittent cyclical etidronate treatment of postmenopausal osteoporosis," *New England Journal of Medicine,* 1990, 323, 73-79.

Weiss, N.S., C.L. Ure, J.H. Ballard, A.R. Williams, and J.R. Darling, "Decreased risk of fracture of hip and lower forearm and postmenopausal use of estrogen," *New England Journal of Medicine,* 1980, 303, 1195-1198.

Whitaker, Dr. Julian, "Your Program for Healthy Bones," *Health and Healing,* January 1994, Vol. 4, No. 1, 4-8.

Will's Biochemical Basis of Medicine, 1989, ch 22, p. 258.

Yoshioka, T., B. Sato, K. Matsumoto, and K. Oso, "Steroid receptors in osteoblasts," *Clin Orthop,* 1980, 148, 297-303.

Zetterberg, C., and G.B.J. Andersson, "Fractures of the proximal end of the femur in Goteberg, Sweden, 1940-1979," *Acta Orthopaed Scand,* 1980, 54, 681-686.

Ziel, H.K., and W.D. Finkle, "Increased risk of endometrial carcinoma among users of conjugated estrogens," *New England Journal of Medicine,* 1975, 293, 1167-1170.

Chapter Nine: Phoenix in the Fire

Beyene, Y., "Cultural significance and physiological manifestations of menopause: a biocultural analysis," *Cult. Med. Psychiatry,* 1986, 10:47-71.

Burrows, Harold, *Biological Actions of Sex Hormones,* 2nd edition, 1949, Cambridge University Press.

Coney, Sandra, *The Menopause Industry,"* Penguin Books, London, 1991.

Cooper, J.C., *An Illustrated Encyclopaedia of Traditional Symbols,* Thames and Hudson Ltd., London, 1982.

DeFazio, J., D.R. Meldrum, J.H. Winer, and H.L. Judd, "Direct action of androgen on hot flashes in the human male," *Maturitas,* 1984, 6:3-8.

Erlik, Y., D.R. Meldrum, and H.L. Judd, "Estrogen levels in postmenopausal women with hot flashes," *Obstet Gynecol,* 1982, 59:403-407.

Feldman, G.M., A. Voda, and E. Gronseth, "The prevalence of hot flashes and associated variables among perimenopausal women," *Res. Nurs. Hlth,* 1985, 8:261-268.

Feldman, J.M., R.W. Postlethwaite, and J.F. Glenn, "Hot flashes and sweats in men with testicular insufficiency," *Arch. Intern. Med.,* 136:606-608.

Ginsburg, J., J. Swinhoe and B. O'Reilly, "Cardiovascular responses during the menopausal hot flush," *Br. J. Obstet. Gynaecol,* 1981, 88:925-930.

Grant, Dr. Ellen, *Sexual Chemistry, Understanding Our Hormones, The Pill and HRT,* Cedar Original, Mandarin Paperbacks, London, 1994.

Greenwood, Dr. Sadja, *Menopause The Natural Way,* Macdonald & Co, London, 1987.

Hudson, Tori, *Gynecology and Naturopathic Medicine,* TK Publications, Oregon, 1992.

Kaufert, Pat, "Anthropology and the menopause: the development of a theoretical framework," *Maturitas,* 1982, 4, 181-193.

Kronenberg, F., "Hot flashes: Epidemiology and Physiology," *Annals of New York Academy of Sciences,* 1990, Vol. 592.

Kronenberg, F., and J. A. Downey, "Thermoregulatory physiology of menopausal hot flashes: A review," *Canadian Journal of Physiology and Pharmacology,* 1987, 65:1312-1324.

Lark, Susan, M., *The Menopause Self Help Book,* Celestial Arts, California, 1990.

Linde, R., G.C. Doelle, N. Alexander, R. Kirchner, W. Vale, J. Rivier, and D. Rabin, "Reversible inhibition of testicular steroidogenesis and spermatogenesis by a potent gonadotropin-releasing hormone agonist in normal men," *New England Journal of Medicine,* 1981, 305:663-667.

Lock, M., "Ambiguities of aging: Japanese experience and perceptions of menopause," *Cult. Med. Psychiatry,* 1986, 10:23-46.

Montreal Health Press, *Menopause, A Well Woman Book,* Second Story Press, Canada, 1990.

Reitz, Rosetta, *Menopause A Positive Approach,* Unwin Paperbacks, London, 1985.

Sherman, B.M., R.B. Wallace, J.A. Bean, Y. Chang, and L. Schlabaugh, "The relationship of menopausal hot flashes to medical and reproductive experience," *J. Gerontol,* 1981, 36:306-309.

Steinfeld, A.D., and C. Reinhardt, "Male climacteric after orchiectomy in patient with prostatic cancer," *Urology,* 1980, 16:620-622.

Steingold, K.A., M. Cedars, J.K.H. Lu, D. Randle, H.L. Judd, and D.R. Meldrum, "Treatment of endometriosis with a long-acting gonadotropin-releasing hormone agonist," *Obstet. Gynecol.,* 1987, 69:403-411.

Studd, John, and Rob Barber, "Mastering the Menopause," Leaflet presented with the compliments of Organon Laboratories Ltd., Cambridge, UK, 1994.

Utian, W.H., "The true clinical features of postmenopause and oophorectomy, and their responses to estrogen therapy," *South African Medical Journal,* 1972, 46:732-737.

Walker, Barbara, G., *The Woman's Encyclopedia of Myths and Secrets,* Harper & Row, San Francisco, 1983.

Chapter Ten: Double Indemnity
(and Chapter Twenty-five: Field and Forest)

American Journal of Clinical Nutrition, 1994, 60, 333-340.

Bavalve, R., et al., "Vegetables inhibit in vivo the mutagenicity of nitrite combined with nitrosable compounds," *Mutation Research,* 1983, Vol. 120, 145.

Business Week, "Breast cancer and PCB's: A Possible Link," April 6, 1992, 36.

Cramer, D.W., et al., "Dietary animal fat and relationship to ovarian cancer risk," *Obstetrics and Gynecology,* 1984, Vol. 63, 6, 833-838.

Dickinson, L.E., et al., "Estrogen profiles of oriental and caucasian women in Hawaii," *New England Journal of Medicine,* 1974, 291, 1211-1213.

Frenkel, K., K. Chrzan, C.A. Ryan, R. Wiesner, W. Troll, "Chymotrypsin-specific protease inhibitors decrease H2O2 formation by activated human polymorphonuclear leukocytes," *Carcinogenesis,* 1987, 8, 1207-1212.

Goldin, B., et al., "Estrogen excretion patterns and plasma levels in vegetarian and omnivorous women," *New England Journal of Medicine,* 1982, 307, 1542-1547.

Hayhow, S., and M. Messina, "The Soy Solution," *Vegetarian Times,* March 1994, 77-84.

Hudson, Tori, et al., "A Pilot Study using Botanical Medicines in the Treatment of Menopause Symptoms," *Townsend Letter for Doctors,* December 1994, 1372.

Khaw, K.T., (ed.), *Hormone Replacement Therapy,* Churchill Livingstein, London, 1992.

McDougall, J., "Balancing the estrogen issue," *Vegetarian Times,* August 1986, 44.

McIntyre, Anne, *The Complete Woman's Herbal,* Gaia Books Limited, London, 1994.

McKenna, T., "Pathogenesis and treatment of polycystic ovary syndrome," *New England Journal of Medicine,* 1988, Vol. 318, 558.

MacMahan, B., et al., "Urine estrogen profiles in Asian and North American women," *International Journal of Cancer,* 1974, 14, 161-167.

Messina, M., V. Messina, K. Setchell, *The Simple Soybean and Your Health,* Avery Publishing Group, New York, 1994.

Nakashima, H., et al., "Inhibitory effect of glycosides like saponin from soybean on the infectivity of HIV in vitro," *AIDS,* 1989, 3, 655-658.

Pizzorno, Joseph E., and Michael T. Murray, *A Textbook of Natural Medicine,* John Bastyr College Publications, Seattle, Washington, 1985.

Ridout, C.L., et al., "UK mean daily intakes of saponins—intestine permeabilizing factors in legumes," *Food Science & Nutrition,* 1988, 42, 111-116.

Schneider, J., et al., "Effects of obesity on estradiol metabolism: Decreased formation of nonuterotropic metabolites," *Obstetrical and Gynecological Survey,* 1980, 38 (10), 616.

Shaffer, Willa, *Midwiffery and Herbs,* Woodland Books, Utah, 1986.

———, *Wild Yam, Birth Control Without Fear,* Woodland Books, Utah, 1986.

Shutt, D.A. and R.I. Cox, "Steroid and phytoestrogen binding to sheep uterine receptors in vitro," *Journal of Endocrinology,* 1972, 52, 299-310.

Snowden, D.A., letter to the editor, *Journal of the American Medical Association,* 1985, Vol. 3, No. 254, 356-357.

Theroux, Paul, "Under the Spell of the Trobriand Islands," *National Geographic,* July 1992.

U.S. Academy of Sciences, *Diet Nutrition and Cancer,* National Academy Press, Washington DC, 1982.

Vines, Gail, "Twilight Zone's New Dawn," *The Guardian,* Sept. 23, 1993.

———, "The Challenge to HRT," *New Scientist,* October 23, 1993.

Walker, Morton, "Soybean Isoflavones Lower Risks of Degenerative Diseases," *Townsend Letter for Doctors,* August/September 1994, 874.

Weed, H.G., et al, "Protection against dimethylhydrazine-induced adenomatous tumours of the mouse colon by the dietary addition of an extract of soybeans containing the Bowman-Birk protease inhibitor," *Carcinogenesis,* 1985, 6, 1239-1241.

Weed, Susun, S., *Menopausal Years, The Wise Woman Way,* Ash Tree Publishing, New York, 1992.

Wilcox, G., et al., "Estrogenic effects of plant foods in postmenopausal women," *British Medical Journal,* 1990, 301 (6757), 905-906.

Williams, D., "The forgotten hormone," *Alternatives for the Health Conscious Individual,* 1991, Vol. 4 (6) 41-46.

Witschi, H., and A.R. Kennedy, "Modulation of lung tumour development in mice with the soybean-derived Bowman-Birk protease inhibitor," *Carcinogenesis,* 1989, 10, 2275-2277.

Chapter Eleven: Order out of Chaos
(and Chapter Twenty-Seven: Seeds of Change)

Abraham, G., "Nutritional factors in the etiology of premenstrual tension syndromes," *Journal of Reproductive Medicine,* 1983, 28, 446-464.

Belleme, John, and Jan Belleme, *Culinary Treasures of Japan,* Avery Publishing Group, New York, 1992.

Burkitt, Denis, *Refined Carbohydrate Foods and Disease,* Academic Press, New York, 1975.

Burkitt, D., and H. Trowell, *Western Diseases: Their Emergence and Prevention,* Harvard University Press, Cambridge, Mass, 1981.

Cohen, A.M., and A. Teitelbaum, "Effect of Dietary Sucrose on Oral Glucose Tolerance and Insulin-like Activity," *American Journal of Physiology,* 1964.

Colgan, Michael, "Pollutants and Food Degradation," *Colgan Institute Lecture Series #3,* Encinitas, CA, 1992.

Craig, Winston J., *Nutrition for the Nineties,* Golden Harvest Books, Michigan, 1992.

Crane, Milton, G., and Gerald Shavlik, "Newstart Lifestyle Program. A Survey of the Results," monograph, Weimar Institute, Weimar, California, 1993.

Crawford, Michael, and Sheila Crawford, *What We Eat Today,* Neville Spearman, 1972.

Facchinetti, F., et al., "Oral Magnesium successfully relieves premenstrual mood changes," *Obstetrics and Gynecology,* 1991, 78, 177-181.

Fontana-Klaiber, H., et al., "Therapeutic effects of magnesium in sysmenorrhoea," *Schweiz Runhdsch Med Prax,* 1990, 79, 491-494.

Foster, Vernon W., *Newstart!,* Woodbridge Press, CA, 1990.

Heaton, K.W., "Food Intake Regulation and Fiber," in *Medical Aspects of Dietary Fiber,* G. Spiller and R.M. Kay (eds), Plenum Press, New York, 1980.

Hur, Robin, *Food Reform: Our Desperate Need,* Heidelberg Publishers, Austin, 1975.

Jenkins, D. J. A., T. M. S. Wolever, and A.L. Jenkins, et al., "Starchy Foods and Glycemic Index," *Diabetes Care,* 1988.

Jenkins, D. J. A., A. L. Jenkins, and T.M. Wolever, et al., "Simple and Complex Carbohydrates," *Nutrition Review,* 1984.

Kamen, Betty, *Hormone Replacement Therapy Yes or No?* Nutrition Encounter Inc, Novato, CA, 1993.

Kenton, Leslie, *Lean Revolution,* Ebury Press, London, 1994.

————, *The New Biogenic Diet,* Vermilion, London, 1995.

Kenton, Leslie, and Susannah Kenton, *The New Raw Energy,* Vermillion, London, 1995.

Lee, John R., *Optimal Health Guidelines,* BLL Publishing, CA, 1993.

Linder, P.G., "'Junk Foods' and medical education," *Obes Bar Med,* 1982.

McCarrison, Sir Robert, *Nutrition and Health,* The McCarrison Society, London, 1953.

National Academy Press, *Recommended Dietary Allowances 10th Edition,* Washington DC, 1989.

Ornish, Dean, *Reversing Heart Disease,* Random Century, London, 1991.

Pritiken, N., *The Pritiken Program for Diet and Exercise,* Grosset and Dunlap, New York, 1979.

Recker, R.R., "The Effect of Milk Supplements on Calcium Metabolism, Bine Metabolism, and Calcium Balance," *American Journal of Clinical Nutrition,* 1968, 41, 254.

Sanders, Hofeldt, Kirk and Levin, "Refined carbohydrate as a contributing factor in reactive hypoglycemia," *Southern Medical Journal,* 1982.

Shurtleff, William, and Akiko Aoyagi, *The Book of Miso,* Ballantine Books, New York, 1991.

Steinman, David, *Diet for a Poisoned Planet,* Ballantine Books, New York, 1990.

Wolever, T.M.S., "The Glycemic Index," *World Review of Nutrition and Diet,* 1990.

Wolf, G., "Is Dietary Beta-Carotene an Anti-Cancer Agent?" *Nutritional Reviews,* 1982.

Worthington-Roberts, B., *Contemporary Developments in Nutrition,* C.V. Mosby, St Louis, MO, 1981.

Wynne-Tyson, Jon, *Food for a Future,* Abacus, 1975.

Chapter Twelve: Body Heat
(and Chapter Twenty-Nine: Second Coming)

Aloia, J.F., et al., "Prevention of Involutional Bone Mass by Exercise," *Annals of Internal Medicine.* 1978, Vol. 89, No. 3, 351-358.

American College of Sports Medicine Position Statement, "The Recommended Quantity and Quality of Exercise for Developing and Maintaining Fitness in Healthy Adults," *Med Sci Sports,* 1979.

Ardawi, M.S., and E.A. Newsholm, *Essays in Biochemistry,* 1985, 21, 1-43.

Bahrke, M.S., "Exercise, Meditation and Anxiety Reduction," *American Corr, Therapy Journal,* 1979, Vol. 33, No. 2, 41-44.

Ballor, D.L., and E.T. Poehlman, *American Journal of Clinical Nutrition,* 1992, 56, 968.

Barry, A., et al., "The Effects of Physical Conditioning on Older Individuals," *Journal of Gerontology,* 1966.

Belloc and Breslow, "Relationship of Physical Fitness and Health Status," *Preventative Medicine,* 1972, Vol. 1, No. 3, 109-121.

Blair, S.N., et al., *Journal of the American Medical Association,* 1989, 262, 2395-2401.

Bortz, W.J., *Journal of the American Medical Association,* 1982, 248, 1203-1208.

Brink, W.D., *The Advisor,* Winter 1994, 2.

Colgan, Michael and Ben Weider, *Bodybuilding for a Healthy Heart,* Published by International Federation of Bodybuilders.

Colgan, M., *Optimum Sports Nutrition,* Advanced Research Press, New York, 1993.

——, *Sexual Potency,* C.I. Publishers, San Diego, CA, 1994.

——, *The New Nutrition—Medicine for the Millennium,* C.I. Publications, Encinitas, CA, 1994.

Eliot, D., et al., *Physician Sportsmedicine,* 1987, 15, 169.

"Exercise and Longevity: A Little Goes A Long Way," *New York Times,* 1989.

Fiatarone, M.A., et al., *New England Journal of Medicine,* 1994, 330, 1769-1775.

Fleck, Steven, J., and William J. Creamer, *Designing Resistance Training Programs,* Human Kinetics Books, Champaign, Illinois, 1987.

Franklin, B.A., E.R. Buskirk, and P.C. Mackeen, "Eighteen Month Follow-Up of Participants in a Physical Conditioning Program for Middle-Aged Women," *Med Sci Sports,* 1978.

Griffin, S.J., and J. Trinder, "Physical Fitness, Exercise, and Human Sleep," *Psychophysiology,* 1978, Vol. 15, No. 5, 447-50.

Griffiths, M., and D. Keast, *Cell Biology,* 1990, 68, 405-408.

Gutin, B., "Effect of Increase in Physical Fitness on Mental Ability Following Physical and Mental Stress," *Research Quarterly,* 1966, Vol. 37, No. 2, 211-220.

Gwinup, G., R. Chelvam, and T. Steinbert, "Thickness of Subcutaneous Fat and Activity of Underlying Muscles," *American International Medicine,* 1971.

Jones, H.H. et al., "Humeral Hypertrophy in Response to Exercise," *Journal of Bone and Joint Surgery,* 1977, Vol. 59, No. 2, 204-208.

Lane, Nancy, "Exercise and Bone Status," *Complementary Medicine,* May/June 1986.

Laragh, J.H., et al. (eds), *Frontiers in Hypertension Research,* Springer-Verlag, New York, 1981.

Larson, L., *Acta Physiol Scand,* 1978, 36, Suppl. 457.

McCarthy, D.A., and M.M. Dale, *Sports Med,* 1988, 6, 333-363.

McCartney, N.A., et al., "Usefulness of Weightlifting Training in Improving Strength and Maximal Power Output in Coronary Heart Disease," *American Journal of Cardiology,* 1991, 67, 939.

Morgan, J., et al., "Psychological Effects of Chronic Physical Activity," *Medical Science Sports,* 1970, Vol. 2, No. 4, 213-217.

Nieman, David C., *The Sports Medicine Fitness Course,* Bull Publishing, CA, 1986.

Oscai, L.B., "The Role of Exercise in Weight Control," in *Exercise and Sport Sciences Reviews,* ed. J.H. Wilmore, Academic Press, New York, 1973.

Pearl, W., *Keys to the Inner Universe. The Encyclopedia on Weight Training*, Bill Pearl Enterprises, Phoenix, Oregon, 1982.

Pollick, M.L., J. Whilmore and S.M. Fox, *Health and Fitness Through Physical Activity,* John Wiley and Sons, New York, 1978.

Prior, J., "Conditioning Exercise Decreases Premenstrual Symptoms: A Prospective, Controlled, 6 Month Trial," *Fertility and Sterility,* 1987, Vol. 47, 402.

Putai, Jin, "Changes in Heart Rate, Noradrenaline, Cortisol, and Mood During Tai Chi," *Journal of Psychosomatic Research,* 1989, Vol. 33, No. 2, 197-206.

Quas, Dr. Vince, *The Lean Body Promise*, Synesis Press, Oregon, 1989.

Ries, L.A.G., et al., (eds), *Cancer Statistics Review,* 1973-1987, National Institute of Health Publications, Bethesda, MD, 1990.

Selvey, N., and P.L. White, (eds), *Nutrition in the 1980s,* Alan R. Liss, New York, 1981.

Shea, S.E., T.J. Benstead, *New England Journal of Medicine,* 1991, 324, 1517-1518.

Stamler, J., et al., *Journal of the American Medical Association,* 1986, 256, 2823-2828.

Swimme, Brian, *The Universe is a Green Dragon,* Bear & Comany, Sante Fe, MN, 1983.

Young, R.J., "Effect of Regular Exercise on Cognitive Functioning and Personality," *British Journal of Sports Medicine,"* 1979, Vol. 13, 3, 110-117.

Chapter Thirteen: Alchemy of Energy

Bellhouse, Elizabeth, "Life's Flowering," unpublished manuscript, 1994.

Bellhouse, Elizabeth, personal correspondence with the author. 1994.

Borho, B., "Therapy of the menopausal syndrome with Mulimen—Results of a multicenter post-marketing survey" *Biological Therapy,* 1972, 10, 226-229.

Borysenko, Dr. Joan, *Fire in the Soul,* Warner Books, 1993.

Burton Goldberg Group, *Alternative Medicine, The Definitive Guide,* Future Medicine Publishing Inc, Puyallup, Washington, 1993 (includes Dr. Robert Jacobs and Ludwig).

Gorman, Teresa, and Malcolm Whitehead, *The Amarant Book of Hormone Replacement Therapy,* Pan Books, London, 1989.

Schrödinger, Erwin, *What is Life? and Mind and Matter,* Cambridge University Press, Cambridge, 1967.

Szent-Györgyi, A., *Bioenergetics,* Academic Press, New York, 1957.

———, *The Living State,* Academic Press, New York, 1972.

Vines, Gail, *Raging Hormones*, Virago, London, 1993.

———, "Twilight Zone's New Dawn," *The Guardian,* September 23, 1993.

———, "The Challenge to HRT," *New Scientist*, October 23, 1993.

Chapter Fourteen: Distant Thunder

Brown, Ellan, and Walker, *Breezing Through The Change,* Frog Ltd, Berkeley, CA, 1994.
Grant, Dr. Ellen, "Long-Term Dangers of Hormonal Treatment," *The Lancet,* April 9, 1994.
———, "Hormonal Mayhem," *What Doctors Don't Tell You,* 1994, Vol. 5, No. 5.
———, "Oral Contraceptives and the Risk of Breast Cancer," *The Lancet,* November 12, 1994.
Menopause News 2(6): *Progesterone: Irrelevant Ingredient,* Nov/Dec 1992.
Poel, W.E., "Progesterone and Tumour Metastasis," *The Lancet,* November 9, 1963.
———, "Progesterone and Mammary Carcinogenesis," *Potential Carcinogenic Hazards from Drugs,* Monograph series Vol. 17, 1967, Springer-Verlag, Berlin.
Rock, John A., et al., "Fetal Malformations Following Progesterone Therapy During Pregnancy: A Preliminary Report," *Fertility and Sterility,* 1985, 44, 1.
Sheehy, Gail, *Silent Passage,* HarperCollins, London, 1993.
Sthoeger, Z.M., et al., "Regulation of the Immune Response by Sex Hormones," *Journal of Immunology,* 1988, 141, 91-98.
Stites, D.P., and P.K. Shteri, "Steroids as Immunosuppressants in Pregnancy," *Immunological Review,* 1983, Vol. 75.
Vessey, M.P., "Female Hormones and Vascular Disease—An Epidemiological Overview," *British Journal of Family Planning,* October 1980, 6, 1-12.

Chapter Twenty-Three: Bad Blood

Abraham, G.E., "Primary Dysmenorrhea," *Clinical Obstetrical Gynecology,* 1978, Vol. 21, 1, 139-145.
Abraham, G.E., "Nutritional Factors in the Etiology of the Premenstrual Tension Syndromes," *Journal of Reproductive Medicine,* 1983, 28, 446.
Abraham, G.E., and J.T. Hargrove, "Effect of Vitamin B on Premenstrual Tension Syndrome: A Double Blind Crossover Study," *Infertility,* 1980, 3, 155.
Biskind, M.S., "Nutritional Deficiency in the Etiology of Menorrhagia, Cystic Mastitis, Premenstrual Syndrome, and Treatment with Vitamin B Complex," *Journal of Clinical Endocrinology and Metabolism,* 1943, 3, 227-334.
Brown, Ellen, and Lynne Walker, *Breezing Through The Change,* Frog Ltd., Berkeley, California, 1994.
Brown, Ellen, and Lynne Walker, *The Informed Consumer's Pharmacy,* Carol & Graf, New York, 1990.
Butler, E. B., and E. McKnight, "Vitamin E in the Treatment of Primary Dysmenorrhoea," *The Lancet,* 1955, Vol. 1, 844-847.
Cohen, J.D., and H.W. Rubin, "Functional Menorrhagia: Treatment with Bioflavonoids and Vitamin C," *Current Therapeutic Research,* 1960, Vol. 2, p. 539.
Coney, Sandra, *The Menopause Industry,* Penguin Books, London, 1991.
Durrant-Peatfield, Barry, "The Premenstrual Syndrome," Monograph. Received December 1994.
Elstein, M., "Minimal/Mild Endometriosis and Infertility: A Review," *British Journal of Obstetrics and Gynaecology,* Vol. 96, No. 4, 454-450.
Endometriosis Association, Milwaukee, "Facts and figures on endometriosis," *U.S. Pharmacist,* February 1993, 42.
Engel, R.W., "The Relation of B Complex Vitamins and Dietary Fat to the Lipotropic Action of Chline," *Journal of Biological Chemistry,* 1941, 37, 140.
Facchinetti, F., et al., "Magnesium Prophylaxis of Menstrual Migraine," *Headache,* 1991, Vol. 31, 298-304.
Facchinetti, F., et al., "Oral Magnesium Successfully Relieves Premenstrual Mood Changes," *Obstetrics and Gynecology,* 1991, 78, 2, 177-181.

Feinstein, A.D., "Conflict over Childbearing and Tumors of the Female Reproductive System: Symbolism in Disease," *Somatics*, 1983, Fall/Winter.

Friedman, A.J., et al., "A Randomized Double-Blind Trial of Gonadotropin...in the Treatment of Leiomyomata Uteki," *Fertility and Sterility*, 1987, Vol. 49, 404.

George, Demetra, *Mysteries of the Dark Moon*, HarperSanFrancisco, HarperCollins, New York, 1992.

Gleicher, Norbert, "Is Endometriosis an Autoimmune Disease?" *Obstetrics and Gynecology*, July 1987, Vol. 70, No. 1.

Goci, G.S., and G.E. Abraham, "Effect of Nutritional Supplement...on Symptoms of Premenstrual Tension," *Journal of Reproductive Medicine*, 1982, 83, 527-531.

Goldin, B.R., et al., "Effect of Diet on Excretion of Estrogen in Pre- and Post-Menopausal Women," *Cancer Research*, 1981, 41, 3771-3773.

Goldin, B.R., et al., "Estrogen Excretion Patterns and Plasma Levels in Vegetarian and Omnivorous Women," *New England Journal of Medicine*, 1982, 307, 1542-1547.

Goodale, I., A. Domar, and H. Benson, "Alleviation of Premenstrual Syndrome Symptoms with the Relaxation Response," *Obstetrics and Gynecology*, 1990, 75, 4, 649-689.

Halme, J., S. Becker, and S. Haskill, "Altered Maturation and Function of Peritoneal Macrophages: Possible Role in Pathogenesis of Endometriosis," *American Journal of Obstetrics and Gynecology*, 1987, Vol. 156, 783.

Halme, J., M.G. Hammond, J.F. Hulka, et al., "Retrograde Menstruation in Healthy Women and in Patients with Endometriosis," *Obstetrics and Gynecology*, 1984, Vol. 64, 13-18.

Hargrove, J.T., W.S. Maxson, A.C. Wentz, and L.S. Burnett, "Menopausal Hormone Replacement Therapy with Continuous Daily Oral Micronized Estradiol and Progesterone," *Obstetrics and Gynecology*, 1989, 73, 4.

Hudson, Tori, *Gynecology and Naturopathic Medicine*, TK Publications, Oregon, 1992.

Hufnagel, V., *No More Hysterectomies*, Penguin Books, New York, 1989.

Hutchins, Francis Jr., "Uterine Fibroids: Current Concepts in Management," *Female Patient*, October 1990, Vol. 15, 29.

Jacobs, Robert H., "Care For Your Self," Seminar given for The Society for Complementary Medicine, 1994.

Kalma, S., et al., "Production of Fibronectin by Peritoneal Macrophages and Concentration of Fibronectin in Peritoneal Fluid from Patients With or Without Endometriosis," *Obstetrics and Gynecology*, July 1988, Vol. 72, 13-19.

Kappas, A., et al., "Nutrition-endocrine interactions," *Proceedings of the National Academy of Sciences*, 1983, 80, 7646-7649.

Kenton, Leslie, and Susannah Kenton, *The New Raw Energy*, Ebury Press, London, 1995.

Kime, Z., *Sunlight Could Save Your Life*, World Health Publications, Penryn, CA, 1980.

Landau, R.S., et al., "The Effect of Alpha Tocopherol in Premenstrual Symptomatology: A Double Blind Trial," *Journal of the American College of Nutrition*, 1983, 2, 115-123.

Lark, Susan M., *The Menopause Self Help Book*, Celestial Arts, California, 1990.

Lee, J.R., M.D., "Clinical Uses of Natural Progesterone," Seminar given at St Thomas's Hospital, London, June 4, 1994.

——, *Optimal Health Guidelines*, Second Edition, BLL Publishing, California, 1993.

——, "Slowing the aging process with natural progesterone," BLL Publishing, CA, 1992.

——, "The Multiple Effects of Progesterone," Seminar given at St Thomas's Hospital, London, June 4, 1994.

——, *Natural Progesterone*, BLL Publishing, California, 1993.

——, Personal communication with the author. 1994.

——, "The Theory of Estrogen Dominance," Seminar given at St Thomas's Hospital, London, June 4, 1994.

——, "Progesterone and Estrogen," Endocrinology Notes, February 1993.

Lubran, M., and G. Abraham, "Serum and Red Cell Magnesium Levels in Patients with Premenstrual Tension," *American Journal of Clinical Nutrition*, 1982, 34, 2364.

Montreal Health Press, *Menopause, A Well Woman Book,* Second Story Press, Canada, 1990.

Nachtigall, L., et al., *Estrogen,* HarperCollins Publishers, New York, 1991.

Norris, Ronald, "Progesterone for Premenstrual Tension," *Journal of Reproductive Medicine,* 1983, 28, 8, 509-515.

Northrup, Christiane, M.D., *Women's Bodies, Women's Wisdom,* Bantam Books, New York, 1994.

Ott, J., *Health and Light,* Pocket Books, New York, 1978.

Parry, B.L., et al., "Morning vs Evening Bright Light Treatment of Late Luteal Phase Dysphoric Disorder," *American Journal of Psychiatry,* 1991, 146, 9.

Peat, R., "Progesterone Safe Antidote for PMS," *McCall's,* October 1990, 152-156.

———, "The Progesterone Deception," *Ray Peat's Newsletter,* May 4, 1986, 44.

———, "Blocking Tissue Destruction," Unpublished Paper.

———, "Progesterone in Orthomolecular Medicine," Booklet.

———, "Progesterone Can Be Taken Orally," Letter to the Editor, *Townsend Letter for Doctors,* November 1994.

———, *Nutrition for Women,* Kenogen, Eugene, Oregon, 1981.

Petersen, Nancy, and B. Hasselbring, "Endometriosis Reconsidered," *Medical Self Care,* May/June 1987.

Pizzorno, Joseph E., and Michael T. Murray, "Premenstrual Syndrome," from *A Textbook of Natural Medicine,* John Bastyr College Publications, Seattle, Washington, 1985.

———, "Fibrocystic Breast Disease," from *A Textbook of Natural Medicine,* John Bastyr College Publications, Seattle, Washington, 1985.

Redwine, David B., "The Distribution of Endometriosis in the Pelvis by Age Groups and Fertility," *Fertility and Sterility,* 1987, Vol. 47, 173.

Reid, R.L., and S.S. Yen, "Premenstrual Syndrome," *American Journal of Obstetrics and Gynecology,* 1981, 139, 86.

Reiter, R.C., P.L. Wagner, and J.C. Gambone, "Routine Hysterectomy for Large Asymptomatic Leiomyomata: A Reappraisal," *Obstetrics and Gynecology,* April 1992, Vol. 79, No. 4, 481-484.

Rossignol, A.M., "Caffeine-Containing Beverages and Premenstrual Syndrome in Young Women," *American Journal of Public Health,* 1985, 75, 11, 1335-1337.

Sampson, John, "Peritoneal Endometriosis Due to the Menstrual Dissemination of Endometrial Tissue into the Peritoneal Cavity," *American Journal of Obstetrics and Gynecology,* 1984.

Snider, B.L., and D.F. Dietman, "Pyridoxine Therapy for Premenstrual Acne Flare," *Archives of Dermatology,* 1974, 110.

Weed, Susun S., *Menopausal Years, The Wise Woman Way,* Ash Tree Publishing, New York, 1992.

Werbach, M.R., *Nutritional Influences on Illness,* Third Line Press, Tarzana, CA, 1988.

Williams, D.G., "The Forgotten Hormone," *Alternatives for the Health Conscious Individual,* 1991, 4(6), 41-46.

Winenman, E.W., "Autonomic Balance Changes During the Human Menstrual Cycle," *Psychophysiology,* 1971, 8, 1, 1-6.

Chapter Twenty-Four: Never Come Morning

Artz, E., S. Fernandez-Castelo, et al., "Immunomodulation by indoleamines: Serotonin and melatonin action on DNA and interferon-y synthesis by human peripheral blood mononuclear cells," *J Clinical Immunology,* 1968, 8(6), 513-520.

Haensel, R., R. Wohlfart, and H. Cooper, "Narcotic action of 2-methyl-3-butene-2-ol contained in hops," *Zhurnal der Natuerforschungen,* 1980, 35c, 1096-1097.

Lutomski, J., E. Signet, K. Szpunar, and K. Grisse, "The meaning of passionflower in the healing arts," *Pharmazie in Unserer Zeit,* 1981, 10(2), 45-49.

Osol, A., and G.E. Farrar, *The Dispensatory of the United States of America,* J.B. Lippincott Co., Philadelphia, 1950.

Peat, Ray, "Insomnia and Hyperactivity," *Townsend Letter for Doctors,* April 1994, 385-386.

Seligmann, Jean, with Carl Robinson, "No More Sag from Jet Lag," *Newsweek,* May 8, 1989, 67.

Shaffer, M., "Melatonin could help elderly sleep better," *Medical Tribune,* July 22, 1993, 15.

Straube, C., "The meaning of Valerian root in therapy," *Therapie der Gegenwart,* 1968, 107, 555-562.

Thrash, Agatha, M., *Health Emphasis,* Revere Publishing, London.

Weed, Susun S., *Menopausal Years the Wise Woman Way,* Ash Tree Publishing, Woodstock, New York, 1992.

Wohlfart, R., R. Haensel, and H. Schmidt, "An investigation into the sedative-hypnotic principle of hops (3)," *Planta Medica,* 1982, 45, 224.

Wohlfart, R., R. Haensel, and H. Schmidt, "The sedative-hypnotic principle of hops (4)," *Planta Medica,* 1983, 48, 120-123.

Wren, R.W., *Potters New Cyclopedia of Botanical Drugs and Preparations,* The C.W. Daniel Company Ltd., Saffron Walden, 1975.

Chapter Twenty-Five (see chapter 10)

Chapter Twenty-Six: Resurrection

Allen, H.E., M.A. Halley-Henderson, and C.N. Hass, "Chemical Composition of Bottled Mineral Water," *Arch Environ Health,* 1989.

Boston Collaborative Drug Surveillance Program Report, "Coffee Drinking and Acute Myocardial Infarction," *The Lancet,* 1972.

Boughman, J., "The Pure Truth," *Health,* 1991.

Brooks, S.M., *The Sea Inside Us: Water in the Life Processes,* Meredith Press, New York, 1968.

"Caffeine Withdrawal Headaches," *Journal of Lab & Clin Medicin,* 1942-1943.

Campion, Kitty, "Water, not a drop to drink," *WDDTY,* Vol. 3, #12.

Cantor, K.P., R. Hoover, P. Hartge, et al., "Bladder Cancer, Drinking Water Source, and Tap Water Consumption: A Case-Control Study," *Journal of the National Cancer Inst,* 1987.

Carpenter, B., S.J. Hedges, C. Crabb, M. Reilly, and M.C. Bounds, "Is Your Water Safe?" *US News & World Report,* 1991.

Colgan, Michael, *Prevent Cancer Now,* CI Publications, San Diego, 1992.

———, "The Importance of Pure Water," *Colgan Institute Seminar Series,* No. 21, 1991.

Craig, Winston J., *Nutrition for the Nineties,* Golden Harvest Books, Michigan, 1992.

deVries, Herbert A., *Physiology of Exercise,* William C. Brown, Dubuque, Iowa, 1966.

Dews, P.B. (ed.), *Caffeine,* Springer-Verlag, Berlin, 1984.

Disler, P.B., S.R. Lynch, et al., "The Effect of Tea on Iron Absorption," *Gut,* 1975.

Fagliano, J., M. Berry, et al., "Drinking Water Contamination and the Incidence of Leukemia: An Ecological Study," *American Journal of Public Health 80,* 1990.

Foster, Vernon W., *Newstart!* Woodbridge Press, CA, 1990.

Gershoff, S.N., "Water, Water Everywhere, But is it Fit to Drink?" *Tufts Univ Diet & Nutr Letter 9,* 1991.

"Getting the Lead Out," FDA Consumer 23. 1989.

Gilber, R.J., *Caffeine. The Most Popular Stimulant,* Chelsea House Publishers, New York, 1986.

Government Printing Office, *Technologies and Management Strategies for Hazardous Waste Control,* Washington, DC, 1983.

Graham, D.M., "Caffeine—Its Identity, Dietary Sources, Intake and Biological Effects," *Nutr Rev,* 1978.

Grossman, M.I., "Physiologic Approach to Medical Management of Duodenal Ulcer," *Am J Dig Dis. New Series,* 1961.

Hager, M., "How Safe is Your Drinking Water?" *Consumers Digest,* 1984.

"How Safe is Your Water?" *Newsweek,* 1982.

Hunt, J., *The Conquest of Everest,* E. P. Dutton, New York, 1954.

Jankelson, O.M., et al., "Effect of Coffee on Glucose Tolerance and Circulating Insulin in Men with Maturity Onset Diabetes," *The Lancet,* 1967.

Lechat, M.F., I. Borlee, et al., "Caffeine Study," *Science,* 207, 1980.

Lefferts, L., "Water: Treat it Right," *Nutrition Action Health Letter,* 1990.

Lymann, G.H., C.G., Lyman, and W. Johnson, "Association of Leukemia with Radium Groundwater Contamination," *JAMA,* 1985.

MacNeal, Herbert P., "Valuable Notes on a Hot Subject," *Resident and Staff Physician,* April 1981.

Morck, T.A., S.R. Lynch, and J.D. Cook, "Inhibition of Food Iron Absorption by Coffee," *American Journal of Clinical Nutrition,* 1983.

Myers, *Medical Pharmacology,* Lange Medical Publication, Los Altos, CA, 1970.

Oglesby, P., "Stimulants and Coronaries," *Postgraduate Medicine,* 1968.

Ostertag, W., E. Duisberg, and M. Sturman,"The Mutagenic Actuary of Caffeine in Man," *Mutation Research,* 1965.

Pearce, Richard, "Body Fluids," *Runners World,* 1982.

Pitts, G.C., et al., "Factors Affecting Work Output in Hot Environments," *American Journal Physiology,* 1944.

Register, U.D., et al., "Influence of Nutrients on Intake of Alcohol," *Journal of the American Dietary Association,* 1972.

Roth, J.L. A., A. C. Ivy, and A .J. Atkinson, "Caffeine & Peptic Ulcer," *JAMA,* 1944.

Sabotka, T.J., "Neurobehavioral Effects of Prenatal Caffeine," *Ann NY Acad Sci,* 1989.

Saketkhoo, K., et al., "Effects of Drinking Hot Water, Cold Water and Chicken Soup on Nasal Mucus Velocity and Nasal Airflow Resistance," *Chest,* 1978.

Sargent, F., and K. Weinman, In *Physiological Measurements of Metabolic Functions in Man,* (eds) C.F. Consolazio et al., McGraw-Hill, New York, 1963.

Slater, D., "Bottled Waters. The Beverage of the Future," *Dairy and Food Sanitation,* 1991.

Smyly, D.S., B.B. Woodward, and E.C. Conrad, "Determination of Saccharin, Sodium Benzoate and Caffeine in Beverages by Reverse Phase HPLC," *J Assoc Off Anal Chem.* 1976.

Special Report, Second International Caffeine Workshop, *Nutrition Review,* 1980.

Stollman, T., *A Manual of Pharmacology,* W.B. Saunders, Philadelphia, 1957.

Taylor, Mary, *Water Pollution: Finding The Facts,* Friends of the Earth, London, 1993.

Thrash, A.M., and C.L. Thrash, *Nutrition for Vegetarians,* Thrash Publications, Scale, AL. 1962.

Travis, C.C., and C.B. Doty, *Environmental Science and Technology,* 1990.

University of California, "In The Heat, Drink Up," *Wellness Letter,* Vol. 1, Berkeley, CA, 1985.

University of California, "Wrap Up: Drink Water," *Wellness Letter,* Vol. 2, 1985.

U.S Dept of HHES Publ., //2(FDA) 81-1081, Caffeine & Pregnancy, 1981.

U.S Food and Nutrition Board, "Water Deprivation and Performance of Athletes," *American Journal of Clinical Nutrition,* 1974.

White, B.C., C.A. Lincoln, et al., "Anxiety and Muscle Tension as Consequences of Caffeine Withdrawal," *Science,* 209, 1980.

Chapter Twenty-Seven (see Chapter Eleven)

Chapter Twenty-Eight: The Professionals

Balch, James F., and Phyllis A. Balch, *Prescription for Nutritional Healing,* Avery Publishing Group Inc., Garden City Park, New York, 1990.

Braverman, Eric R., with Carl C. Pfeiffer, *The Healing Nutrients Within,* Keats Publishing Inc., New Canaan, Connecticut, 1987.

Davies, Dr. Stephen, and Dr. Alan Stewart, *Nutritional Medicine,* Pan Books, London, 1987.

Dean, Ward, John Morgenthaler, and Steven W. Fowkes, *Smart Drugs II, The Next Generation,* Health Freedom Publications, Menlo Park, California, 1993.

Garrison, Robert H., and Elizabeth Somer, *The Nutrition Desk Reference,* Second Edition, Keats Publishing Inc., New Canaan, Connecticut, 1985.

Jacobs, Robert H., "Care For Yourself," Booklet published by The Society for Complementary Medicine, London, 1994.

Kirschmann, John D., with Lavon J. Dunne, *Nutrition Almanac,* Second Edition, McGraw-Hill, New York, 1984.

Lee, J. R., M.D., *Natural Progesterone,* BLL Publishing, California, 1993.

Pearl, Bill, *Keys to the Inner Universe,* Bill Pearl Enterprises, Phoenix, Oregon, 1982.

Werbach, Melvyn, R., *Nutritional Influences on Illness,* Second Edition, Third Line Press, Tarzana, California, 1993.

Chapter Twenty-Nine (see Chapter Twelve)

Chapter Thirty: Magnum Force

Alvarado, Donna, "Hormone Use Cuts Risk of Heart Disease," *Press Democrat,* November 18, 1994.

Cowan, L.D., and L. Gordis, et al., "Breast Cancer Incidence in Women with a History of Progesterone Deficiency," *American Journal of Epidemiology,* 1981, 114, 209-217.

Dalton, Dr. K., "The Premenstrual Syndrome" *British Medical Journal,* 1953, 1, 1007.

Durrant-Peatfield, Barry J., "Hypothyroidism and You," Monograph. Received December 1994.

——, "The Menopause," Monograph. Received December 1994.

——, "The Menopause and Natural Progesterone," Monograph. Received December 1994.

Gaby, Alan R., "Progesterone: Oral versus Transdermal," *Townsend Letter for Doctors,* August/September 1994, 850.

Hargrove, Joel T. "Progesterone: Safe Antidote for PMS," *McCalls,* October 1990.

Hargrove, Joel T., Wayne S. Maxon, and Anne Colston Wentz, "Absorption of Oral Progesterone is Influenced by Vehicle and Particle Size," *American Journal of Obstetrics and Gynecology,* October 1989.

——, and Lonnie Burnett, "Menopausal Hormone Replacement Therapy with Continuous Daily Oral Micronized Estradiol and Progesterone," *Obstetrics and Gynecology,* April 1989, 606-612.

Kradjian, Robert M., *Save Yourself from Breast Cancer,* The Berkeley Publishing Groups, New York, 1994.

Lee, J. R., M.D., *Natural Progesterone,* BLL Publishing, California, 1993.

——, "Dr. John Lee speaking at the Chelsea Hotel, London, June 5th 1994," Video.

——, "The Theory of Estrogen Dominance," Seminar given at St Thomas's Hospital, London June 4, 1994.

——, "Clinical Uses of Natural Progesterone," Seminar given at St Thomas's Hospital, London, June 4, 1994.

————, "Endocrinology Notes: Progesterone and Estrogen," Monograph, February 6, 1993.

Peat, Raymond F., "Progesterone in Orthomolecular Medicine," Blake College Booklet, Eugene, Oregon.

————, "The Progesterone Deception," *Ray Peat's Newsletter,* May 4, 1986, 44.

————, "Progesterone Can Be Taken Orally," Letter to the Editor, *Townsend Letter for Doctors,* November 1994.

Prior, J. C., "Progesterone as a Bone-Trophic Hormone," *Endocrine Review,* 1990, 11, 386-398.

Williams, David G., "The Forgotten Hormone," *Alternatives,* December 1991, 4, 6.

If you wish to be kept informed of Leslie Kenton's books, videos, workshops, and other activities, please write to the Publicity Director, Hay House, Inc., P.O. Box 5100, Carlsbad, CA 92018-5100.

American Holistic Medical Association
4101 Lake Boone Trail, Suite 201, Raleigh, NC 26707
(703) 556-9728 or (703) 556-9245
The American Holistic Medical Association is composed of medical doctors (MDs), osteopaths (DPs), and naturopaths (NDs) who share a common philosophy of encouraging personal responsibility for health and emphasizing the whole person.

American Association of Naturopathic Physicians
(206) 298-0125
601 Valley St., Suite 105, Seattle, WA 98109
The American Association of Naturopathic Physicians (AANP) is the professional organization of licensed naturopathic physicians.

PERSONAL GROWTH

Esalen Institute
Esalen Hot Springs, Big Sur, CA 93920
(408) 667-3000

The Hendricks Institute
401 East Carrillo, Suite A2, Santa Barbara, CA 93101
(800) 688-0772

Omega Institute
(914) 266-4444

Open Center
(212) 219-2527

The Foundation for Shamanic Studies
P.O. Box 1939, Mill Valley, CA 94942
(415) 380-8282   Fax: (415) 380-8416
This organization provides worldwide training in shamanic practices offering more than 180 courses to over 4,500 individuals annually. For a list of shamanic practitioners who do soul retrieval in your particular country, write to Sandra Ingerman, author of *Soul Retrieval*, at the address above.

SOURCES OF NATURAL HORMONE PRODUCTS

Karuna Corporation
42 Digital Drive, Suite 7, Novato, CA 94949
(800) 826-7225
(888) PHYTOGEST (749-8643)—Progesterone cream orders only

PharmWest, Inc.
520 Washington Blvd. #401, Marina Del Rey, CA 90292
(310) 301-4015   Fax: (310) 577-0296

Transitions for Health, Inc.
621 S.W. Alder, Suite 900, Portland, OR 97205-3627
(800) 888-6814 (regular customers)   (800) 861-5009 (professionals)
Fax: (503) 226-6455   (503) 226-1010

Women's International Pharmacy
5708 Monona Drive, Madison, WI 53716-3152
(800) 279-5708   (608) 221-7800

SOURCES OF SALVARY HORMONE TESTS

Aeron Lab
1933 Davis St., Suite 310, San Leandro, CA 94577
(800) 631-7900   Fax: (510) 729-0383

Diagnos-Techs, Inc.
6620 192nd Place, Suite J-104, Kent, WA 98032
(800) 878-3787   Fax: (425) 251-0637

RECOMMENDED ALTERNATIVE HEALTH NEWSLETTERS

Alternatives **(Dr. David G. Williams) One year, 12 issues, $69**
Mountain Home Publishing
2700 Cummings Lane, Kerrville, TX 78028
(830) 367-4492

Nutrition and Healing **(Drs. Alan Gaby and Jonathan Wright) One year, 12 issues, $49**
Publishers Management Corporation
P.O. Box 84909, Phoenix, AZ 85071
(800) 528-0559   Fax: (602) 943-2363

Self-Healing **(Dr. Andrew Weil) One year, 12 issues, $29**
Thorne Communications, Inc.
42 Pleasant St., Watertown, MA 02172
(617) 926-0200

Wisdom for Women **(Dr. Christiane Northrup) One year, 12 issues, $49**
Phillips Publishing, Inc.
7811 Montrose Rd., Potomac, MD 20854
(800) 777-5005

INFORMATION—HERBS

American Association of Naturopathic Physicians
601 Valley St., Suite 105, Seattle, WA 98109
(206) 298-0125
The American Association of Naturopathic Physicians (AANP) is the professional organization of licensed naturopathic physicians.

American Botanical Council
P.O. Box 201660, Austin, TX 78720
(512) 331-8868   Fax: (512) 331-1924
A nonprofit organization dedicated to education. Co-publishes the *HerbalGram* with the Herb Research Foundation. Provides excellent reference materials, including a series of Classic Botanical Reprints.

American Herb Association
P.O. Box 1673, Nevada City, CA 95959
(916) 265-9552   Fax: (916) 274-3140
Membership includes a subscription to the *AHA Quarterly*, which is devoted to providing information on medicinal herbs.

American Herbalist Guild
P.O. Box 1683, Soquel, CA 95073
A nonprofit membership organization. Members receive a quarterly journal and discounts to seminars and workshops.

American Holistic Medical Association
4101 Lake Boone Trail, Suite 201, Raleigh, NC 26707
(703) 556-9728 or (703) 556-9245
The American Holistic Medical Association is composed of medical doctors (MDs), osteopaths (DPs), and naturopaths (NDs) who share a common philosophy of encouraging personal responsibility for health and emphasizing the whole person.

American Society of Pharmacognosy
Chicago School of Pharmacy
555 31st St., Downers Grove, IL 60515
A nonprofit membership organization. Members receive the *Journal of Natural Products.*

The Herb Research Foundation
1007 Pearl St., Suite 200, Boulder, CO 80302
(303) 449-2265   Fax: (303) 449-7849
The foundation provides accurate and reliable information on herbs. Co-publisher of the *HerbalGram.* Offers research and educational services.

LIVE HERBS

Amazon Herb Co.
725 North A1A, Suite C-115, Jupiter, FL 33477
Professional/wholesale only. Herbs from the South American rain forest, including Suma and pau d'arco. Providing this work for rain forest natives helps halt the destruction of the area by cattle raisers.

Bioessence
220 Harmony Lane, Garberville, CA 95542
Fresh, wild crafted echinacea extract, pau d'arco, citrus seed and other extracts, and chlorella and wild blue-green micro algae.

East Earth Trade Winds
P.O. Box 493151, Redding, CA 96049
(800) 258-6878
Chinese herbal preparations and major tonic herbs

Elixir
8612 Melrose Avenue, Los Angeles, CA 90069
(888) 486-6427
Reputable dealer of quality ginseng.

Gaia Herbs
108 Island Ford Road, Brevard, NC 28712
(800) 831-7780

Health Center for Better Living
6189 Taylor Road, Naples, FL 33942
Individual and combinations of Western herbs in bulk and various preparations

Herbalist & Alchemist, Inc.
P.O. Box 553, Broadway, NJ 08808
(800) 611-8235　Fax (908) 689-9071
PCM Phytocalm: Scullcap, Oat, Hops, Passionflower, Valerian, California Poppy
VVCC Vitex/Vervain Compound: Chastetree berry, Blue Vervain, Motherwort, Kava Kava
WOF Woman's Formula: Motherwort, Helonias Root, Wild Yam Root, Raspberry leaf, Ginger, Chastetree berry
WOC Woman's Transition Compound: Chastetree berry, Dang Gui root, Blue Vervain, Black Cohosh, Cactus stem
FLM Full Moon Plus: Wild Yam, Black Haw Bark, Roman Chamomile Flowers, PA free Petasites root, Cyprus root, Jamaican dogwood
Plus: A couple hundred single herb extracts, all made in the ancient alchemist, Spigeric way, as well as many Chinese herbs and extracts

Sandy Mush Herbs
Surrett Cove Road, Leicester, NC 28748-9622
(704) 683-2014 for catalog

Spirit of the Forest
P.O. Box 126, Maryland, NY 12116
(607) 638-9729
A reputable dealer for quality ginseng

FOOD AND HERB SEEDS

Abundant Life Seed Foundation
P.O. Box 772, Port Townsend, WA 98368
Grains, beans, perennial woody plants, wildflowers; all untreated non-hybrid heirloom varieties; also books

Bountiful Gardens
18001 Shafer Ranch Road, Willits, CA 95490
(707) 459-6410
Open-pollinated heirloom seeds of vegetables, herbs, flowers, and grains; also beneficial insects, fertilizers, and books

Japonica Seeds
P.O. Box 729, Oakland Gardens, NY 11364
Seeds of Oriental herbs and vegetables

Johnny's Selected Seeds
310 Foss Hill Road, Albion, ME 04910
Wide variety of mainly untreated, organic, high-quality seeds

Native Seeds/Search
(Southwestern Endangered Aridland Resource Clearing House)
2509 N. Campbell Avenue #325, Tucson, AZ 85719
Southwest desert traditional and wild seeds preserving gardening heritage of Southwest drought-resistant varieties.

Nichols Garden Nursery
1190 N. Pacific Highway, Albany, OR 97321
Good variety of herb seeds

Peace Seeds
2385 S.E. Thompson St., Corvallis, OR 97333
Planetary gene pool service and resource center; organic nonhybrid herb, vegetable, and flower seeds; and trees.

ORGANIC FOOD

Organic produce is becoming much more available in the U.S. these days, and can be purchased at many major markets across the country, and for certain at most health food stores. To order directly, try these superb companies:

Diamond Organics
P.O. Box 2159, Freedom, CA 95019
(888) ORGANIC (674-2642)
They have all kinds of fresh produce, sprouts, flowers, bread, pasta, dried fruit, nuts, seeds, and nut butters; and all kinds of canned and bottled foods, vinegars, oils, and herbs.

Jaffe Brothers

P.O. Box 636, 28560 Lilac Road, Valley Center, CA 92082
(760) 749-1133   Fax: (760) 749-1282
They offer many different varieties of nuts, seeds, dried fruits, nut and seed butters, pastas, grains, vegetable oils, sprouting seeds, and many canned goods.

Walnut Acres Organic Farm

Walnut Acres Road, Penns Creek, PA 17862
(800) 433-3998
An excellent selection of all kinds of organic foods, condiments, and herbal drinks of many varieties.

Paradise Farm

1000 Wild Iris Lane, Moscow, ID 83843
(208) 882-6590

UNREFINED FOODS

Gold Mine Natural Foods

3419 Hancock St., San Diego, CA 92110
(800) 475-3663   Fax: (619) 296-9756

Green Earth Farm

P.O. Box 672, Saquache, CO 81149
Quinoa and herbal products

Mountain Ark Trading Company

799 Old Leicester Hwy, Asheville, NC 28806
(800) 643-8909   Fax: (704) 252-9479

Pronatec International

P.O. Box 193, Peterborough, NH 03458
Producers of unrefined dried sugar cane juice, the first commercially available whole sugar in the West.

South River Miso Company, Inc.

South River Farm, Conway, MA 01341
Unpasteurized, organic, handmade misos.

SEAWEEDS

Maine Coast Sea Vegetables
R.R. 1, Box 78, Franklin, ME 04634
(207) 565-2907

ENERGY SUPPLEMENTS

The Synergy Company
HC 64 Box 2901, Castle Valley, UT 84532-6913
(800) 723-0277 or order through Hay House: (800) 654-5126
Pure Synergy™ is a superfood product that surpasses all others! It contains 62 of nature's finest, most nourishing ingredients. These ingredients are organically grown or ethically wild crafted from pristine areas, tested for freshness and purity and sanctioned by the FDA. There are 11 species of algae, 7 types of grass juice powders, a variety of Chinese and Western nutritional herbs, as well as 5 Asian mushrooms and other exotics, like royal jelly. Hermetically sealed, amber glass bottles preserve this highly vital food source. Pure Synergy does not contain inexpensive fillers or fibers of any kind. For those who want to feed themselves and their families only the very best; eat Pure Synergy from the Synergy Company for your supreme health and ongoing well-being.

Please inquire about their other nature-based products, including men's or women's multivitamin/mineral supplements, an antioxidant formula, and probiotics. Also available are water and air filters, as well as other life-enhancing products.

Bach Flower Remedies
Flower Essence Services
P.O. Box 1769, Nevada City, CA 95959
(800) 548-0075
These can be purchased at many health food stores across the country, or ordered directly from the huge variety offered.

Vita Fons II
Vita Florum Products, Box 85, Station "A," Toronto, M5W 1A2, Canada
This company, which is owned by a charitable trust, offers a full range of Vita Fons II energy products including the water, tablets, ointment, lotion, massage oil, talcum powder and salve, as well as Vita Fons II for animals and plants.

Vita Fons II Water is primarily used in the form of doses—5 drops: neat, on food or in any beverage. It is also used in conjunction with hydrotherapy, and ocular, vaginal and colonic irrigation. It can be ordered in a spray bottle—the best for both external and internal use.

Vita Fons II Tablets are for those who prefer tablets to liquid. A compound of gypsum, calcium phosphate, kelp, sago flour, and palm oil, each tablet equals one dose and may be chewed, swallowed, or allowed to dissolve on the tongue.

Vita Fons II Ointment is one of the most generally useful of the preparations for external use. It contains water, hamamelis water, almond oil, wax, and Vita Fons II.

Vita Fons II Talcum Powder is the most potent Vita Fons II product for external use. It can be used all over the exterior of the body. Dust on top of any other Vita Fons II product to obtain increased effect.

For animals, use the same products and application systems as for people. For all mammals, regardless of size, the dose is 3 drops. For birds, reptiles, fish, and insects, the dose is one drop.

For plants, Vita Fons II Foliar Spray (or Dusting Powder) may be used on leaves, branches, and trunks with a view to increasing crop weight, disease/parasite-resistance, helping transplanted plants and reviving wilted plants. A Seed Dressing and a Root Powder are also available.

OILS

Flora, Inc.
P.O. Box 73 or 805 E. Badger Road, Lynden, WA 98264
(800) 446-2110
Oils pressed without heat, air, or light.

Home Health Products, Inc.
1160 A Millers Lane, Virginia Beach, VA 23451
(800) 284-9123   Fax: (800) 285-8155
Cold-pressed, cold-processed castor oil.

Omega Nutrition
165-810 West Broadway, Vancouver, BC, V5Z 4C9, Canada
Fresh, unrefined, cold-pressed flax oil

Spectrum Naturals
Wholesale only
133 Copeland St., Petaluma, CA 94952
Fresh, unrefined, cold-pressed flax and wheat-germ oils, extra virgin olive oil, and a variety of other refined and unrefined oils (a number of their oils are not recommended by this book).

KITCHENWARE, SPROUTING SUPPLIES, HOUSEHOLD GOODS

Miracle Exclusives
P.O. Box 8 or 64 Seaview Blvd., Port Washington, NY 11050
(800) 645-6360   Fax: (516) 621-1997
Juicers, grain mills, wheat-grass juicers, sprouters, food mills, cookware

Real Goods
555 Leslie St., Ukiah, CA 95482
Order: (800) 762-7325   Administration: (707) 468-9292
Products for energy independence, home solar-powered electrical systems and
devices, many environment-preserving household items including water purifiers,
and books

The Sprout House
40 Railford St., Great Barrington, MA 01230
Sprout bags, newsletter, books, audiocassette classes, juicers, composters, food
dehydrators

BALANCED SPECTRUM LIGHTING

Lights of America
611 Reyes Drive, Walnut, CA 91789
(800) 321-8100
Color-corrected fluorescent lamps can be purchased in the U.S. from all major
lighting companies, and at most hardware stores. Industrial lamps may be purchased here.

USEFUL PUBLICATIONS AND ORGANIZATIONS

Earthsave
706 Frederick St., Santa Cruz, CA 95062
Information including newsletter based in part on John Robbins's book, *Diet for a
New America,* which promotes vegetarianism and exposes the meat industry as a
major contributor to pollution and disease.

Natural Health
P.O. Box 57320, Boulder, CO 80322
A magazine on Eastern and Western alternative approaches to health and well-being, including in-depth information on food and cooking.

Food First
145 Ninth St., San Francisco, CA 94103
Information on business practices and politics that cause inequalities in food distribution, especially among Third World peoples.

Herb Research Foundation
1007 Pearl St., Suite 200, Boulder, CO 80302
(303) 449-2265   Fax: (303) 449-7849
Information on well-researched therapeutic herbs, an herb magazine, *Herbal-Gram,* and a large list of herb seed sources.

Price Pottenger Foundation
P.O. Box 2614, La Mesa, CA 92041
Books on the subject of physical degeneration in various cultures from refined foods.

People for the Ethical Treatment of Animals (PETA)
P.O. Box 42516, Washington, DC 20077

Vegetarian Resource Group
P.O. Box 1463, Baltimore, MD 21203
Vegetarian Journal, and educational resources promoting vegetarianism; designed for use in schools.

World Research Foundation
15300 Ventura Blvd., Suite 405, Sherman Oaks, CA 91403
Both computerized and manual library searches on current health information and treatments available around the world. Often used by health-care practitioners as well as individuals, for finding wider options than standard medical sources provide.

Methods of Measuring Levels of Progesterone
and Estrogen in the Blood

Here is what a typical lab analysis in Britain looks like.

Estradiol	<37 pmol/L
Ref. range (Follicular)	(110–440)
Ref. range (Mid-cycle)	(550–1300)
Ref. range (Luteal)	(365–770)
Ref. range (Post-menopause)	(35–175)
Progesterone	2.4 nmol/L
Ref. range (Follicular)	(0.3–5.0)
Ref. range (Luteal)	(8.0–90) (For implantation, 30)
Ref. range (Post-menopause)	(0.1–2.0)
* thyroid-stimulating hormone	0.2 mU/L (0.33.5)
Growth hormone	5.4 mU/L (Adult <10 : Child <20)

However, in whichever country, serum progesterone levels are expressed in terms of concentration, i.e., X amount of progesterone per Y amount of serum.

My *Merck Manual* lists it as ng/ml (elsewhere I have seen picograms per deciliter [µµ/dl]) and as nmol/L. A mol is the amount of a given chemical substance equivalent to its molecular weight in grams. One nmol = 1 nanomol = one-billionth (10^{-9}) of a mol of some substance. For progesterone, you can convert ng/ml into nmol/L by multiplying by 3.1.

One picogram = one-trillionth (10^{-12}) of a gram. A ml = one-thousandth (10^{-3}) of a liter and a dl = a deciliter, or one-tenth (10^{-1}) of a liter.

Thus, the luteal range for progesterone could be written as 7-28 ng/ml or 21-84 nmol/L, and the non-ovulating level is often as low as 0.3 ng/ml or 0.9 nmol/L.

Amenorrhea—absence of menstruation.

Amino acid—organic acids that are the building blocks of protein.

Analgesic—something that relieves pain.

Androgens—hormones secreted by the testes that produce secondary male characteristics.

Anovulatory—suspension or cessation of ovulation.

Antioxidant—a chemical or compound that inhibits reactions caused by free radicals.

Arteriosclerosis—deposits of cholesterol, lipid material, and cellular debris in the inner lining of arteries.

Atrophic vaginitis—thinning and inflammation of the vagina.

Auto-immune—the production of reactivity by an organism to its own tissues.

Autonomic—self-controlling. Refers to parasympathetic and parasympathetic nervous systems.

Bacteria—single-celled organisms of the plant kingdom.

Bioflavonoids—brightly colored substances in plants that are concerned with maintaining a normal state in blood vessel walls.

Carcinogen—a cancer-producing substance.

Catalyst—a substance that affects the rate of a chemical reaction.

Cervix—mouth of the womb.

Chelating agents—soluble organic compounds that can fix certain metallic ions into their molecular structure.

Collagen—the main protein of connective tissue—skin, bone, tendon, and cartilage.

Compression fracture—break in a weakened bone that is unable to support weight and therefore becomes crushed.

Conjugated—one compound combined with another.

Corpus luteum—small yellow glandular mass in the ovary formed after ovulation.

Corticosteroid—hormones produced by the adrenal cortex.

Diuretic—a substance that promotes the secretion of urine.

DNA—the acid of which chromosomes are made.

Dysmenorrhea—painful menstruation.

Endocrine—system composed of organs (glands) that make and secrete substances (hormones) directly into the bloodstream.

Endogenous—developing or originating within the body.

Endometriosis—mysterious condition where the tissue that forms the lining of the womb (the endometrium) grows outside the uterine cavity in other areas of the pelvis, sometimes causing pain and infertility.

Endometrium—the inner secretory lining of the uterus.

Endorphin—polypeptide hormone of the central nervous system.

Enzyme—any of numerous complex proteins that act as catalysts in specific biochemical reactions.

Essential fatty acids—organic acids, including linoleic and linolenic acids, required by the body for health.

Estrogen—the ovarian hormones that initiate the body's preparation for possible fertilization and pregnancy.

Exogenous—originating outside the body.

Follicle—a small excretory sac or gland—e.g., the ovarian follicle that produces the ovum.

Follicle-stimulating hormone (FSH)—neuropeptide hormone secreted by the pituitary that stimulates the follicle in the ovary to grow.

Free radical—a compound with unbalanced electrons, capable of causing destabilizing oxidation reactions.

Gene—the biological unit of heredity, a segment of DNA.

Genetic—referring to reproduction, birth or heredity.

Gonadotrophic releasing hormone (GnRH)—the hormone made by the hypothalamus that stimulates the pituitary gland to produce gonadotrophins.

Gonadotrophin—a hormone that can stimulate the sex glands.

Half life—the time it takes for an active element or substance to lose half its potency.

Homeostasis—the body's ability to maintain a stable internal environment.

Hormone—a substance that usually circulates in the blood and produces a specific effect on the activity of cells.

Hypoglycemia—low blood-sugar level.

Hypothalamus—neural nuclei in the limbic brain just above the pituitary.

Hysterectomy—surgical removal of the uterus.

Limbic brain—brain cortex below the *corpus callosum* and above the pituitary that contains neural nuclei controlling autonomic functions, homeostasis, emotional sensation and responses, and regulates immune responses.

Luteinizing—refers to maturation of ovarian follicles for ovulation.

Luteinizing hormone (LH)—hormone produced in the pituitary that triggers the maturation of ovarian follicles. A big surge of this hormone precedes ovulation by 2 to 24 hours each month.

Menopause—cessation of menstrual cycles.

Menorrhagia—irregular menstruation.

Metabolism—the biochemical process of living organisms by which substances are produced and energy is made available to the organism.

Microgram—one millionth of a gram.

Micron—one thousandth of a millimeter.

Milligram—one thousandth of a gram.

Mitochondria—small organelles within the cytoplasm that are the site of converting sugar into energy.

Molecule—a combination of two or more atoms that form a specific chemical substance.

Nanogram—one billionth of a gram.

Oocyte—the cell that produces the ovum.

Oophorectomy—surgical removal of an ovary or ovaries.

Osteoblast—bone cell that forms new bone.

Osteoclast—bone cell that resorbs old bone.

Osteocyte—a bone cell that may become an osteoclast or an osteoblast.

Peptide—a class of low molecular weight compounds composed of several amino acids.

Perimenopausal—the period in a woman's life that precedes menopause.

Phyto—relating to plants.

Polyunsaturated fatty acid—a fatty acid with more than one double bond in its carbon chain.

Precursor—specific nutrient or body chemical required for the manufacture of a particular substance within the body.

Premenopausal—before menopause—perimenopausal.

Progesterone—natural ovarian hormone made by the corpus luteum to sustain the endometrium and support the fertilized ovum.

Progestogen—a synthetic compound with progesterone-like action—a progestin.

Prostaglandin—hormone composed of essential fatty acids with effects on smooth muscle contraction; regulates cell behavior and inhibits hormones.

Radical—a group of atoms that enter into and go out of chemical combinations without change, and that form one of the basic constituents of a molecule.

Resorption—the loss or dissolving away of a substance.

RNA—ribonucleic acid.

Saturated fatty acid—fatty acid with full complement of hydrogen (i.e., no double bond).

Steroid—any compound based on and derived from the cholesterol molecule—includes sex hormones and corticosteroids.

Sterol—compounds with single hydroxyl group, soluble in fat, for example cholesterol.

Synthesis—the building of a chemical compound by the union of its elements.

Trans—compounds that have been altered from their natural state as in trans-fatty acids.

Triglyceride—a fat composed of glycerin and 3 fatty acids.

Unsaturated fatty acid—fatty acid with at least one double bond in the carbon chain.

Xeno—meaning "strange," or denoting relationship to foreign material, as in xenoestrogens.

I have given approximate measurements in the recipes as cupfuls (an ordinary cup holds about 8 fluid ounces or 225 ml), tablespoons, teaspoons, and so on. Where measuring is important, I have given the imperial measurement as well as the metric. Most of the recipes are designed to feed four people. As the quantities are approximate, the amounts can easily be adjusted to suit your own particular needs.

Weight
1 oz. = 28 grams
1/4 lb. = 112 grams
1 lb. = 450 grams
2.2 lb. = 1 kilogram

Volume
1 pint = 570 ml
1 3/4 pints = 1 liter
1 gallon = 4.5 liters

Length
1 inch = 2.5 cm
1 foot = 30 cm
39 inches/3.3 feet = 1 meter/100 cm
1 mile = 1.6 kilometers

About the Author

Award-winning writer, television broadcaster, and author of numerous bestsellers, **Leslie Kenton** is described by the press as "the guru of health and fitness" and "the most original voice in health." A shining example of energy and commitment, she is highly respected for her thorough reporting. Leslie was born in California, and is the daughter of jazz musician Stan Kenton. After leaving Stanford University, she journeyed to Europe in her early 20s, settling first in Paris then in Britain, where she has since remained. She has raised four children on her own by working as a television broadcaster, novelist, writer, and teacher on health. For 14 years she was an editor at Harpers & Queen.

Leslie's writing on mainstream health is internationally known and has appeared in *Vogue,* the *Sunday Times, Cosmopolitan,* and the *Daily Mail,* and she is the author of many other health books. Former consultant to a medical corporation, Leslie's writing has won several awards. In recent years, she has become increasingly concerned, not only with the process of enhancing individual health, but also with reestablishing bonds with the earth as part of helping to heal the planet.

BOOKS

EMERGING WOMEN: The Widening Stream, by Julie Keene and Ione Jenson

EMPOWERING WOMEN: Every Woman's Guide to Successful Living, by Louise L. Hay

LOVE YOUR BODY, by Louise L. Hay

WOMEN ALONE: Creating a Joyous and Fulfilling Life, by Julie Keene and Ione Jenson

AUDIOS

ELDERS OF EXCELLENCE, by Louise L. Hay

EMPOWERING WOMEN, by Louise L. Hay

LOVE YOUR BODY, by Louise L. Hay

REFLECTIONS ON A WOMAN'S BOOK OF LIFE, by Joan Borysenko, Ph.D.

WOMEN'S BODIES, WOMEN'S WISDOM, by Christiane Northrup, M.D.

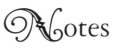

Notes

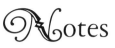

Notes

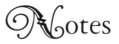

Notes

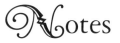

Notes

We hope you enjoyed this Hay House book.
If you would like to receive a free catalog
featuring additional Hay House books and products,
or if you would like information about the
Hay Foundation, please contact:

Hay House, Inc.
P.O. Box 5100
Carlsbad, CA 92018-5100

(760) 431-7695 or **(800) 654-5126**
(760) 431-6948 (fax) or **(800) 650-5115 (fax)**

Please visit the Hay House Website at: **www.hayhouse.com**